THE ULTIMATE GUIDE TO

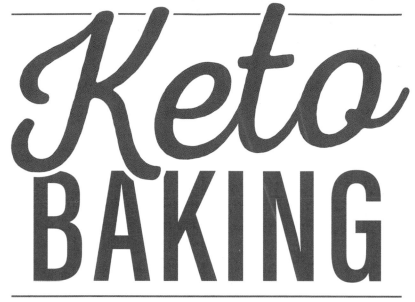

Keto
BAKING

MASTER ALL THE BEST TRICKS FOR LOW-CARB BAKING SUCCESS

Carolyn Ketchum

D1580668

VICTORY BELT PUBLISHING INC.
Las Vegas

First published in 2020 by Victory Belt Publishing Inc.

ISBN-13: 978-1-628603-84-2

Front and back cover food styling by Marcella Capasso

Front and back cover photography by Lance Friemuth, Kat Lannom, and Justin-Aaron Velasco

Author photos by Brad Self/JBSelf Photography

Cover design by Kat Lannom

Interior design by Charisse Reyes and Crizalie Olimpo

TC 0220

CONTENTS

Preface

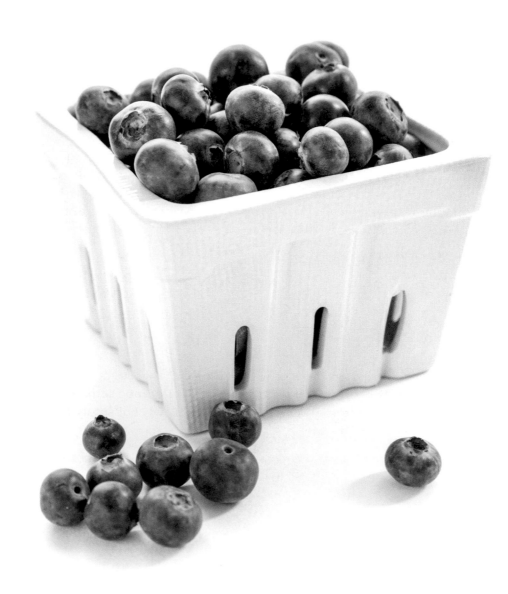

That girl. You know the one I'm talking about. She's your coworker, or maybe she sits next to you in class. Perhaps she's your neighbor or your friend. However you happen to know her, she's always the first one to volunteer to bring treats to a function, be it a work meeting, a study group, or a block party. She views every birthday as an excuse to make some sort of elaborate cake. Like an eager puppy, her ears perk up and her eyes brighten at the very thought of a gathering where people might eat her creations. And she's positively gleeful when her goodies are met with murmurs of approval. She loves to bake and she loves to share, and you know she will never come over to your house empty-handed.

I was that girl. I still am that girl.

The only thing that's really changed are the ingredients I use. I've traded in wheat flour and sugar for almond flour, coconut flour, and alternative sweeteners. And in the process, I've traded in the carb-heavy treats that took my blood sugar for a wild ride and substituted keto-friendly sweets that keep my glucose perfectly stable.

Maybe that's not such a small change after all. In fact, it's quite a monumental change when you think about it. And it certainly wasn't one I embraced readily at the beginning. Truth be told, I would say that I came to the keto diet kicking and screaming.

See, I was mourning a very important part of my identity: my baking self. A self who, when staring down the barrel of type 2 diabetes, thought that she would never be able to enjoy baking again. Perhaps that sounds like a trivial concern in the face of a chronic disease, but it wasn't trivial to me. My love of baking was a huge part of who I was—how could I be me without it?

Clearly, I couldn't. I quickly delved into the weird and wonderful world of sugar and flour alternatives with abandon. I read everything I could get my hands on about baking with nut flours and coconut flour. I spent a small fortune on new-to-me ingredients. And I tried. And I tried. And then I tried again.

I entered the keto baking world in its nascent stages, when there weren't a lot of resources out there, and I had to go it alone much of the time. I made some serious blunders, thinking my new flours and sweeteners should behave the way my old ones did. But with every mistake and every failure, I learned something new, and I filed it all away in my baking-obsessed brain. And slowly but surely, I started to have more and more success.

It wasn't long before I was taking beloved conventional recipes and making them over with keto-friendly ingredients. And then I began to let my imagination run wild, dreaming up all-new recipes and getting into the kitchen to see if I could bring them to fruition. Slowly but surely, people started paying attention, making my recipes and asking me if I could make over their favorites, too.

I daresay I have become a much better baker in the process. In my past life, I never really paid attention to what made a recipe work or why it might fail. I didn't understand the difference between baking soda and baking powder or the role that gluten plays in helping baked goods rise or hold together. And it wasn't until I had to go without that I came to understand that sugar does so much more than simply sweeten foods. My technical baking skills have vastly improved, and I am far more creative in the kitchen than I used to be, developing new recipes on an almost daily basis.

That baking self I was so afraid of losing? She's very much alive and kicking. I may have changed *how* I bake, but I haven't changed *why* I bake: that deep and abiding passion to create something utterly delectable that will elicit ooohs and aaahs from the crowd. I still get that eager gleam in my eye at the very thought of warming up my oven and greasing my pans. I still view every get-together as an opportunity to indulge my inner domestic goddess. I am still that girl.

Since you are holding this book in your hands, chances are that you are also that girl, or that guy. Chances are that you too embarked on the keto lifestyle, apprehensive about what it might mean for your favorite pastime. Well, friends, I am here to tell you that you can still be that girl or guy. You can still bake, and you can still enjoy the fruits of your labor.

My deepest wish is that *The Ultimate Guide to Keto Baking* becomes your indispensable keto kitchen companion. Come along with me for a journey into this strange but delicious world and enjoy everything the keto lifestyle has to offer.

Let's face it, a good creamy chocolate cake
does a lot for a lot of people.

— *Audrey Hepburn*

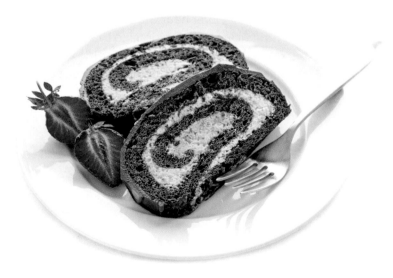

BAKERS GONNA BAKE

Why is it that some of us love to bake so much? And by "some of us," I mean the millions and millions of us across the globe who love to indulge in this ancient pastime, who can't get enough of mixing and stirring, beating and whipping. Those of us who feel compelled to wake up in the morning, turn on the oven, and get to work to create some mouthwatering masterpiece.

A love of baking has far less to do with a love of eating than the uninitiated might realize. I bake cookies not so that I can stuff my face with cookies but for the deep sentiments that those cookies represent: warmth, comfort, home, family, and love. Do I enjoy eating the cookies when they're done? Of course I do, but I love the process of creating and sharing them even more.

Baking affords me a sense of well-being that is hard to put into words. There really is nothing quite like it, but I am going to try my best to capture the essence and beauty of the baking experience.

Baking is magic. It is the modern equivalent of alchemy, the bringing together of various materials to create something altogether new, something that is far more than the sum of its parts.

Baking is sensual. It involves all five senses. Taste, sight, and smell are obvious, but hearing and touch are also involved. The whisk brushing against the side of the bowl, the hum of a preheating oven, and the whoosh of an electric mixer are all part of the symphony of baking. It is an incredibly tactile experience, rolling out dough, patting out scones, forming cookies by hand. If you didn't get your hands dirty, you didn't do it right.

Baking is luxurious. It requires time and effort, and perhaps a little money, too. You can easily follow a keto diet without baking tasty treats, but it is much more satisfying and feels far less restrictive if you can indulge a little.

Baking is relaxing. Ever hear the term "stress-baking"? It's a real thing; a number of studies and articles have legitimized this concept. Baking requires mindfulness and presence, putting the rest of your life on hold as you read the recipe and pay close attention to the steps. It can be incredibly soothing and a wonderful way to slough off stress and tension.

Stressed spelled backwards is desserts.

Loretta LaRoche

Baking is creative. Baking is often referred to as a science, but it's also a creative process. Even when following someone else's recipe to the letter, you are creating something with your own hands. And when you become comfortable with baking, you often put your own little spin on a recipe, switching up the flavor profile or adding something like chocolate chips. Decorating your baked goods can be quite an artistic endeavor as well.

Baking is nostalgia. Many of us grew up baking with our mothers and grandmothers. Or we enjoyed family celebrations that revolved around homemade cakes and cookies. Baking is a throwback to childhood, to cozy kitchens and joyous gatherings. And sometimes it feels like a step back to simpler times, when all foods were homemade.

Baking is an act of love. Food is nourishment, and to bake delicious treats for others is an expression of how much you care. You are seeking to nurture, to take care of people, and your baked goods are a tangible (and edible!) demonstration of your love.

Baking is most certainly part of my love language. Is it part of yours, too?

Cookies are made of butter and love.

———————————————————— *Norwegian proverb*

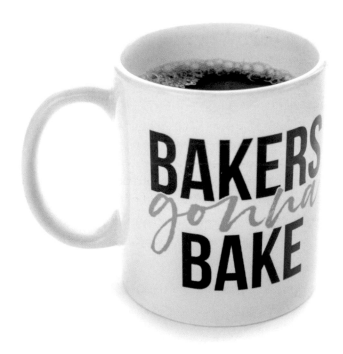

HOW TO USE THIS BOOK

At the beginning, keto baking can make you feel a little like Alice in Wonderland. You've fallen down the rabbit hole and have landed in a topsy-turvy world where nothing behaves quite like it should. Going it alone can end in frustration and wasted ingredients. Trust me, I've been there.

The Ultimate Guide to Keto Baking is so named for a reason. Consider this your guidebook to a foreign land, with me as your tour guide and interpreter. I have written this book to be as comprehensive as possible and have done my utmost to touch upon everything that contributes to success in baking.

I want you to get the most out of your time in the kitchen, so I have included many handy tips and other features throughout the book.

Chapter 1 is a must-read for keto bakers new and old, as it includes important tips that everyone should keep in mind. Be sure to keep the Baking Rockstar Checklist handy—it's a great reminder of all the best baking practices. Also look for the smaller tips included in the recipes.

Chapter 2 takes an in-depth look at keto ingredients and how they behave, as well as all the pantry staples you want to keep on hand. I make no apologies for the length of this chapter, as the ingredients you use are by far the most important factors in your success. Chapter 3 discusses essential and nonessential baking tools, as well as including a guide to scaling recipes.

Chapters 4 through 15 include a wide array of keto baking recipes. Keep in mind that this is more than just a dessert cookbook. The recipe chapters comprise everything from easy savory crackers to showstopper layer cakes. I included anything and everything that could possibly be baked in an oven—even pizza!

I had so many cookie and cake recipes I wanted to share that I split them into two chapters each. "Everyday Cookies" and "Everyday Cakes" are simple recipes that come together easily and are great served any time. "Fancy Cookies" and "Special Occasion Cakes" are recipes that take a little more time and effort and are perfect for serving at parties and during the holidays. But of course, "just because" is a good enough reason to make these recipes, too.

The final recipe chapter, "Extras," includes some of the fundamentals for other recipes—pie crust doughs, pizza doughs, pastry cream filling, and frostings. Plus, I've included a recipe for my favorite vanilla ice cream because it goes so well with baked goods.

I also tried to include a wide variety of methods and ingredients. I pushed myself to experiment and get outside my comfort zone, testing new products and techniques so that I could speak more knowledgeably about what works and what doesn't. My hope is that this book will give you a jumping-off point to try out your own ideas.

Do keep in mind that the keto world is ever-evolving. Even as I write this, someone is developing some new sweetener or other product that I haven't had a chance to test. But I have given you an array of recipes to play with and learn from so that you can venture into your own experiments.

For each recipe, you will find the following information.

Nutritional Information

Every recipe includes key nutritional information per serving, including optional ingredients:

NUTRITIONAL INFORMATION

CALORIES: 292 | FAT: 24.3g | CARBS: 8.5g | FIBER: 4.4g | PROTEIN: 7g

---

Carbs are listed as **total grams of carbohydrate**. If you prefer to count net carbs, simply subtract the grams of fiber from the grams of carbs.

Please note that the sweeteners I use in this book technically contain carbohydrates, but they have zero carb impact for most people. They are metabolized and exit the body without raising blood glucose or insulin, so for the purposes of the keto diet, they should not be counted in the total carbohydrates.

I calculated all the nutritional information using MacGourmet, a paid software program that relies on the USDA National Nutrient Database. I strive to be as accurate as possible, but these numbers are often only estimates based on the average size of certain ingredients. I encourage you to calculate your own nutritional information whenever you can.

Swaps and Substitutions

While I recommend following the recipes as written, I understand that food allergies, intolerances, and ingredient availability might warrant the occasional substitution. I have done my best to recommend swaps wherever possible, but keep in mind that the nutritional information was calculated using the ingredients listed. Swapping one ingredient for another may change those counts, so be sure to recalculate them based on the specific ingredients you use.

Time Management Guidelines

Baking is a process and not something to be hurried. To use your time in the kitchen most efficiently, be sure to take note of the prep and cook times listed at the top of each recipe.

To help you strategize, the prep times listed in this book include the active prep time followed by additional information about long chilling, cooling, or resting times. They also indicate clearly when the time to make a subrecipe, such as a crust or frosting, is not included in the overall time. You will need to remember to factor in the time to make those subrecipes.

Cook times always give the upper limit of the entire cooking and baking time, including anything you might need to make on the stovetop or in the microwave. But be sure to make note of the range of baking time in the recipe instructions. Since every oven is different, it's best to start checking your baked goods at the lower end of the range.

Almost all baked goods need to cool to some extent before serving. This is particularly important for keto baked goods, as many of them continue to firm up as they cool. Because cooling is a nearly universal step, only particularly long cooling times—45 minutes or longer—are noted in the listed prep times. Standard cooling times are listed in the recipe method, so be sure to make note of these as well.

Quick Reference Icons

To help you find exactly the types of recipes you're looking for, I've included some easy visual reference icons in the recipes.

For those people with food allergies, I have noted which recipes are free of coconut, dairy, eggs, and/or nuts. I also have noted which recipes include options to make them free of these potential allergens.

I also have marked the recipes that are great for beginners and those that are best suited to advanced keto bakers.

For easy access, the chart on pages 404 to 407 summarizes which of these categories each recipe falls into. You'll also find a fabulous visual recipe index on pages 408 to 415. Feel like making cookies but not quite sure what kind you want? Check this index to quickly spot what tempts your tummy.

Additional Baking Information

Finally, I have included other helpful resources, such as a Metric Equivalency Chart for the most common ingredients (see pages 398 and 399). And be sure to check out the Resource Guide on pages 400 to 403, which includes recommended reading and places to source interesting keto ingredients.

Chapter 1:
THE ART AND SCIENCE OF KETO BAKING

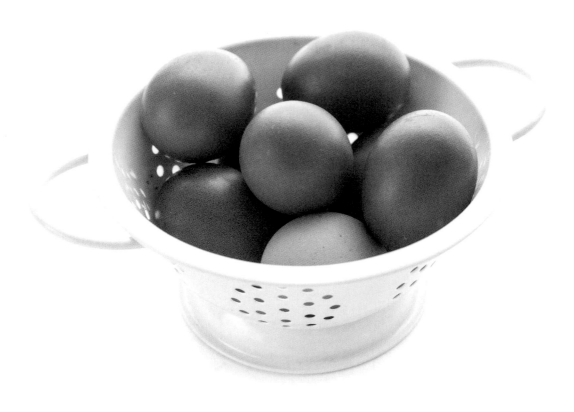

Baking is often referred to as a science, which implies that if one follows the formula exactly as written, the results will always be the same. However, I've always felt that baking is far more intuitive than this scientific approach would imply.

While the success of your baked goods does rely a great deal on physics and chemistry, it's very difficult for a home baker to be as precise as a scientist can be. Everything makes a difference, from the softness of your butter to the fineness of your flour to the quality of your baking pans. Unless you are baking in a climate-controlled environment with the exact same ingredients and tools every time, your results will vary. But who bakes in a laboratory?

I must have made the chocolate chip cookies from *Joy of Cooking* a few hundred times while I was growing up. And every time I made them, they turned out slightly differently. Sometimes they were flat and crisp, and other times they were puffier and chewier. Maybe my butter was softer one day, or I used a different brand of flour. Or maybe I was using a new oven or a different cookie sheet. Who knows exactly what contributed to the differences in texture? The cookies always tasted delicious.

When it comes to keto baking, the variances can be even greater. There is far less standardization in ingredients such as almond flour, coconut flour, and low-carb sweeteners, making it even trickier to be precise.

This is where intuition comes in. Is the batter too wet? Add a little more flour. Too dry? Add a little more liquid. Admittedly, this ability to make adjustments comes with experience. Because keto ingredients don't always behave the way you might expect, it may take you a little while to become familiar and comfortable with this brave new world, and there may be a few mishaps along the way.

Nevertheless, I am going to give you as many tips and tricks as I can to help you avoid costly errors. Keto ingredients aren't cheap, and I want you to succeed.

In addition to the larger tips I give you here, be sure to look for the tips in the recipes.

It's all about a balancing act between time, temperature, and ingredients: That's the art of baking.

— *Peter Reinhart*

KETO BAKING TIPS

Leave Your Expectations at the Door

So you think you know how to bake. You've been baking all your life, and you're pretty confident in the kitchen. How hard can it be to switch to keto baking?

Okay, stop right there, hotshot. I was you about ten years ago, and my first few attempts at low-carb, sugar-free baking almost brought me to my knees. It's a completely different world, and while some of your previous experience will be helpful, your expectations of how things should look, feel, and act may be a detriment.

Low-carb batters and doughs simply are not the same as their high-carb counterparts. They may be thicker, more fragile, less elastic, more absorbent, take longer to cook, rise less, and so on and so on. If you cling to your previous experience and adjust your batter or dough to look similar to a conventional one, you are bound to meet with failure. If you think to yourself, "Surely the recipe can't take that many eggs or that much baking powder," your muffins or cake will be flat and crumbly.

So I ask you to set all your expectations aside for now. Put your faith in these well-tested recipes and try them as written. And enjoy the journey.

Get to Know Your Oven Intimately

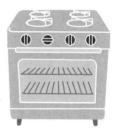

No two ovens are exactly the same, and no oven is perfect when it comes to exact temperatures. Similar to the furnace that heats your home, ovens are based on thermostats, so the heat is constantly going on and off, attempting to keep the temperature inside the oven near the target temperature. And that thermostat is probably somewhere in the back of your oven, not in the center where you typically place baked goods.

Most ovens run a little too hot or too cool. The best fix is an accurate oven thermometer, one that hangs somewhere in the center of your oven and can tell you the exact temperature in that spot, so that you can adjust accordingly.

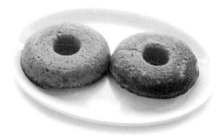

It's also good to know if your oven has hot spots, as most ovens do. My oven has one at the very back on the right-hand side, and I know that any baked goods in the corner of my large baking sheet will get more browned than the rest. So I always set a timer for halfway through the baking time and rotate the pan so that my treats bake more evenly.

Pay Special Attention to Ingredient Temperatures

Recipes always specify the temperature your ingredients should be: softened, room temperature, chilled, cold, or melted. These instructions are not to be dismissed, as they are critical to the outcome. Adding cold eggs or liquid to nicely beaten butter will cause it to clump up again. Subsequently, you won't be able to smooth out your batter no matter how hard you beat it.

- **What "room temperature" really means:**
  Room temperature means 70°F, give or take a few degrees. If your house is particularly warm or chilly, your ingredients won't be at the correct temperature, so keep this in mind when preparing to bake. You can gently warm ingredients to bring them up to temperature or chill them for a few minutes in the fridge.

- **How soft is softened butter?**
  Many recipes call for softened butter or cream cheese. You will know that it is softened properly if you can press a finger into it and leave a dent. But it shouldn't be so soft as to squish all over the place under the pressure.

- **Melted but not hot:**
  Some recipes call for melted butter or oil. While it should be completely liquefied, you don't want it to be hot to the touch. Hot butter or oil can curdle any eggs included in the recipe, so make sure to let it cool to lukewarm before adding it.

Humidity can play a role, too, although perhaps not as much as it does in conventional baking. Dry ingredients can absorb moisture from the air if not stored properly in sealed bags or containers. Since almond flour, as well as other nut and seed meals, already contains far more moisture than wheat flour, humidity isn't nearly as much of a concern. But do keep an eye on your keto baked goods, as they may need a bit longer in the oven to cook through.

Coconut flour, on the other hand, is like a sponge, soaking up every bit of moisture it can. If you're working in a very humid environment, you may need to reduce the amount of liquid in a recipe by a tablespoon or two. If you've never worked with coconut flour, it's hard to know what the right consistency is for your batter or dough, so look for the visual and tactile cues in the recipes. After a time, you will get a feel for how coconut flour works and will be able to adjust accordingly.

What's in a Brand Name?

Because there can be such variation among brands of keto flours and sweeteners, it is best to use the same brands that I do. I fully recognize, however, that this isn't always possible because you may not have access to these products. Just keep in mind that any effort to limit the variability will help.

Substitute at Your Own Risk

In keeping with the theme of limiting variability, try not to make ingredient substitutions unless they are suggested in the recipe. These recipes were carefully developed and tested for the specific ingredients listed. Changing even a single ingredient can throw off the rest of the recipe. To make sure you have everything you need, read the recipe in full before you start.

Consider Your Bakeware

Investing in good bakeware may seem like an extravagance, but it really makes a difference and saves you money in the end. Thin, flimsy pans don't conduct heat as evenly or efficiently as heavy-gauge pans do, and your baked goods may end up cooking unevenly or even burning in spots.

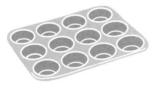

The color and material of the bakeware are also important considerations:

- Metal pans are much better conductors of heat than glass or ceramic dishes, so they heat up more quickly and efficiently. Dark-coated metal pans tend to brown the bottoms and sides of baked goods faster. Light-colored pans are better for most recipes.

- Glass and ceramic dishes take longer to heat up, but they also hold on to heat longer after they come out of the oven.

  Conventional wisdom holds that you should reduce your oven temperature by 25°F and consider taking foods out of the oven earlier if you're using a glass or ceramic baking dish. However, I've found that for keto recipes, things actually take *longer* to bake through. I've baked my Chewy Keto Brownies (page 178) in both metal pans and ceramic dishes, and they needed about 10 minutes more at the same temperature to cook through properly in the ceramic dish. This likely has something to do with the differences between keto and regular flours.

- Silicone bakeware doesn't conduct heat well at all and doesn't brown foods very well, but it does protect baked goods from burning more than other kinds of pans.

Unless a recipe specifies using a dish of another material, you should use good metal bakeware. See my recommendations for the best baking pans in the Tools chapter.

Grease Is the Word

The majority of the recipes in this book require you to grease your pans. Be prepared to put a little elbow grease into it (pun intended!). I recommend using a solid fat, like butter or coconut oil, and really working it into the creases. With cakes that need to come out of the pan perfectly, I often grease the pan twice, once with a solid fat and once with avocado or coconut oil cooking spray.

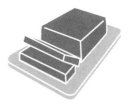

Some recipes call for only a light greasing, and a spray works well in these cases. But do note that sprays and liquid oils tend to pool as they sit. You can take a pastry brush and brush the oil around the sides and bottom of the pan if it pools. You can also wait to grease the pan until just before you add the batter.

Repurposing "Mistakes"

Did something come out not quite perfect? Perhaps it's a bit dry or it got stuck in the pan. Wait! Before you tip the whole lot into the trash, stop and think about how you might use it in some other way.

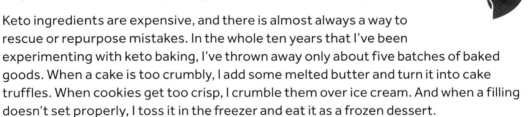

Keto ingredients are expensive, and there is almost always a way to rescue or repurpose mistakes. In the whole ten years that I've been experimenting with keto baking, I've thrown away only about five batches of baked goods. When a cake is too crumbly, I add some melted butter and turn it into cake truffles. When cookies get too crisp, I crumble them over ice cream. And when a filling doesn't set properly, I toss it in the freezer and eat it as a frozen dessert.

Unless the flavor is completely unpalatable to you, it's worth figuring out another use for those imperfect baked goods.

So the pie isn't perfect? Cut it into wedges.
Stay in control and never panic.

— *Martha Stewart*

Don't Rush It

Don't bake when you're short on time. Baking is a process that requires patience and mindfulness, and you should make time to enjoy it. Baking when you're in a hurry often results in mistakes. Who among us hasn't turned around after popping something into the oven and seen the butter/sweetener/baking powder we forgot to add to the batter? So take a deep breath, be present, and step through the recipe carefully. It can be quite therapeutic.

KETO BAKING FOR BEGINNERS

If you are completely new to baking with keto ingredients, it's best to start simple. Pick out a few easy recipes that are noted as beginner level, such as muffins, brownies, or an easy one-layer cake. This affords you the opportunity to get used to these unfamiliar ingredients and to get a feel for how they behave. It will help build your confidence and prepare you to tackle more complicated baking projects.

Look for the Beginner Level icon to find the recipes that are best for inexperienced bakers.

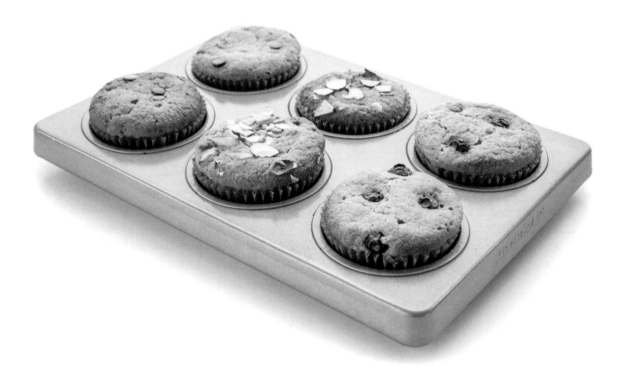

BAKING ROCKSTAR CHECKLIST

No matter whether you are baking with flour and sugar or with keto-friendly alternatives, there are some basic steps that you should always take before starting, during baking, and after things come out of the oven. Following this checklist will help you get the most out of your keto baking experience.

BEFORE YOU START:

1. Read the whole recipe through to the very end. Boring, I know, but important nonetheless. Doing so gives you at least a rough idea of how things will proceed, and you won't be caught out by an unexpected step or the lack of a required ingredient.

2. Prep your ingredients. The recipe may call for room-temperature ingredients or for something to be finely chopped or cut into cubes. Because baking can require precise timing, preparing everything in advance helps you avoid falling behind and having to scramble.

3. Preheat your oven. Baked goods often need a blast of heat right at the beginning to rise and crisp up. Most ovens take at least 10 minutes to come to the proper temperature.

4. Prep your pans. Should they be greased? Lined with parchment paper? Dusted with flour or sweetener? All of these steps are best done before you start mixing and stirring.

DURING BAKING:

1. Measure ingredients accurately. Whether you use weight or volume (see page 21 for more on these two approaches to measuring), make sure you use the correct tools to get the exact amount needed of each ingredient.

2. Add the ingredients in the order listed. Trust me, we recipe developers are not just making things complicated for our own self-aggrandizement. Creaming butter with sweetener before adding eggs helps create the air bubbles that make baked goods rise. Adding eggs one at a time to cheesecake batter allows them to mix in properly. Dumping ingredients in willy-nilly could have a negative impact on the outcome of your recipe.

3. Scrape the beaters and bowls as you go. A good flexible rubber or silicone spatula is a must for this task. Many ingredients, such as butter, stick to the bottom of the bowl during the beating process. Leaving it unincorporated could affect the consistency of your baked good.

4. Set your timer for the lowest amount of baking time. Baking recipes usually give a time range, since different ovens and pans can affect how long things take to cook. Always go with the lowest amount and check on your baked goods frequently. When I am following an unfamiliar recipe, I usually set my timer for at least 5 minutes *less* than what is stated, just in case.

5. Rotate your pans halfway through baking for more even browning unless the recipe instructions state that the oven door should not be opened during baking.

6. Follow the visual and tactile cues for doneness. I cannot stress this point enough. Baking times are only guidelines; it is these other measures that really tell you when baking is complete.

AFTER BAKING:

1. Have patience! Let baked goods cool as directed, and be sure to follow any chilling instructions. Many keto baked goods tend to firm up and hold together better once they are completely cool. And cookies and crackers simply will not be crisp when they are still warm.

2. Wait to frost cakes until they are completely cool—unless you enjoy having melted frosting run down your cake and onto your countertop!

3. Read the serving and storage information. Many baked goods, keto or not, dry out quickly when exposed to air, so don't cut them into bars or slices until you're ready to serve them. Wrap up leftovers tightly, covering the exposed edges with plastic wrap, parchment paper, or foil. Other goodies that are designed to be very moist are best kept refrigerated. See the section "How to Store Keto Baked Goods" on pages 23 to 25 for more information.

4. Dig in and enjoy your treats. Share or don't share...that part is up to you!

BAKING AT ALTITUDE

Confession: I have never, ever baked at any significant altitude, so I have no hands-on experience in adjusting recipes for altitude. However, my understanding from those who do is that many of the same rules apply for keto baking as conventional baking.

Lower atmospheric pressure at altitude means that baked goods rise more quickly and lose moisture faster than at sea level. If you don't account for these differences, your cakes will rise rapidly but fall when they come out of the oven. They might also be more dry and crumbly because of faster evaporation.

There are a number of ways to offset this, including adding more liquid and/or eggs to the batter, decreasing the amount of leavening agents like baking powder, increasing the oven temperature, and shortening the baking time. There are detailed formulas to follow based on how many feet above sea level you are, so be sure to look those up and make the necessary changes.

One very detailed article I found comes from King Arthur Flour, a trustworthy source of information about baking: www.kingarthurflour.com/learn/high-altitude-baking.html.

ACCURATE MEASURING FOR KETO BAKING

No factor is more important in successful baking than measuring your ingredients accurately. Baking is both a science and an art, and it relies on precise measurements for the best results—even more so when you are unfamiliar with keto ingredients, which behave so very differently from regular flour and sugar. So it would be remiss of me not to discuss the most accurate ways to measure ingredients.

Volume Versus Weight: Which Is Better?

There's no question that the American system of cups and tablespoons is archaic and far less accurate than measuring by weight. Nevertheless, it is still widely used, and many of us feel more comfortable with it. It is, therefore, the primary system of measurement used for the recipes in this book.

I grew up in Canada, which uses the metric system for almost everything outside the kitchen. But every cookbook I owned, even the Canadian ones, gave volume measurements. *Canadian Living,* Canada's foremost lifestyle magazine, still publishes recipes in cups and tablespoons. Metric was not something I used for cooking until more recently.

However, I fully recognize the advantage of metric weight measurements for accuracy, especially when it comes to ingredients such as nut flours and coconut flour. Because these flours can vary so much from brand to brand in terms of grind, measuring by the cup can lead to inaccuracies. A cup of Bob's Red Mill almond flour can vary significantly in weight from a cup of almond flour from Trader Joe's, whereas 100 grams of either brand is always going to equal 100 grams.

Since I always use Bob's Red Mill brand for almond and coconut flour, my volume measurements are pretty accurate. But not everyone has access to the same brands, and I have a worldwide audience of readers. For that reason, I give the amount of almond and coconut flour by weight in grams as well as by volume in cups in every recipe in all of my cookbooks.

And because I want everyone to be highly successful at keto baking, no matter where they live or what system of measurement they use, I am also including a Metric Equivalency Chart for the most commonly used keto ingredients; see pages 398 and 399.

Measuring Accurately by Volume

If you prefer to measure ingredients by volume, there are ways to be more accurate and reduce inconsistencies. Here are some things to keep in mind:

Scoop and level dry ingredients: Unless a recipe specifies otherwise, avoid packing your ingredients into the cups. Simply dip your measuring cup into the container and then use a straightedge, like a knife, to level it off. Don't press down on the ingredient with your hand as you scoop, as this can pack more in than you intend.

> **PRO TIP:**
>
> If you have just opened your bag of almond or coconut flour, give it a stir and fluff it up a bit before scooping. The flour can get rather compressed in the bag during shipping and storage. I like to transfer my flours to stainless-steel canisters for less compression and easier scooping.

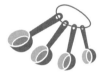

Use dry for dry and liquid for liquid: There are two kinds of measuring cups. The nested cups that have a single measurement on them are meant for dry ingredients like flour and sweetener. The clear glass or plastic cups with multiple markings on them are for liquids. They are not interchangeable.

Dry measuring cups are meant to be filled to the top and leveled off, as outlined above. But it's difficult to pour liquid right to the top of the cup without spilling. And it's difficult to even out dry ingredients to line up with the markings in a liquid measuring cup. Have a set of both and use them accordingly.

Read liquid measuring cups from the side: Remember science class, where you were taught to measure liquids in glass beakers and to look at the beakers from the side to read the measurements? The process for measuring baking ingredients is exactly the same. Set your liquid measuring cup on the counter so that it's perfectly level. Get low enough so that the markings are at eye level as you pour in the ingredient.

Pay careful attention to the way ingredient prep instructions are written: The way ingredients are described in the ingredient list gives you important information. Look at the order of the words. The meaning of "1 cup chopped strawberries" is very different from "1 cup strawberries, chopped." In the first instance, the strawberries should be chopped before being measured. In the second, they should be chopped after measuring. This can make a significant difference in the overall amount of an ingredient. Many more chopped strawberries can fit in a cup compared to whole strawberries.

Don't sweat the small stuff: Tablespoons and teaspoons are much smaller than cups, and mismeasurement is not nearly such an issue. While you should use the scoop-and-level approach with measuring spoons as well as cups, the volume that fits in a measuring spoon is small enough that any errors are minor and not likely to cause serious issues.

You can use the same measuring spoons for both wet and dry ingredients.

What about measuring semisolid ingredients like nut butters and coconut oil? Unlike most dry ingredients, you want to pack semisolid ingredients into dry measuring cups. You need to pack them in to make sure that any gaps or air bubbles are pressed out, then level the top. For sticky nut butters, lightly grease the measuring cup first so that the butter slides right out after measuring.

HOW TO STORE KETO BAKED GOODS

The majority of baked goods are best served fresh, but many recipes serve upwards of twelve people. Unless you have a very large family or are baking for a party, you may need to store your leftover goodies for a period of time. On the whole, keto baked goods store just as well their high-carb counterparts, but there are a few things to consider when choosing the best storage options.

Countertop or Refrigerator?

Sugar has a preservative effect on foods, so it helps inhibit mold growth. And because it is hygroscopic, it also helps keep foods moist. This means that baked goods made with alternative sweeteners are at a bit of a disadvantage when left at room temperature.

That said, I find that many keto baked goods are just fine on the counter for up to three days, as long as they are wrapped up tightly or stored in an airtight container. Unless you live in a very hot, humid environment, muffins, cookies, and even many cakes will fare well and taste just as good the next day. And the day after that, too.

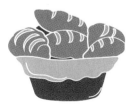

Consider the texture and consistency. If the baked good in question is dry to the touch on the outside, like a muffin or a cookie, it should be fine on the counter. However, if it's creamy, is deliberately underbaked, or is particularly moist on the inside, it should probably be refrigerated. Anything that will be hanging around for more than a few days should be refrigerated. Most items will keep in the fridge for up to a week.

It is interesting to note that I have many followers who find that they enjoy the flavor and texture of their baked goods more after a day in the fridge, regardless of original texture. However, I prefer most muffins and scones at room temperature. You might try both ways and see what appeals more to you.

The only exceptions to this rule are foods like crackers and biscotti. Because they are baked to the point of being hard and dry, they can be stored at room temperature for up to two weeks. The humid environment of a fridge can actually cause them to lose their crispness.

Let all baked goods cool completely before storing them. They are still cooking and releasing moisture as they cool, and wrapping them up too early will trap the moisture and make them soggy.

Freezing Baked Goods

A great many keto baked goods freeze really well and are ideal for meal prep and planning ahead. As with any other food, you want to let them cool completely before putting them away. To reduce the chance of freezer burn, make sure they are tightly wrapped in plastic wrap or placed in freezer bags or airtight containers. If using freezer bags, remove as much of the air as possible before sealing.

Again, texture is the giveaway here. Bready and cakey baked goods freeze nicely, but custards and very creamy dishes may not fare as well. The consistency can change and become very grainy. I also don't recommend freezing baked items made with fathead dough, as they become very dense and too chewy. You can, however, roll out the dough as a pizza crust and freeze it, unbaked, in that form.

Consider cutting larger baked goods into individual servings prior to freezing. This way, you can thaw as much or as little as you need. Even cheesecake can be portioned into slices and each slice wrapped up individually.

For more fragile items that might be crushed, such as sugar cookies, consider flash-freezing them first. Simply set them on a cookie sheet lined with parchment or waxed paper, not touching, and place in your freezer for a few hours. Once they are solid, you can place them all together in one bag or container.

Cakes are best frozen unfrosted or unglazed. If you must freeze a cake after it is frosted, expect the consistency of the frosting to change a little. Slow defrosting the cake in the fridge can help, as the temperature change is not as sudden. Chocolate glaze may "bloom," meaning that it takes on a grayish color. This discoloration usually disappears as the glaze thaws, but not always.

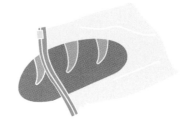

Some raw cookie doughs freeze really well. Cookies that are rolled into balls before baking can be frozen after rolling. Simply flash-freeze them on a cookie sheet first, making sure they don't touch one another so that they don't stick together, and then transfer them to a resealable freezer bag and squeeze out as much air as possible. Thaw on the counter before baking.

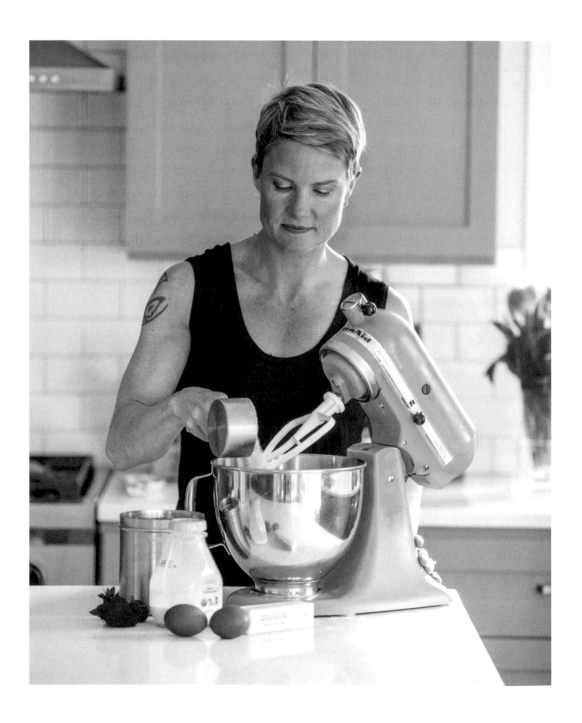

Chapter 2:
THE INGREDIENTS

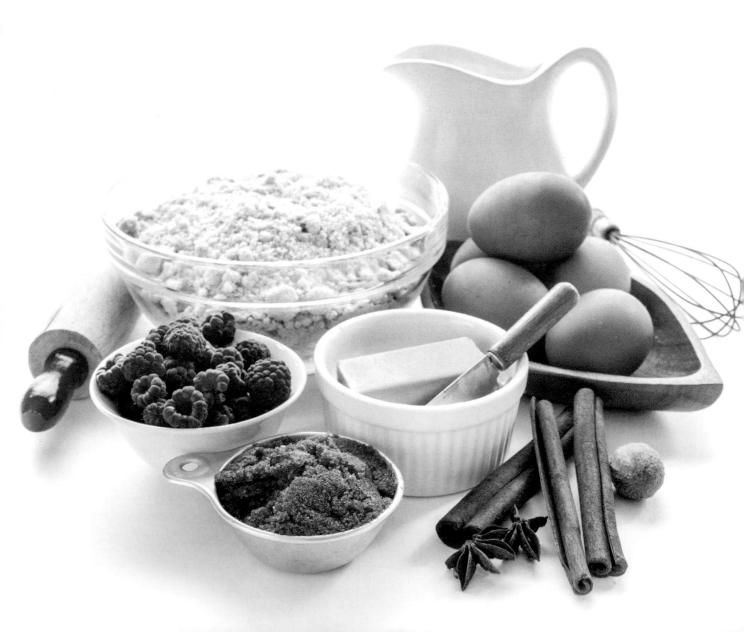

Just as in conventional baking, every ingredient plays a role in giving keto baked goods their structure, flavor, and consistency. Many of them make a greater contribution to the final product than you may realize. Skipping or swapping a key ingredient could spell disaster for your cake or cookies. So it's imperative to understand your ingredients and the roles they play in keto baking.

Some are more integral than others, of course. We're going to take a deep dive into these integral ingredients, looking closely at how they behave and how they interact with the other players on the baking stage.

ALL ABOUT KETO FLOURS

While most people associate the word *flour* with wheat, the rise of low-carb and gluten-free diets has challenged this notion to the extreme. If a food substance can be ground finely enough, someone out there is going to make flour with it. And someone like me is going to try to bake with it—with varying degrees of success.

There are a few wheat-based flour products on the market that have somehow magically been decarbified. At the beginning of my keto journey, I tried these products a number of times, and I can't say that they live up to their promise. They don't taste very good, they don't rise or hold together well, and you have to ask yourself: what sort of processing do they go through to reduce the carb count so much?

For the purposes of this book, we are going to stick with real whole-food flour alternatives like nut flours, seed flours, and coconut flour, with a few other notable options. It may be difficult to believe now, but I promise that with one or more of these keto flours, you can create baked goods that rival their high-carb counterparts in taste and consistency.

I am often asked if there is a basic formula for substituting keto flours for wheat flour, and I wish it were that simple. But it really depends on what you are making. Cookies are dense and crunchy, whereas cakes should be light and fluffy, and they are going to require very different ratios of keto flours to other ingredients.

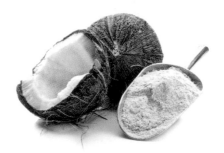

THE ROLE OF GLUTEN IN BAKING

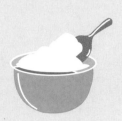

Most keto baking is, almost by default, gluten-free. And most keto dieters choose to avoid gluten and grains entirely. So it may seem strange to devote a whole section of this book to the "G word."

However, one of the keys to mastering gluten-free baking is having an in-depth understanding of the role that gluten normally plays. Wheat-based flour is such an accepted part of standard baking practices that we rarely stop to consider what it actually does in various recipes. Only by breaking down all the properties of gluten can we begin to figure how best to replace it.

If you've been baking with wheat flour all your life, you've been availing yourself of all the amazing properties of gluten, perhaps without ever really knowing how it works. While it may not be the healthiest food on the planet, gluten is a remarkable substance with many valuable qualities. That's why it's often such a surprise to find that you can't simply substitute a cup of almond or coconut flour for a cup of wheat flour.

WHAT IS GLUTEN?

You may be surprised to learn that gluten is a protein, even though people tend to associate it with high-carb foods. It's made up of two protein molecules, glutenin and gliadin, found naturally in wheat and other grains such as barley and rye.

These molecules are essentially inactive in the dry flours made from these grains. But the moment they come into contact with liquid, they begin to change rather dramatically. The individual molecules bind together to create long strands known as gluten. These strands then link up to create a fine network that is both strong and elastic. The more you work the dough through kneading or mixing, the longer and stronger those strands become.

Okay, enough with the science lesson. What does gluten actually do? A better question might be, what doesn't it do?

- **Elasticity:** That elastic strength is the hallmark of traditional baking. The network of gluten strands traps gases given off by leavening agents like yeast, baking powder, or baking soda. Like a balloon, it expands but does not break, allowing the dough to rise during the baking process.

- **Structure:** That network of fine strands also gives traditional baked goods their structure. Once baked, the gluten network hardens and firms up so that the final product doesn't collapse as it cools. And the air bubbles created by the leavening agent and trapped by the gluten bake into place.

- **Moisture:** Gluten also absorbs and holds moisture, so traditional baked goods don't dry out too much in the oven. When properly stored and wrapped, they can also stay moist for days.

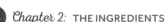

HOW DO WE REPLACE GLUTEN IN KETO BAKING?

Given all that gluten does for conventional baking, you may be wondering how on earth to bake without it. The truth is that no single keto ingredient can do everything that gluten does. But there are ways and means to account for most, if not quite all, of its properties. What and how much you use depends very much on the consistency you are trying to achieve.

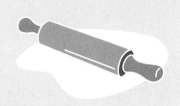

Eggs can be great binders for cakes, muffins, and quick breads. The addition of dry protein powders like whey or egg white protein also helps them rise and hold their shape. Other binding agents like glucomannan, xanthan gum, and psyllium husk can create bonds that mimic gluten protein strands. Adding a bit of gelatin to cookie dough helps create that chewy quality. Even mozzarella cheese can help, as it produces an unrivaled stretchiness in keto pizza dough.

Read on to see how all these ingredients work in keto baking!

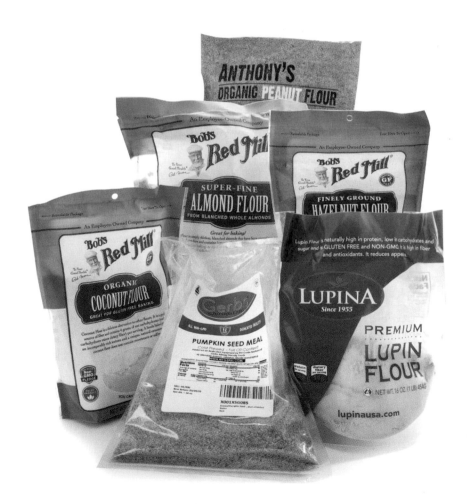

Almond Flour

Almond flour is by far the most widely known and commonly used low-carb flour, and I find it to be one of the most versatile for keto baking. Thanks to the popularity of Paleo and gluten-free diets, as well as the steady rise of keto, it is readily available at most grocery stores.

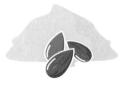

Almond flour is really just ground almonds, but the grind and consistency can vary dramatically from brand to brand. You want to look for one that is quite finely ground without larger particles in it, which will result in cakes and cookies with a better, more cohesive crumb. I prefer Bob's Red Mill but also have had good luck with Honeyville and the Costco store brand, Kirkland.

Many nuts can be ground into flours of sorts, but almonds have a distinct advantage in that they can be blanched and the skins entirely removed before being ground into flour. The color is lighter, the grind is finer, and the flavor is more neutral than that of other nut flours, so the resulting baked goods resemble their wheat flour counterparts a little more closely.

That said, it's never going to be as simple as making a 1:1 substitution of almond flour for wheat flour, and you can see why if you give it a little thought. Being made from nuts, almond flour has a much higher fat content and isn't nearly as fine and powdery as wheat flour. It also contains more protein, but the proteins in almonds don't create any sort of bond the way gluten does.

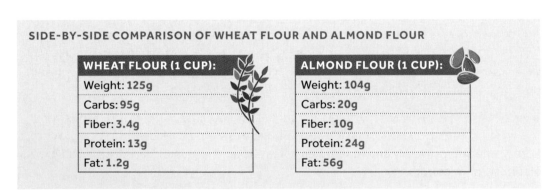

SIDE-BY-SIDE COMPARISON OF WHEAT FLOUR AND ALMOND FLOUR

WHEAT FLOUR (1 CUP):	ALMOND FLOUR (1 CUP):
Weight: 125g	Weight: 104g
Carbs: 95g	Carbs: 20g
Fiber: 3.4g	Fiber: 10g
Protein: 13g	Protein: 24g
Fat: 1.2g	Fat: 56g

Other Nut Flours

There are a number of other nut flours out there, but they aren't as widely available and can be costly. I love using hazelnut flour and pecan flour for the unique flavor they add to keto baked goods. Check out the Chocolate Hazelnut Torte (page 120) and the Salted Caramel Tart with Chocolate Glaze (page 322) for recipes that include these ingredients.

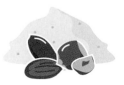

I've also seen walnut flour, cashew flour, and even Brazil nut flour. All of these other nut flours tend to be slightly heavier and more coarsely ground because the skins are included. Since cashews are much higher in carbs than other nuts, cashew flour should be used sparingly, if it all, in keto baking.

Macadamia nuts are an ideal keto snack, but they don't make great flour because they are so high in fat that they tend to turn into butter before they can be ground finely enough.

CAN YOU GRIND YOUR OWN NUT FLOURS?

Yes and no. You can make nut "meals" at home by grinding nuts in a food processor or other chopper. But you will never get them as fine or as uniform as the commercially ground versions. Homemade nut meal can be serviceable for some purposes, like breading chicken, but it's not going to produce stellar results for cakes. I don't recommend it for most baked goods.

Coconut Flour

Coconut flour is another very popular keto flour that is widely available in most grocery stores. Although I don't find it quite as versatile as almond flour, it's still incredibly useful and makes some of the best nut-free keto cakes and muffins. My favorite chocolate cupcakes (see page 78) are made entirely with coconut flour.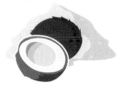

If you have never baked with coconut flour before, you are in for a wild ride. I only ask that you set aside all your experience with conventional flour before attempting to use it. It's about as different from wheat flour as any "flour" can be, and it's also very different from nut flours. While coconut flour is quite useful and can produce beautiful results, it takes some time to get used to.

Coconut flour is the by-product of coconut milk production. After the milk has been extracted, the leftover coconut meat is dried at a low temperature and then ground. It is very fine and powdery and resembles wheat flour in appearance, although it smells distinctly of coconut.

The most distinctive characteristic of coconut flour is the rather astonishing way it soaks up moisture and liquids. In this way, it differs from all other flours, gluten-free or otherwise. It's like a sponge in powder form, taking in a remarkable amount of eggs, oil, and other wet ingredients and still staying as thick as porridge until it finally reaches saturation. But be careful: add too much liquid and you'll end up with a soggy baked good that won't cook through. It's a delicate balance.

The trick to working with coconut flour is accepting the fact that it requires quite a few eggs to give it structure and body. It can be a little shocking to see half a dozen to a dozen eggs in a recipe, but as you try it out, you will see that it works. The end results are rarely too eggy or rubbery.

You will also be surprised to see how little coconut flour is used in most recipes. It's incredibly dense, but it expands remarkably with the addition of eggs and liquid, so you typically need only about a third of the amount you would need with conventional flour or nut flours.

As with almond flour, different brands of coconut flour vary quite a bit in consistency and absorbency, which can affect the outcome of your baked goods. I always use Bob's Red Mill coconut flour because it gives me consistent results. If you use a different brand, you need to be ready to add either a little more coconut flour or a little more liquid to your batter.

Sunflower Seed Flour

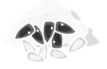

One of the best nut-free alternatives to almond flour is sunflower seed flour. It has a similar texture and consistency, as well as a similar nutritional profile, so it can be subbed cup for cup, which makes it easy to adapt recipes to be nut-free.

Here's where it gets weird, though. Sunflower seeds react with leavening agents such as baking powder and baking soda and turn an odd shade of green after baking. Nothing has gone bad; it's simply a chemical reaction. Adding a tablespoon or so of an acid, such as lemon juice or apple cider vinegar, can offset this reaction. Recipes that include cocoa powder are usually fine, too, since the brown color masks the green.

If you or any of your loved ones has a severe nut allergy, make sure the sunflower seed flour you buy was not processed in a facility that also processes nuts. The brand GERBS is totally allergen free, so it's a good choice. I purchase it on Amazon.

Pumpkin Seed Flour

I've only just begun to play around with pumpkin seed flour, but it's another good nut-free alternative. Like sunflower seed flour, it seems to work as a cup-for-cup replacement for almond flour. Since it has a greenish color, however, it is not ideal for all recipes. But again, it would be an excellent substitute in a cocoa-based recipe like brownies or chocolate cake.

Pumpkin seed flour can have a slightly bitter taste when used alone, so you may want to up the amounts of sweetener and perhaps flavorings like vanilla extract to mask it.

Peanut Flour

This useful and tasty flour is a little harder to define, since the way it is made varies so much from brand to brand. It can simply be ground peanuts, in which case it's light in color and rather coarse. Or the peanuts can be roasted and the flour partially defatted, in which case it is darker in color and very fine and powdery. The latter type is more commonly available, and I typically recommend either Protein Plus or Anthony's. Both products work well.

Because it's so fine and powdery, peanut flour is more absorbent than almond flour, and you may need a lot of liquid to thin it out. It can also produce a bit of a dry mouthfeel when used alone. I often use it in combination with other keto flours.

You might also see it referred to as peanut powder or peanut butter powder. Be careful here, though, as some peanut flours/powders contain added sugars.

Sesame Flour

This flour is very dry and powdery, and it's not quite as low in carbs as other flour alternatives, with 10 grams of carbs per ¼ cup and very little fiber to speak of. It also has a strong sesame flavor, which can be good or bad, depending on your perspective. I don't think it makes a great keto flour on its own, but it can be used in combination with other flours, such as in my Toasted Sesame Crackers (page 298).

Lupin Flour

Something of a newcomer on the scene, lupin flour is gaining in popularity among many keto dieters. Readers have begun to ask me to develop recipes with it, so I have used it in a few of the baked goods in this book. Lupin flour is made from lupin beans, which are legumes related to peanuts and soybeans, so be aware if you have allergies to these foods.

It is a bit high in carbs (12 grams per ¼ cup) but about 90 percent of that is fiber. Still, I advise caution here since it's hard to know how much of the fiber is soluble, some of which is absorbed into the bloodstream.

Lupin flour also has a distinct taste that, while not unpleasant, can take a little getting used to. I think it's probably best used in savory recipes and in combination with other keto flours.

Oat Fiber

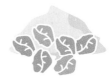

This is not to be confused with oat flour, which is made from ground oats and is not at all keto-friendly. Oat fiber is made from the husk that surrounds the oat (the kernel) itself. It is quite high in carbs, with about 27 grams per ¼ cup, but almost all of that is fiber. Again, I advise caution since it's unclear how much of this fiber is absorbed into the bloodstream.

My thought on oat fiber is that it's rather flavorless and dry, although it can help give some baked goods a more bready consistency. On its own, it doesn't make great treats; it works best in combination with other keto flours.

Ground Pork Rinds

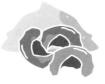

It might seem crazy to think that fried pigskin could be used as a flour, but it really can in some applications. And it's hands down the lowest-carb option out there, having zero carbs per serving. The keto community has been using ground pork rinds as a breading for chicken and fish for a long time. Why not use them in baked goods, too?

Because it's hard to grind them super finely, pork rinds aren't ideal for finer baked goods like cakes. And the high collagen content makes them a bit too gummy and soft for cookies and the like. But I decided to play with them in a few recipes and even created delicious breadsticks (page 274) with ground pork rinds as the only "flour."

You can easily grind your own at home in a food processor. Just be sure to measure them after grinding, as they reduce in volume significantly. I also have been using the preground pork crumbs from Pork King Good and have had great success with that product.

Combining Keto Flours

As you work your way through these recipes, you will notice that I often combine flours like almond and coconut. Over the years, I've found that these two flours produce great results when used in tandem, particularly for cakes. A little of the dry coconut flour can help offset the moister almond flour and reduce the carb count a little.

I encourage you to experiment as you become more adept at keto baking. You may discover your own preference for flour combinations along the way.

ALL ABOUT KETO SWEETENERS

A book about keto baking wouldn't be complete without an in-depth discussion of sweetener options. But the topic of keto-friendly sweeteners is a big one and getting bigger every moment. In an effort to get a little piece of the growing sugar-free market, companies are coming out with new sugar substitutes seemingly by the day. And since all of them are formulated slightly differently, it can be difficult to figure out which ones to use when.

I am going to give it my best shot at tackling this monumental subject. It's beyond the scope of this book to try to account for every single sugar alternative out there, but I hope to give you enough information about how these sweeteners behave that you can deduce which would work best in any given situation.

I have experimented with a great many of these sweeteners, and I can tell you that none of them behaves exactly like sugar. I want to be very clear about that. There really is no such thing as a perfect sugar substitute; they all have very different properties.

That said, there are some that really do bake quite well. The trick is to harness the various properties of different sweeteners and use them to your advantage. Before you can do that, you need to have an understanding of how each of them works. Most of the popular sweeteners on the market are made with a few ingredients in varying amounts, so I will break them down into their ingredients.

For the purposes of this book, we are going to stick with naturally derived keto sweeteners. You are free to substitute artificial sweeteners like sucralose and aspartame if you wish, but they are generally not recommended for a keto (or any other) diet.

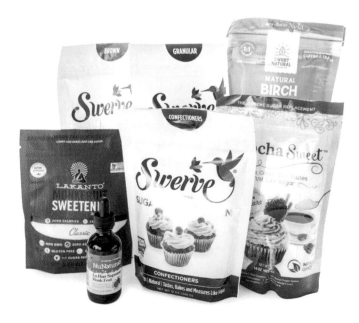

THE ROLE OF SUGAR IN BAKING

Sugar does more than sweeten conventional baked goods. Just as understanding how gluten works gives us insight into how to bake gluten-free, understanding how sugar works will give us great insight into baking sugar-free.

The unique chemical makeup of sugar performs a number of critical functions in traditional baking, such as:

- **Leavening:** The crystalline structure of sugar helps whip air bubbles into softened butter during the creaming process. These air bubbles then trap the gases given off by leavening agents, helping the baked goods rise in the oven.

- **Stabilization:** Whipping sugar into egg whites helps to stabilize them and keeps them from collapsing during baking, giving certain cakes and cookies additional volume and structure.

- **Moisture:** Sugar is hygroscopic, meaning that it attracts and locks in moisture, so baked goods don't dry out too quickly.

- **Browning and crisping:** Sugar caramelizes easily when exposed to high heat. It also undergoes a chemical reaction called the Maillard reaction when combined with proteins. Both of these reactions help produce a deeper flavor and a golden-brown exterior for baked goods and helps cookies crisp up.

- **Spreading:** Because sugar melts during the baking process, it helps baked goods like drop cookies spread out.

- **Inhibits microbial growth:** Sugar interferes with the growth of microbes, which is why it's often used in preserving and curing foods. It helps keep baked goods shelf stable longer.

- **Tenderizing:** Sugar also interferes with the development of gluten, so it keeps baked goods from becoming too tough. But because there is no gluten in keto flours, this property isn't of much concern for us!

Erythritol

Erythritol is one of the most popular keto sweeteners on the market, and it is a common ingredient in many packaged keto snacks, as well as in many sweetener alternatives. It is a sugar alcohol that is naturally present in some fruits and fermented foods. For mass production, it is made by fermenting glucose syrup with yeast.

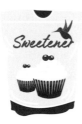

Sugar alcohols are actually neither sugars nor alcohols but have a chemical makeup that is similar to both. There are a number of sugar alcohols on the market, and you will see many of these polyols in "sugar-free" products. But not all sugar alcohols are created equal, as you will soon realize.

What makes erythritol unique among sugar alcohols is that it has zero carb impact. By this, I mean that it does not raise blood sugar at all—most of it is absorbed into the bloodstream in the small intestine and then excreted virtually unchanged in the urine. Our bodies simply do not recognize erythritol as a carbohydrate. And because erythritol is absorbed before it enters the colon, it does not have the laxative effect that other sugar alcohols do.

The same cannot be said for other sugar alcohols, and you would be wise to steer clear of anything containing sorbitol or maltitol. Xylitol is a decent choice, but it has a slightly higher glycemic index and may have a small impact on blood glucose (more on xylitol below).

ERYTHRITOL IN BAKING

Erythritol-based sweeteners are some of the most popular for keto baking, and I myself am partial to Swerve Sweetener. But like any sugar substitute, erythritol has its pros and cons.

Erythritol mimics sugar in its crystalline structure, so it functions similarly for whipping air into fats and egg whites. It also browns and crisps up nicely, and with a little extra coaxing, it will even caramelize.

It comes in a powdered version, perfect for making frostings, and a granular version; several brands have good "brown sugar" varieties as well. These products are extremely useful for replacing sugar in many applications.

But erythritol differs from sugar in several important ways. It is only about 70 percent as sweet as sugar when used on its own, which is why so many brands combine it with other ingredients to enhance the sweetness.

In addition, erythritol Is nonhygroscopic, which means that unlike sugar, it does not attract or hold onto moisture. If you were simply to substitute it for the sugar in a conventional recipe, the baked good would dry out and become stale much faster. For our purposes, this isn't as much of an issue, as keto baked goods often have a much higher fat content, which helps keep them moist longer. But erythritol doesn't melt as easily during baking, so keto cookies don't spread nicely the way cookies made with sugar do.

Perhaps one of the biggest disadvantages of erythritol is its propensity to recrystallize in liquid applications, causing sauces and custards to become gritty or harden after they cool. I find that the more heat that is applied during the cooking of a sauce or custard, the more the erythritol recrystallizes as it cools.

Finally, many people experience a mouth-cooling sensation when consuming erythritol, similar to sucking on a mint. Not everyone experiences this sensation, and some of the formulations of erythritol-based sweeteners can minimize or even eliminate it. I personally experience it with plain erythritol but not with Swerve Sweetener, which is why Swerve has become my favorite keto sweetener.

 Bulk sweetener, crystalline structure, promotes browning, caramelizes

 Only 70% as sweet as sugar, recrystallization, some people experience a cooling sensation

ERYTHRITOL-BASED SWEETENERS

Because erythritol isn't as sweet as sugar, many manufacturers combine it with another more concentrated sweetener, such as stevia or monk fruit, in order to make it a cup-for-cup sugar replacement. This makes it much more straightforward to convert a conventional recipe to a keto one. But each sweetener blend is formulated a little differently, and you may find that you prefer the taste of one over another.

BRANDS (US): Swerve Sweetener, Lakanto, Pyure, So Nourished, ZSweet

OUTSIDE THE US: Natvia, Sukrin

Xylitol

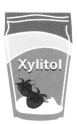

Xylitol is also a sugar alcohol, and it is a common ingredient in sugar-free gums and mints. It is naturally present in some fruits and vegetables, as well as in wood and corn. Commercially, it is usually manufactured from corn or birch trees.

Xylitol is low on the glycemic index, although not as low as erythritol. About 50 percent of the xylitol is absorbed by the intestines into the bloodstream and metabolized. Because it is incompletely digested, xylitol can cause some gastrointestinal discomfort when consumed in large amounts. Additionally, some people with diabetes, myself included, notice an increase in blood sugar when they consume xylitol.

Perhaps one of the biggest issues with xylitol is that it is extremely toxic to dogs. Even tiny amounts can cause hypoglycemia, seizures, and liver failure, so consider other sweeteners if you have a beloved canine at home. A recent study in the *Journal of Veterinary Pharmacology and Therapeutics* indicates that xylitol does not have the same adverse effects in cats.

XYLITOL IN BAKING

Because of its crystalline structure, xylitol can whip air into butter and egg whites. It comes in a powdered version as well as a granular one, but at the time of the writing of this book, there do not appear to be any xylitol-based brown sugar substitutes.

Xylitol is as sweet as regular cane sugar, so no additional additives are needed to make it measure like sugar.

Compared to erythritol, xylitol is far more hygroscopic, so it attracts and holds on to moisture. This can be both good and bad in keto baking and cooking. It's good in liquid applications, as xylitol helps sauces stay soft and pourable, and they don't recrystallize. It's great for ice cream as well.

Xylitol doesn't caramelize or crisp up the way erythritol does, however, so baked goods that should have a more crisp texture, like cookies, end up soft and cakey when it is used as the sweetener. Meringues made with xylitol are a total disaster—they stay gooey and soft, like marshmallows, and stick to the parchment paper.

Powdered xylitol makes good frosting, but I've found it troublesome for thinner glazes, as it absorbs the liquid quickly and doesn't thicken up easily as powdered erythritol.

 As sweet as sugar, crystalline structure, more hygroscopic, doesn't recrystallize

 Causes some GI distress, may raise blood sugar, toxic to dogs, doesn't crisp up or caramelize

Bocha Sweet

This unique sweetener has been around for a while but is gaining in popularity lately. It is derived from the kabocha squash, a type of winter squash also known as Japanese pumpkin. It's a pentose sugar, meaning that five atoms make up each molecule. But don't panic when you see that it's a sugar. Like erythritol, it has little to no impact on blood glucose.

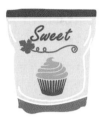

Xylose, from which xylitol is made, is also a pentose sweetener. Not surprisingly, then, Bocha Sweet has some of the same benefits and limitations in baking as xylitol does. It's as sweet as sugar, can be measured cup for cup like sugar, and has no apparent aftertaste for some people. But it can cause gastrointestinal upset when consumed in larger quantities.

And, like xylitol, Bocha Sweet doesn't caramelize or crisp up. It's great in baked goods like cakes or muffins, and it's particularly useful in sauces, custards, and ice creams that need to retain a creamy texture. I have started using it in all of my ice cream recipes, as they stay soft and scoopable right out of the freezer. But cookies made with Bocha Sweet will be cakey and soft.

Meringues are the ultimate test of a sweetener's ability to crisp up. I tried making meringues with mostly Swerve and a single tablespoon of Bocha Sweet, hoping the combo would give me the ideal meringue texture. Alas, they turned out like gooey marshmallows, and my kids simply ate them with a spoon right off the parchment.

 As sweet as sugar, crystalline structure, more hygroscopic, doesn't recrystallize

 Causes some GI distress, doesn't crisp up or caramelize

Allulose

This "rare sugar" is a relative newcomer to the keto baking scene. It is a monosaccharide found in minute amounts in dried fruits such as figs, jackfruit, and raisins. It really is a sugar, but again, one that is only partially metabolized. Like erythritol, it is absorbed in the small intestine, and the majority is excreted in the urine without affecting blood glucose levels.

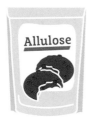

Because allulose is so new on the scene, there are relatively few clinical trials in humans, but thus far, studies indicate that it doesn't cause spikes in blood sugar or insulin. In fact, it may even help lower blood sugar when other carbs are eaten along with it.

However, I caution you from personal experience that allulose may cause serious gastrointestinal distress. Not everyone has problems with it, apparently, but some people experience severe diarrhea, abdominal pain, and headaches. One study I found indicates that almost everyone will have some issues when consuming more than 0.4 gram of allulose per kilogram of body weight in a single serving.

Let me put that into perspective for you. I weigh 120 pounds, or about 54 kilograms. According to the formula above, I should consume no more than 21 grams of allulose, which is about 5 teaspoons.

Allulose is only about 70 percent as sweet as table sugar, so it takes more to sweeten baked goods. And being rare in nature means that it's also quite expensive, although new techniques allow for more efficient large-scale production.

As for baking properties, allulose caramelizes quite well, but it doesn't crisp up at all; baked goods made with it stay soft and cakey. Using even a small amount of allulose in addition to an erythritol-based sweetener will keep your baked goods very cakelike. Not a great choice if you want crispy cookies.

I also have found that allulose makes some baked goods very brown on the outside. They aren't burnt, but the parts of the cake touching the sides of the pan get very dark; see the Rum Cake (page 104) for an example. This effect isn't always appealing for cakes or muffins that should be light in color.

 Crystalline structure, more hygroscopic, doesn't recrystallize, will caramelize

 Only 70% as sweet as sugar, causes some GI distress, doesn't crisp up in cookies

Stevia and Monk Fruit Extracts

I am lumping these two sweeteners together because they have similar properties for keto baking. They are both naturally derived high-intensity sweeteners, hundreds of times sweeter than sugar. Stevia comes from the *Stevia rebaudiana* plant, which is native to South America. Monk fruit, also known as lo han guo, comes from a fruit grown in Southeast Asia.

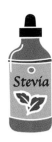

These sweeteners are extremely concentrated, and a tiny amount (think ¼ teaspoon) can sweeten a whole recipe. While that may sound like a good thing, it can have serious implications for baking.

Such concentrated sweeteners have no bulk, which means that they don't have much in the way of weight or volume. They can't whip air bubbles into butter or egg whites, and they don't contribute to the texture or consistency of baked goods. They also don't caramelize or crisp up at all. They really don't add anything to a recipe except sweetness.

Substituting a non-bulk sweetener like stevia or monk fruit in a recipe that calls for a bulk sweetener could affect the outcome significantly. Your baked good may rise less and be more fragile, or, in the case of custard, it may not set properly.

Because bulk is such an important factor in baking, some companies "bulk up" stevia and monk fruit by mixing them with ingredients like maltodextrin. I'd steer clear of these sweetener blends since maltodextrin is a glucose derivative and tends to spike blood sugar.

Other brands combine stevia or monk fruit with erythritol. Many of these, such as Lakanto, say "Monkfruit Sweetener" on the front of the package, but don't be fooled. They are, in reality, erythritol-based sweeteners and should be treated as such for baking because erythritol is the primary ingredient. The giveaway here is that the package will say that the sweetener measures cup for cup like sugar. Flip the bag over and look at the ingredients; erythritol almost always comes first.

Combining Sweeteners

As with keto flours, keto sweeteners sometimes work best in combination. It really depends on the texture you want to achieve. When I want something to be softer or gooier or to avoid recrystallization, I often use a mix of Swerve and Bocha Sweet. When I want something to be crisp or crunchy, I use only Swerve.

Also, if you experience a strong aftertaste with a particular sweetener, combining it with another can help reduce that effect.

I experimented a great deal with the recipes in this book. In some cases, where the type of sweetener won't affect the outcome too much, I give you the choice of using whichever sweetener you like best. In other recipes, I specify exactly what and how much sweetener you should use. And in others, I simply provide tips to guide your choices.

BROWN SUGAR SUBSTITUTES

The development of Swerve Brown has been an absolute game-changer for me. There are other keto "brown sugars" out there, such as Lakanto Golden and Sukrin Gold, and they are all erythritol based. To my knowledge, no one has developed a brown sugar substitute based on anything else.

The Swerve version is far superior, in my opinion. It smells, tastes, and even feels more like real brown sugar, because it's moist and quite dense and tends to pack into the measuring cup as you scoop it out. I find myself reaching for it regularly because it gives certain baked goods a true brown sugar flavor.

For the recipes in this book, I simply say "brown sugar substitute" so that you can use what you like best. If you can't get your hands on any such thing, you can simply use a granulated erythritol sweetener and 1 to 2 teaspoons of molasses or yacón syrup. While these are both sugars, they will add only about 11 grams of carbs to your full recipe. Divided among 12 or so servings, that is less than 1 gram per serving.

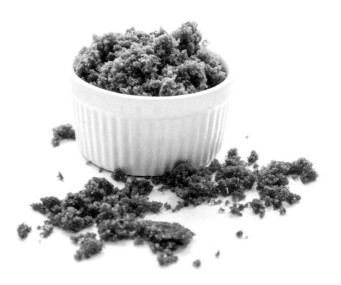

ALL ABOUT EGGS

Eggs play an important role in baking, providing structure, moisture, fat, and helping baked goods rise. For many grain-free baked goods, which lack gluten, the binding power of eggs helps keep them from crumbling into dust.

You should use large eggs for all recipes unless otherwise specified. This is standard across most baking, not just for the keto diet. The size of the eggs matters more than you might realize. It can make the difference between your goodies being overly eggy and moist or falling apart in your hands.

If you purchase eggs from a farmer's market, the sizes can vary quite a bit. Not to worry, it's easy to weigh them. The average size of a large egg in the shell is 2 ounces. If yours are very different from this standard, simply use fewer or more eggs, as applicable. It does not need to be exact but should be close.

How to Separate Eggs

- Eggs are easiest to separate while they are cold, although it is better to whip them at room temperature. Plan ahead and separate your eggs as soon as you take them out of the fridge.

- You can use an egg separator, which is a small spoon-shaped gadget that sits over a bowl or cup, with slits that allow the egg white to slip through while the yolk stays inside.

- You can also use the broken halves of the eggshell, holding them over a bowl and transferring the egg back and forth between the halves. The egg white will slip off into the bowl while the yolk remains in the shell. Be careful with this method and try to keep the yolk from catching on the sharp shell edge.

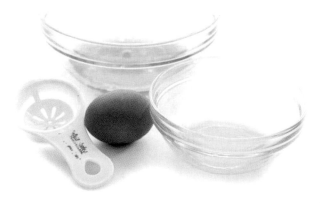

How to Whip Egg Whites

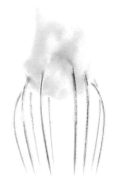

- The bowl and beaters must be very clean and dry and free from oil. Stainless-steel bowls are best, as they are the cleanest and help the egg whites billow up.

- Even a single drop of yolk, oil, or water can keep the whites from whipping properly.

- If you are separating multiple eggs at a time, use three bowls. Use one bowl to catch the egg white and then transfer it to the bowl in which you plan to whip them. That way, if one yolk breaks while you are in the process of separating the eggs, you haven't ruined all of your egg whites. The third bowl is for the yolks.

- Cream of tartar and salt both help stabilize the whites as they whip. You usually need only about ¼ teaspoon cream of tartar and/or a pinch of salt.

Love and eggs are best when they are fresh.

— *Russian proverb*

ALL ABOUT LEAVENERS

Have you ever forgotten to add baking powder to a cake or muffin batter? Then you know the importance that leavening agents have in baking. They help baked goods rise and be lighter and fluffier. Without them, your goodies would be incredibly dense.

How it works: Leavening agents like baking soda and baking powder create carbon dioxide when mixed with liquids and then heated. The released gas is then trapped by the structure of the dough or batter, causing the entire volume to expand and lift.

Most keto recipes rely on baking powder or baking soda for leavening. These are not interchangeable, so be sure to use the one your recipe calls for.

Baking soda is straight sodium bicarbonate. It requires an acid to start reacting and creating carbon dioxide. This reaction begins the moment it comes in contact with the acid, so you need to work quickly and get your batter into the oven soon after mixing.

Baking powder is baking soda mixed with a dry acid (often cream of tartar) and a little starch. The starch inhibits the sodium bicarbonate and the acid from combining and reacting in dry form. It's not until baking powder comes in contact with a liquid that the reaction begins. Baking powder is more stable than pure baking soda and works more slowly, so you don't need to rush as much to get things into the oven.

Yeast is also a biological leavener, although it's not frequently used in keto baking. However, I wanted to include a yeast bread recipe (page 272) in this book because of its unique bready flavor.

Yeast is a single-celled organism that lies dormant until it comes in contact with moisture. It needs sugar to feed on and grow. In conventional recipes, the starches in the flour provide enough sugar, but for grain-free recipes, you do need to add a little honey or sugar (only 2 teaspoons or so). The sugar is completely digested by the yeast, and there is no residual sugar in the resulting baked good.

ALL ABOUT BUTTER, FATS, AND OILS

Butter and oils are more than just added calories in baked goods. They provide tenderness, moisture, and flavor, and they help bind other ingredients together. They even make a contribution to leavening power. Beating a crystalline sweetener into a semisolid fat such as butter or coconut oil creates tiny air pockets, which help trap the gases given off by baking soda or baking powder, providing a better rise and a fine-textured crumb.

Some recipes call for melted butter or coconut oil. Melting the fat simplifies the recipe, making it easier to mix the ingredients together. You may not get quite the same rise, but melted fats are useful for muffins, quick breads, and snack cakes.

A number of liquid oils are useful in keto baking, such as avocado oil, olive oil, and cold-pressed nut oils. Avoid highly processed man-made oils like canola oil, safflower oil, and other vegetable oils. These simply aren't healthy alternatives.

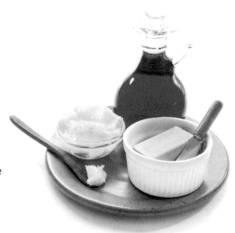

In this book, and for most baking, unsalted butter is the standard. Since the salt content of salted butter can vary brand to brand, using unsalted butter allows you to control the saltiness of the final product.

Substituting for Butter

It may come as a surprise that butter is not a pure fat. It contains water and milk solids as well, so substituting another fat or oil could affect the flavor and quality of your baked goods.

If a recipe calls for softened butter, don't replace it with a liquid oil. The softened state of the fat is important to the recipe for rising or tenderness. The best substitutes are softened coconut oil and softened ghee.

However, if the recipe calls for melted butter (or melted coconut oil, for that matter), you should be able to substitute a liquid oil. It comes down to flavor in many cases. Some oils, like extra-virgin olive oil and certain nut oils, may impart strong flavors to the finished product. Avocado oil is quite neutral in flavor, so it makes a good substitute.

Because butter contains some water, baked goods made with other oils may seem greasier as they come out of the oven. I find that this excess oil usually reabsorbs into the baked goods as they cool. However, you can also cut back on the substituted oil by a tablespoon or two and add a tablespoon or two of water to make up the liquid.

ALL ABOUT CHOCOLATE

Oh chocolate, how I love thee! I could probably write a whole cookbook devoted entirely to chocolate. Perhaps that should be my next book project. (Publisher, take note!) But I digress...

There are many different kinds of chocolate, and using the right one is critical for both the structure and flavor of your recipe. They really aren't interchangeable unless the chocolate is just an "addition," such as a decoration on top of a cake or chocolate chips in a cookie.

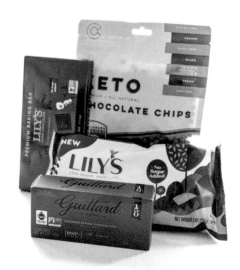

Chocolate is ground from the beans of happiness.
— *Terri Guillemets*

Cocoa Powder

Cocoa powder is really just the cocoa solids with most of the fat (also known as cocoa butter) removed. The solids are ground to a powder and can be "natural," which means that the powder is left untreated and is more acidic and bitter, or "Dutch process," which is treated with an alkaline solution to neutralize the acidity. Dutch process cocoa powder is also darker in color than the natural variety.

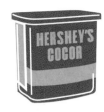

For the most part, the two types can be used interchangeably. But recipes that call for baking soda as the leavener may be relying on the acid in natural cocoa powder to activate the soda. Read the recipe in full to see if this is the case. (There are no such recipes in this book.)

If not, then it comes down to personal taste. Most American grocery store brands, such as Hershey's and Ghirardelli, are natural cocoa powder. Hershey's Dark is a mix of both to impart a darker color and flavor. I often use Ghirardelli, but I also like Guittard and Rodelle, which are both Dutch process.

I don't recommend substituting raw cacao powder. Cocoa powder is made from roasted cocoa beans, so it has a richer, more chocolatey flavor. I find that raw cacao powder tends to clump up in batters, leaving little bits of cacao in the finished product.

Unsweetened Chocolate

Also known as baking chocolate, unsweetened chocolate is the cocoa solids and the cocoa butter together with no sweeteners, dairy, or other additives. Most people find it far too bitter to be palatable on its own, but it adds a rich chocolate flavor to sweetened baked goods and desserts. It can be tricky to work with at times and is prone to seizing, so it needs to be treated carefully.

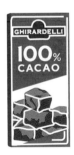

The quality of the unsweetened chocolate you use makes a big difference in the finished product. I prefer Ghirardelli, Guittard, and Dagoba in recipes that call for unsweetened chocolate.

Unsweetened chocolate is not available in some countries, including Australia and the UK. In a pinch, you can use 3 tablespoons of cocoa powder and 1 tablespoon of unsalted butter or coconut oil for every ounce of unsweetened chocolate called for in a recipe. Half an ounce of cocoa butter is an even better substitute, since cocoa butter is a fat that's actually found in unsweetened chocolate.

Sugar-Free Chocolate

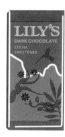

This absolutely should not be confused with unsweetened chocolate. Sugar-free chocolate is sweetened with something other than sugar, be it stevia, erythritol, or some other sweetener. It usually has other additives as well to give it a smoother, creamier mouthfeel. It comes in many varieties, from milk chocolate to very dark chocolate, and different products contain varying amounts of cacao.

Sugar-free chocolate is useful in keto baking; I often melt it down for coatings, drizzles, and other chocolatey decorations. I generally don't recommend using it in place of unsweetened chocolate, since the different cacao content can affect the texture of your baked goods and the added sweetener can alter the taste. Tart fillings and custards may not set properly and will be overly sweet if you make this mistake.

I also advise steering clear of sugar-free chocolate that is sweetened with maltitol, which can spike blood sugar and cause tummy upset. I prefer Lily's, but Lakanto and ChocZero are also popular choices.

Sugar-Free Chocolate Chips

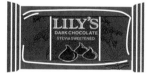

Baking—low-carb or otherwise—just wouldn't be the same without chocolate chips. When I embarked on my low-carb baking journey, the only option was Hershey's sugar-free chips, which are sweetened with maltitol. Thankfully, there are now a few brands that are sweetened with erythritol and stevia instead. My favorite is Lily's. They've recently come out with milk chocolate chips for those of you who prefer.

I recently discovered keto mini chocolate chips from a company called Explorado Market. They're very good, and I wish I'd discovered them before completing the recipes in this book. They would be perfect sprinkled over the Cannoli Icebox Cake (page 118), for example.

In a pinch, you can always chop up a sugar-free chocolate bar and use that in place of chocolate chips.

ALL ABOUT DAIRY (AND DAIRY-FREE SUBSTITUTES)

Dairy has always played a significant role in baking, and the fats in dairy products lend tenderness and moisture to baked goods. Sometimes dairy is the primary fat source for a whole recipe, and other fats and oils are entirely or mostly absent.

Don't panic if you are dairy-free. These days, there are a number of fantastic alternatives to dairy. Many of the recipes in this book were tested with both dairy and dairy-free products.

Heavy cream: Regular milk really has no place in keto baking because of its relatively high carb count, but cream is a welcome addition to many recipes. I call for "heavy whipping cream" in my recipes. This is simply how many companies label heavy cream these days. It is distinguished from whipping cream only in that it has a higher milk fat content (36 to 40 percent). Whipping cream (30 to 36 percent) works just as well for the recipes in this book.

Dairy-free alternative: To replace heavy cream in many recipes, you can use full-fat coconut milk or, better yet, coconut cream. Typically, a can of coconut milk separates, and the denser, creamier portion rises to the top. Scooping this cream off the top and not allowing it to mix with the watery portion will give you a closer substitute in terms of fat content. However, since coconut cream is almost solid at room temperature, you may need to warm it up a bit if it's meant to be added as a liquid.

Cream cheese: Keto dieters do love their cream cheese, and I am no exception. It's great in cheesecakes and frostings, and it can help bind baked goods and give them a wonderful texture and flavor. Check out the Cream Cheese Cutout Cookies (page 152) to see how I used it in an egg-free cookie recipe.

Dairy-free alternative: It used to be that all dairy-free cream cheese was soy based, but thankfully things have changed. There are a few good cream cheese alternatives now, and my favorite by far is from Kite Hill. It's almond milk based, and it works just as well as dairy cream cheese in most recipes, without a loss of flavor or texture. One of my recipe testers used it for the Cream Cheese Cutout Cookies and found that it worked perfectly. It's just as low in carbs as regular cream cheese, too, so it subs right in.

Ricotta cheese: Ricotta is a mild fresh cheese, and I feel like I've only just started to realize its potential for baking. The Ricotta Cheesecake with Fresh Berries on page 116 may rank up there as one of my favorite cheesecakes ever—and I eat a lot of cheesecake! For keto baking, stick to the full-fat variety, both for consistency and for the lower carb count.

Dairy-free alternative: Kite Hill also makes an almond-based ricotta. While you may not be able to use it for a full cheesecake, I think it would work well in the Fresh Herb Ricotta and Scones on page 248.

Sour cream: This is cream that has been fermented by the addition of certain bacteria so that it thickens and becomes quite tangy. Full-fat sour cream is incredibly rich and thick, and I love the tenderness it gives cakes and muffins. If you prefer, you can use full-fat Greek yogurt in its place.

There are a few dairy-free alternatives to sour cream, but I have never tried them in baking and cannot speak to their success as a replacement.

Almond and nut milks: I call for unsweetened almond milk in some of my cakes and other recipes. This is really to add moisture without too many carbs, since a cup of cow's milk has 12 grams of carbs but a cup of almond milk has only 2 grams. If you prefer, you can replace the almond milk with half heavy cream and half water. Using just cream often makes the batter too thick.

Nut-free alternative: Unsweetened hemp milk is a good low-carb alternative to almond milk.

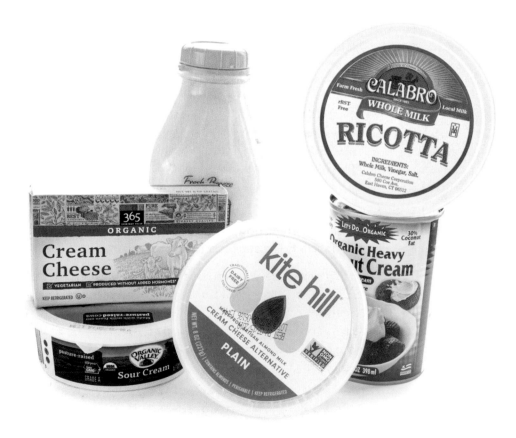

OTHER KETO PANTRY STAPLES

If you had all of the above items in your pantry, you would be well on your way to keto baking success. But beyond the basics, here are some other ingredients that can take your recipes from pretty good to absolutely spectacular.

In my many years of experimenting with keto baking, I have found that using a protein powder, such as whey or egg white protein, creates lighter and fluffier cakes, muffins, and quick breads. It helps replace the protein bonds formed by gluten, trapping gases more readily for a better rise.

I don't use protein powder in all of my cakes, as it depends on the rest of the ingredients and the texture I'm aiming for, but you will see it featured quite often. I recommend the unflavored variety so that it doesn't add sweetness or overpowering flavor to your recipes.

Please note that I do not recommend using collagen peptides or collagen protein powder as a replacement for whey or egg white protein. I've tried this many times, and the baked goods always become quite gummy and difficult to cook through.

Gelatin and collagen peptides: Grass-fed gelatin is an extremely useful ingredient for keto baking, and I recommend always having it around. In addition to the gelling power it provides for fillings, it gives many baked goods a chewiness they would not otherwise have. I've started to add it to many of my cookie recipes, and it's changed the game for me. It's also a key ingredient in my Chewy Keto Brownies (page 178).

I don't often use collagen in my baked goods, because of the gumminess mentioned above. But I do add it to the Granola Bars (page 206), and it gives them a great chewy consistency. Without it, the bars tend to be harder and more crisp, but also more fragile. The choice to include the collagen or leave it out is yours.

Gums/thickeners: Glucomannan and xanthan gum are both very useful for thickening batters and fillings in the absence of starches. I find that I can use them almost interchangeably for thickening power. Xanthan gum has the added benefit of inhibiting recrystallization in foods like sauces and ice creams.

Extracts and flavorings: This is where you can have a little, or perhaps a lot of, fun with your keto baking. Some of our old favorite treats are off-limits because the fruits and other additions don't fit well with the keto diet. But I say fake it 'til you make it, my friends. I love having a fun collection of extracts in my cupboard so I can play with different flavors. Think beyond the basic vanilla, peppermint, and lemon to things like pineapple, apple, and cherry.

There are even truly astonishing flavors out there like cornbread and oatmeal cookie. Check out the Resource Guide on pages 400 to 403 for where to source these kinds of unusual ingredients.

Herbs and spices: Another great way to amp up the flavor of your baked goods, both sweet and savory, is to use herbs and spices. Having a fully stocked spice cabinet can be the difference between ho-hum and absolutely fabulous.

Keep in mind that spices lose their flavor over time. Six to twelve months is really the longest you should keep any ground spice in your cupboard. If it's something you will use frequently, such as cinnamon, purchase it in bulk. But if it won't see much use, buy the smallest quantity, even though the cost per ounce is higher. In the end, you will save money by not tossing an almost-full bottle or bag of something that you needed for only one or two recipes.

Some recipes call for chopped fresh herbs. If you can get them fresh, that's preferred. But the rule of thumb for substituting dried herbs for fresh is 3:1. Dried herbs have a more concentrated flavor, so for every tablespoon of fresh, you want only 1 teaspoon of the dried form.

Nuts and coconut: Recipes often call for toasted and/or chopped nuts as an addition to a batter or as a garnish or decoration. I have all sorts of nuts in various forms (sliced, chopped, and whole), and I keep them in my freezer for longevity. Unless otherwise specified in the recipe, use raw and unsalted nuts.

Both shredded and flaked coconut are also useful. Do read the labels carefully, because the coconut products often found in the baking aisles of many grocery stores are sweetened. The unsweetened versions may be in the natural foods aisle, the gluten-free aisle, or sometimes in the bulk foods section.

Salt: Do not skip the salt! Salt adds flavor and brings out the best in any baked good, keto or not. Usually, you need only ¼ to ½ teaspoon for something that serves 12 to 20 people. But believe me, if it's not in there, you would notice. Desserts and sweets can taste mighty flat without the addition of a little salt.

Fine-grained salts are better for baking, as they distribute more evenly and dissolve more readily in batters and doughs. Regular table salt and fine sea salt are your best options. Some recipes call for coarse sea salt, usually as a garnish.

Cocoa butter (aka cacao butter): This isn't a must, but I find cocoa butter, the fat that is pressed out of cocoa beans, to be highly useful for keto desserts. It's becoming common enough as an ingredient that stores like Whole Foods tend to carry it in the baking aisle.

For the most part, I use cocoa butter to help sugar-free chocolate melt more smoothly and thinly for dipping and drizzling. You can use coconut oil for this purpose, too, but it can make the chocolate too thin. Butter tends to make it thicken up.

Cocoa butter can also help you achieve a white chocolate flavor in baked goods like the White Chocolate Macadamia Nut Blondies (page 184).

Note: When I was developing these recipes, there were no companies in the U.S. that sold decent sugar-free white chocolate. But in the intervening months, not one but *two* brands have developed keto-friendly white chocolate chips. See page 402 for more information.

Food coloring: I don't use food coloring often in keto baking, because I tend to prefer the natural and rustic look to my cakes and cookies. But there are few decent natural options available if you do want to play with colored batters and frostings. I like the vegetable color powders from Color Kitchen. Be forewarned, they are potent. The package states that a full envelope colors a single recipe, but I find that I need only a quarter to half of an envelope to achieve a pretty pastel shade. When I use more powder than that, I end up with something that's neon bright.

Psyllium husk powder: Psyllium husk powder is a soluble fiber made from the husks of the seeds from the psyllium plant. It's a common ingredient in many laxatives, but some smart individual decided to try using it in gluten-free baking. It acts as a binding agent and gives baked goods a bready quality. I don't use it frequently, but it plays an important role in my Keto Yeast Bread (page 272). I give props to *Cook's Illustrated,* which provided me with the tip that a little psyllium can help trap the gases given off by the yeast.

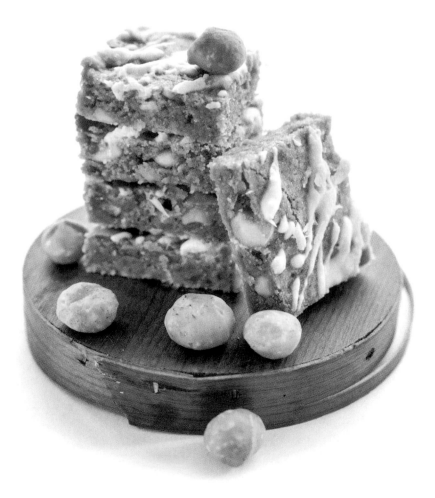

Chapter 3:
THE TOOLS

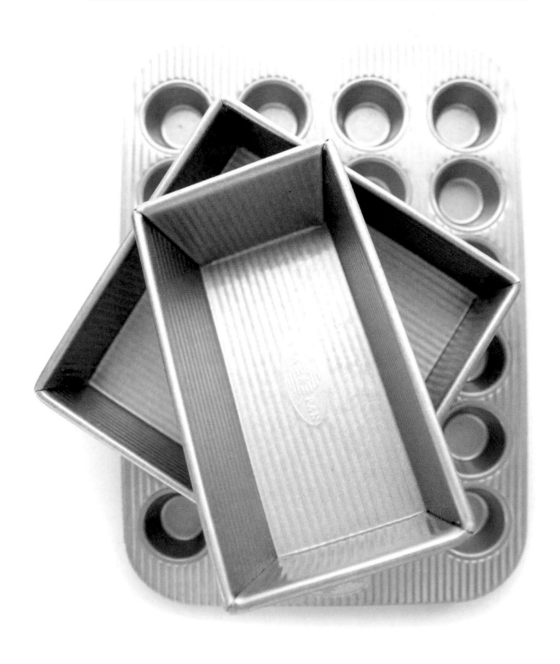

The tools you use to bake with are almost as important as the ingredients. You don't necessarily need the fanciest top-of-the-line equipment, but you do need to have some basics. Putting a little thought into what you use can help save time, effort, and the heartache of a baking failure.

BAKEWARE

There is a bewildering array of bakeware out there these days—everything from basic cookie sheets to Twinkie pans to castle-shaped cake pans. Trying to figure out what you really need can be overwhelming, and stocking up can be costly. My best advice is to steer clear of single-use items and purchase bakeware that can handle multiple jobs.

I have far more bakeware than the average home baker—perhaps too much. And still I find myself reaching for the same pans over and over again. There are a few items in my arsenal that have never even seen the light of day.

When choosing new bakeware, select light-colored nonstick metal pans with nontoxic coatings. (See why this is important in the "Keto Baking Tips" section on pages 14 to 18.) My favorite brand is USA Pan.

The Basics

Round cake pans: 8- or 9-inch metal pans with straight sides that are at least 2 inches deep. For layer cakes, you should have at least two of these pans in the same size.

Square baking pan: 8- or 9-inch metal pan with straight sides that are at least 2 inches deep. Perfect for brownies, bars, and snack cakes. I prefer my 8-inch pan for most recipes, as it makes deeper, more impressive-looking bars.

Rectangular baking pan: 9 by 13-inch metal pan with straight sides, useful for brownies, bars, and snack cakes.

Loaf pan: Loaf pans are usually either 9 by 5 inches or 8 by 4 inches, with 3-inch sides. Both sizes are fine: 8 by 4-inch pans make taller, more impressive-looking loaves, but they may take longer to cook through properly. Metal loaf pans are best to promote browning.

Standard muffin pan: A nonstick metal muffin pan with 12 wells, each with about a ½-cup capacity. Silicone muffin pans and muffin cups also work well for keto baking.

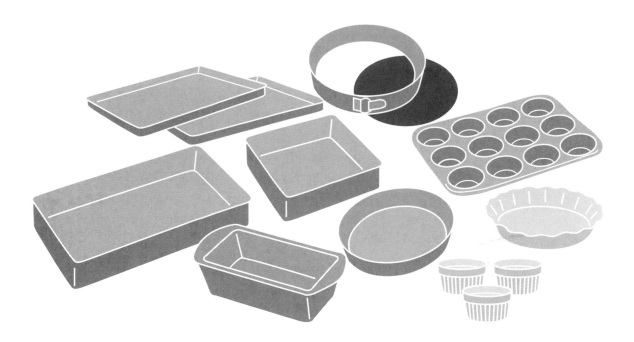

Rimmed baking sheets (aka sheet pans): Rectangular metal pans that come in various sizes, with sides that are about 1 inch high. Common sizes are 18 by 13 inches and 17 by 11 or 12 inches. These pans are useful for everything from cookies to cake rolls. It's good to have several in different sizes.

Springform pan: An 8- or 9-inch metal pan with a removable bottom and tight-fitting ring that locks in place is ideal for full-size cheesecakes and other delicate cakes that can't be flipped out of a regular cake pan. I always use a 9-inch springform pan for my cheesecake recipes.

Glass pie plate: A 9-inch glass or ceramic pie plate is better for keto crusts than its metal counterpart. It is less likely to burn the delicate nut or coconut flour. Also great for crustless pies and custards.

4-ounce ramekins: These ceramic dishes come in a variety of shapes and sizes, but I find the small, steep-sided 4-ounce ramekins to be the most versatile. They are ideal for soufflés, baked custards, and other small desserts.

GLASS OR CERAMIC BAKING DISHES

On the whole, I recommend baking in metal pans, since ceramic dishes take longer to heat up and hold heat longer, which affects baking time (see more in "Keto Baking Tips" on pages 14 to 18). For a few recipes, however—think eggy dishes like custards and soufflés and more acidic foods like fruit crisps—glass or ceramic dishes are a better choice because they are nonreactive.

When a recipe simply calls for a baking *pan*, assume the pan is metal. *Dish* usually refers to ceramic. All the recipes in this book specify when a glass or ceramic dish is required.

Wish List Items

4-inch tart pans: I have a set of four of these small metal tart pans with removable bottoms, and I used them for the Dairy-Free Coconut Cream Tarts (page 324). But you can make one full-size tart instead.

9- or 10-inch tart pan: A fluted tart pan makes for an elegant presentation, but you can almost always use a pie plate instead. I own several tart pans. The metal pans with the removable bottoms make serving easy, but I also love my white ceramic tart pan: it looks so nice that you can serve straight from it.

10- to 12-cup Bundt pan: Bundt pans add instant elegance to cakes. I recommend sticking with the metal fluted pans that don't have all sorts of deep ridges or nooks and crannies. The fancier shapes can make it much more difficult to get the cake out intact.

16-cup nonstick tube pan: This large, high-sided metal pan with a removable bottom is typically used for angel food cake. I never owned one until I decided to write this book (see the Chiffon Cake on page 108). Angel food and chiffon cakes require this specific pan, but you could certainly bake other kinds of cake in it.

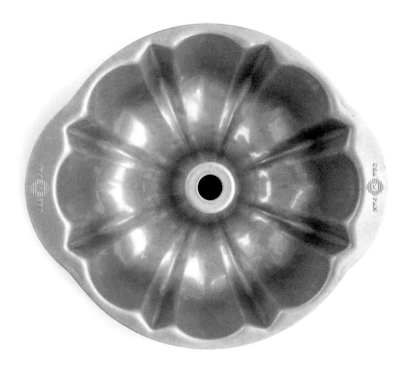

Cast-iron skillet: Baking in a skillet can give some recipes a fun rustic look. Any ovenproof skillet will do, but if you can get your hands on cast iron, all the better. It gives the edges of the baked goods a delicious crispy quality that you just can't get with nonstick pans.

Cookie sheets: You can always use rimmed baking sheets for cookies, but rimless pans allow more air to circulate around the cookies. I have one very large (15 by 20-inch) cookie sheet that is insulated on the bottom to help keep cookies from burning. It's my go-to pan for any cookie.

Donut pan: While you can't make keto donuts without a donut pan, you can always make muffins from the same batter. But donut pans are so fun, and it's really wonderful to indulge in a donut now and again. Some donut pans have 12 cavities and some only have 6 cavities. The donut recipes in this book make 10 to 12 donuts, so if you only have a 6-well pan, you may need to work in two batches.

Jelly roll pan: This is really just a rimmed baking sheet, but it's a specific size of 15 by 10 by 1 inch. It's great for the Flourless Swiss Roll (page 100), but you could make that dessert in another size of sheet pan. The baking time would change, depending on the size.

Mini muffin pan: A nonstick metal muffin pan with 24 wells, each with about a 2-tablespoon capacity. Fun for mini muffins, mini cupcakes, and tartlets. Everything is somehow more delicious in miniature, but you can always scale things up for full-size versions.

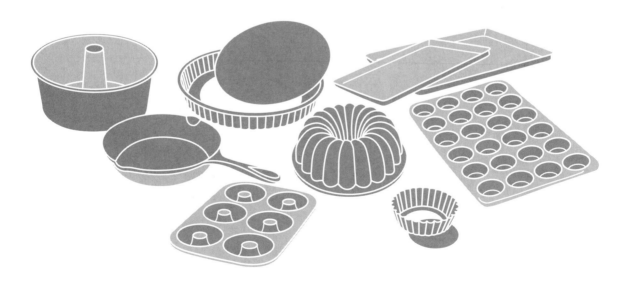

OTHER EQUIPMENT

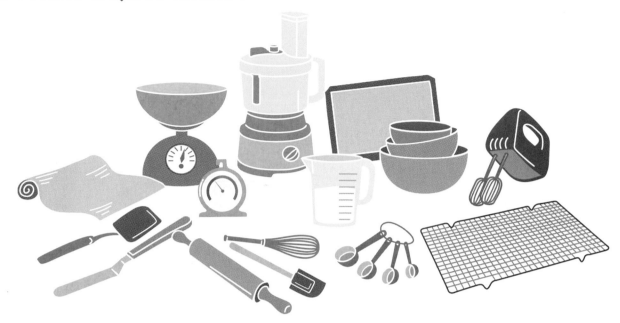

The Basics

Dry measuring cups and spoons: The American system of cups and tablespoons may be archaic, but it is still what most people use when measuring dry ingredients. Thus, while I include weight measurements for many ingredients (see the chart on pages 398 and 399), volume is the main form of measurement used in this book. See pages 22 and 23 for more on measuring dry ingredients accurately.

Liquid measuring cups: Do not use dry measuring cups for liquid ingredients (or vice versa!). They're simply not as accurate. Look for clear glass measuring cups with red or black lines denoting the volume of liquid.

Electric mixer: It doesn't have to be a big stand mixer, although those are useful. A handheld mixer will do the job well enough too.

Food processor: From making shortbread to grinding nuts and pork rinds, there is no substitute for a good food processor. You want one with a capacity of at least 11 or 12 cups so that it can handle the volume of larger recipes.

Mixing bowls: A set of stainless-steel and/or glass mixing bowls in various sizes is a must. Glass is wonderful because it is microwaveable, for melting butter and coconut oil. I also prefer it for creating a double boiler to melt chocolate. But glass is heavier and more fragile than stainless steel. If you can choose only one, go with metal bowls.

Metal/silicone lifters: Also known as spatulas, turners, or flippers. Look for thin, somewhat flexible blades that can get under cookies on a cookie sheet or under brownies or bars in a baking pan.

Offset spatulas: Another baking implement I reach for almost constantly. I like the little 4-inch ones, which are ideal for spreading frosting, spreading thick batters into pans, and getting under fragile doughs.

Rolling pin: Any wooden or silicone rolling pin will do.

Rubber/silicone spatulas: I rarely reach for wooden implements for mixing and stirring anymore because silicone spatulas are much more versatile. Skip the implements with wooden handles and look for all-silicone spatulas with metal cores, which can go straight into your dishwasher. Make sure to get one or two that have very thin, flexible blades for folding mixtures together, scraping batters out of bowls, and gently releasing cakes and breads from pans.

Whisks: Such simple and yet vital baking tools, and inexpensive to boot, whisks are perfect for mixing and breaking up clumps in dry ingredients. They are also ideal for incorporating sauces and custards. Look for metal whisks with wires that are coated with silicone so you can use them on any surface, including nonstick.

Cooling racks: The best ones are stainless steel with narrow grids so that smaller items don't slip through. Large racks are great for setting larger sheet pans right on top to let air circulate underneath.

Parchment paper: Parchment is a keto baker's best friend, and you would do well to load up on it. It's great for lining cookie sheets and cake pans, allowing easier release of your baked goods. And large sheets of parchment are necessary for rolling out dough.

Parchment muffin cups are great, too, as keto muffins and cupcakes tend to stick to the regular paper cups too much. I also purchase 8- or 9-inch round sheets for lining my round cake pans.

Silicone baking mats: You can always use parchment paper, but I find baking mats better for cookies, biscuits, scones, and other baked goods that might get too dark on the bottom. Silicone adds more protection from the heat of your baking sheets. And it means you won't go through expensive parchment at a rapid rate.

Kitchen scale: Even if you plan to measure most of your ingredients by volume, a scale is a vital piece of equipment. Some items, like almond and coconut flour, chocolate, cocoa butter, and shredded cheese, are best measured by weight (grams or ounces). See more on using weights for measuring on page 21.

Oven thermometer: Ovens are as idiosyncratic as people are, and knowing whether yours runs hot or cold makes for better baking. An oven thermometer can also help you figure out if your oven has hot spots that you'll need to work around, like mine does (see page 14).

Wish List Items

High-powered blender: Put this one at the top of your wish list because it is ever so useful for the keto diet. I use mine frequently in baking to whip batters to a finer consistency (see the Lemon Ricotta Muffins on page 218, for example).

Cookie/biscuit cutters: If you love roll out cookies, you're going to want at least a basic set of cookie cutters. I use my plain 2-inch round biscuit cutters for Chocolate Wafers (page 146) and fancier shapes for Cream Cheese Cutout Cookies (page 152).

Cookie scoops: Spoons work well enough, but cookie scoops are great for measuring dough more precisely. I also love the spring release feature for getting the dough out of the scoop easily. A scoop that holds 1½ tablespoons of dough is about right for most keto cookie recipes.

Pastry brush: This type of brush is inexpensive and great for brushing butter or other fats over baked goods, both before and after baking. It's also useful for greasing pans.

Piping bags and decorating tips: It's up to you how fancy you want to get with your cakes and cookies. I am a terrible cake decorator, but I still love using these tools to make things look a little more elegant. For drizzles and other easy glazes, you can always use a regular zip-top plastic bag with one corner snipped off.

Silicone muffin liners: Parchment paper is great, but I've fallen in love with my silicone muffin liners. I use them for almost every muffin recipe I make now. Muffins practically fall right out of them.

SCALING RECIPES: HOW TO ADJUST FOR DIFFERENT PAN SIZES

Perhaps you're having company over and you want to double a recipe. Or maybe you want to take a layer cake batter and bake it in a 9 by 13-inch pan for ease. Or possibly you don't have quite the right size of bakeware and don't want to buy another pan. What to do, what to do?

Grab your calculator, because it's time to do a little basic math. Calculating the area of the pans will help guide you in how to scale a recipe up or down. And keep in mind that bakeware is always measured across the very bottom of the pan. Many pans flare outward toward the top so you risk some inaccuracy if you take the dimensions elsewhere.

Square/Rectangular Pans

For example, a recipe might call for an 8-inch square baking pan, which has an area of 64 square inches. If you'd like to double the recipe, you need to know which size pan to use instead. The area of a 9 by 13-inch pan is 117 square inches. While it's not perfectly double the area of the 8-inch pan, it's close enough that you can use it for a double batch of batter. The batter will be somewhat deeper in the rectangular pan, so you should expect it to take a little longer to bake through.

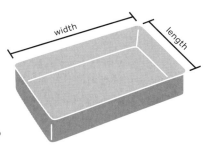

Keep in mind that while 8-inch and 9-inch square pans look pretty similar to the naked eye, they are actually quite different in terms of area. A 9-inch pan is 81 square inches, which is more than 25 percent larger than an 8-inch pan (64 square inches). That means you have two choices: either scale your recipe up or down by 25 percent or be prepared to bake it for a different length of time.

Whenever you use a pan that is a different size than the one your recipe calls for, I recommend watching your baked good very carefully while it's in the oven. Check on it early and continue to check it in 3- to 5-minute increments after that. You simply don't know how long it will take to bake.

Round Pans

But what about those pesky round pans? Well, that involves figuring out the radius of the pan, squaring the radius, and then multiplying it by pi (3.14). So the area of an 8-inch round cake pan would be 4 x 4 x 3.14, which is 50.24.

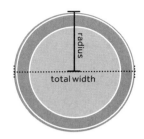

But I will be honest, for round cake pans, I just head on over to Google, type in "area of a circle," and enter the radius. Google does all the work for me. So obliging, that Google.

Assuming two layers, an 8-inch layer cake is a total of 100 square inches. It is going to be a little thin if you spread it into a 9 by 13-inch pan, so you're going to want to bake it a little less and watch it carefully. See where I'm going with this?

Fractions of Eggs

If you've decided to scale a recipe up or down to fit your pan of choice, you clearly need to adjust all the ingredients accordingly. For most ingredients, this task is fairly straightforward, but what about eggs? What if you have a three-egg recipe and you need to scale it up by 50 percent? How does one measure out 4.5 eggs?

It's not as hard as it sounds. Grab your kitchen scale and set the unit to grams. Weigh a bowl on your scale and then zero out the scale again. Break the egg into the bowl and whisk it to combine the yolk and white. Place the bowl back on the scale to weigh it, and add only half of that weight to your recipe for the ½ egg quantity. You can do the same thing for just the whites or just the yolks.

You can measure partial eggs by volume as well by whisking the egg and measuring it out in tablespoons. Weight would be slightly more accurate, but most recipes won't suffer for an extra teaspoon or so of egg.

Chapter 4:
EVERYDAY CAKES

A party without cake is really just a meeting. —Julia Child

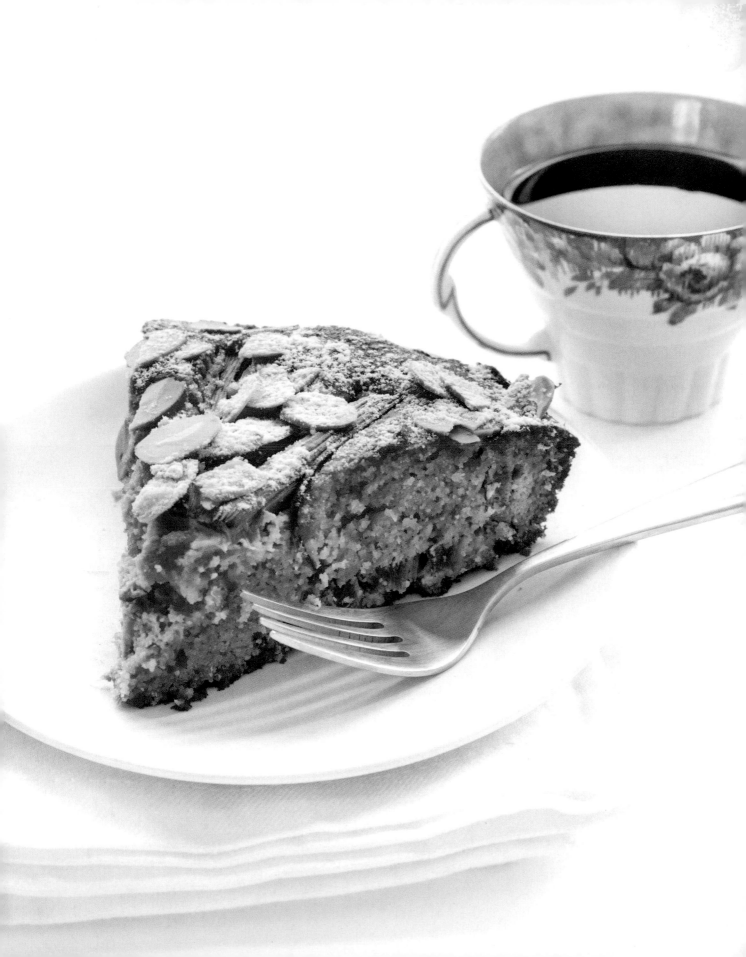

CHOCOLATE ZUCCHINI SHEET CAKE

Yield: 20 servings Prep Time: 15 minutes, plus 1 hour to drain zucchini (not including time to make frosting) Cook Time: 22 minutes

Sheet cakes are wonderful for serving a crowd, and they bake quickly. And since the cake is so thin, it's got a great cake-to-frosting ratio.

2 cups shredded zucchini, loosely packed

¾ teaspoon salt, divided

¾ cup (83g) coconut flour

⅔ cup granulated erythritol sweetener

½ cup cocoa powder

1 tablespoon baking powder

1 teaspoon espresso powder (optional)

8 large eggs, room temperature

½ cup (1 stick) unsalted butter, melted but not hot

½ cup water, room temperature

1 teaspoon vanilla extract

1½ recipes Chocolate Buttercream Frosting (page 382)

1. Put the shredded zucchini in a sieve in the sink or over a bowl. Sprinkle with ½ teaspoon of the salt and toss to combine. Let drain for 1 hour, then squeeze out as much moisture as possible.

2. Preheat the oven to 325°F and grease a 10 by 15 by 1-inch jelly roll pan. Line the bottom with parchment paper and grease the paper.

3. In a large bowl, whisk together the coconut flour, sweetener, cocoa powder, baking powder, espresso powder (if using), and remaining ¼ teaspoon of salt.

4. Whisk in the eggs, melted butter, water, vanilla, and squeezed zucchini until well combined. Spread the batter evenly in the prepared pan.

5. Bake for 18 to 22 minutes, until the top of the cake is firm to the touch. Remove from the oven and let cool completely in the pan.

6. Spread the frosting over the cooled cake and cut into squares to serve.

DAIRY-FREE OPTION:

Use melted coconut oil or avocado oil in place of the butter and frost the cake with the Dairy-Free Chocolate Frosting (page 384).

TIPS: *A standard jelly roll pan is 10 by 15 inches. You can use a larger rimmed baking sheet (aka sheet pan) instead, but I wouldn't go larger than 11 by 17. The cake will be thinner and will take only about 15 minutes to bake.*

The addition of espresso powder does not make this cake taste like coffee at all. It simply intensifies the chocolate flavor. A small amount of espresso or instant coffee can help bring out the chocolate flavor in many desserts.

NUTRITIONAL INFORMATION

CALORIES: 248 | FAT: 21.4g | CARBS: 7.1g | FIBER: 3.5g | PROTEIN: 5.5g

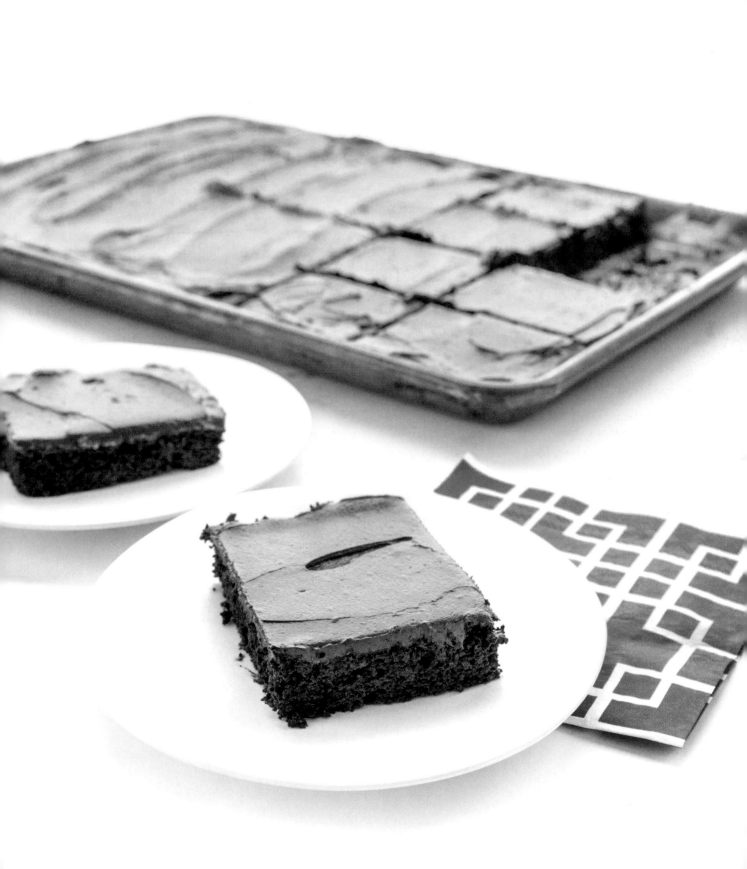

DAIRY-FREE LEMON CAKE

Yield: 12 servings   Prep Time: 10 minutes   Cook Time: 45 minutes

A simple lemon cake can be more enticing than even the most decadent multi-layer frosted cake. This version is deceptive in its simplicity, with true lemon flavor bursting through every bite.

Cake:

3 cups (300g) blanched almond flour

¾ cup granulated erythritol sweetener

¼ cup unflavored egg white protein powder

2 teaspoons baking powder

¼ teaspoon salt

Grated zest of 1 lemon

3 large eggs

½ cup melted (but not hot) ghee or palm shortening

¼ cup fresh lemon juice

¼ cup water

1 teaspoon lemon extract

½ teaspoon vanilla extract

Glaze:

¼ cup powdered erythritol sweetener

2 tablespoons fresh lemon juice

TO MAKE THE CAKE:

1. Preheat the oven to 325°F and grease a 9-inch round cake pan. Line the bottom with parchment paper and lightly grease the paper.

2. In a large bowl, whisk together the almond flour, sweetener, protein powder, baking powder, and salt. Stir in the lemon zest.

3. Add the eggs, melted ghee, lemon juice, water, and extracts and stir until well combined.

4. Spread the batter in the prepared pan and bake for 35 to 45 minutes, until the edges are golden brown and the top is firm to the touch. Remove from the oven and let cool in the pan, then flip out onto a serving platter. The bottom of the cake becomes the top.

TO MAKE THE GLAZE:

5. Whisk together the sweetener and lemon juice until smooth and drizzle over the cooled cake.

TIP: *You can use coconut oil in this recipe, but virgin coconut oil has a strong coconut flavor that may overpower the lemon. Ghee is technically a dairy product but has no milk solids, so it is appropriate for most people with dairy intolerances.*

NUTRITIONAL INFORMATION
CALORIES: 282 | FAT: 25.2g | CARBS: 7g | FIBER: 3g | PROTEIN: 9g

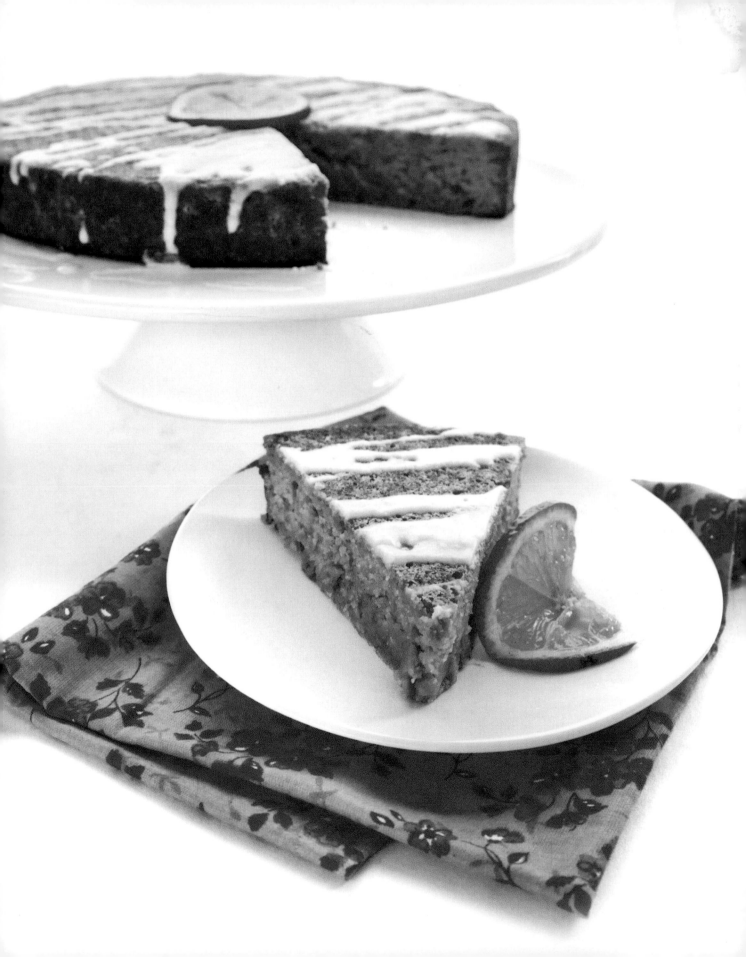

NEW YORK CRUMB CAKE

Yield: 16 servings   Prep Time: 15 minutes   Cook Time: 40 minutes

A sweet and tender coffee cake in the style of New York crumb cake. It is perfect paired with a cup of coffee.

Crumb Topping:

1 cup (100g) blanched almond flour

¼ cup (28g) coconut flour

¼ cup brown sugar substitute

¼ cup granulated erythritol sweetener

¾ teaspoon ground cinnamon

¼ teaspoon salt

½ cup (1 stick) unsalted butter, melted

Cake:

1½ cups (150g) blanched almond flour

½ cup granulated erythritol sweetener

2 tablespoons coconut flour

1½ teaspoons baking powder

¼ teaspoon salt

¼ cup (½ stick) unsalted butter, melted but not hot

1 large egg

1 large egg yolk

1 teaspoon vanilla extract

¼ cup heavy whipping cream

¼ cup water

1. Preheat the oven to 325°F and grease a 9-inch square baking pan.

TO MAKE THE CRUMB TOPPING:

2. In a medium bowl, combine the almond flour, coconut flour, sweeteners, cinnamon, and salt. Stir in the melted butter until well combined. The batter will be thick and crumbly.

TO MAKE THE CAKE:

3. In a large bowl, whisk together the almond flour, sweetener, coconut flour, baking powder, and salt. Stir in the melted butter, whole egg, egg yolk, vanilla, cream, and water until thoroughly combined.

4. Spread the batter in the prepared pan and smooth the top. Crumble the topping mixture with your fingers into pea-size pieces and sprinkle evenly over the top of the batter.

5. Bake for 35 to 40 minutes, until the topping is golden and a tester inserted in the center of the cake comes out clean. It won't be firm to the touch because the topping is so tender.

SERVING SUGGESTION: *Dust with a little powdered sweetener before serving.*

NUTRITIONAL INFORMATION
CALORIES: 237 | FAT: 21.7g | CARBS: 5.7g | FIBER: 2.9g | PROTEIN: 4.9g

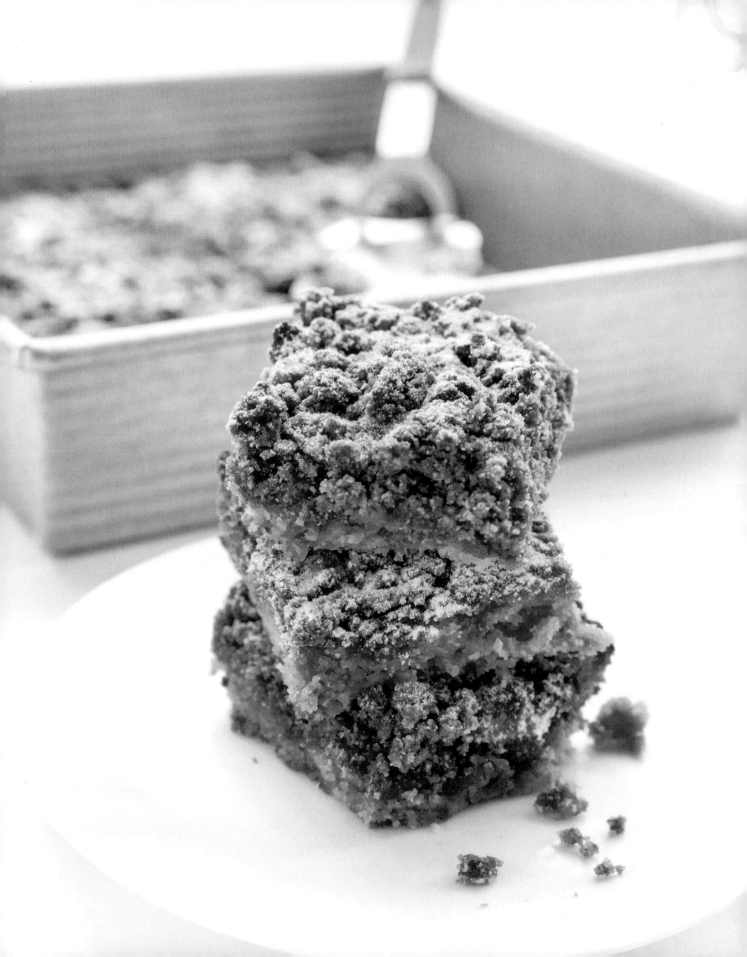

DAIRY-FREE BLUEBERRY CREAM CHEESE COFFEE CAKE

OPTION

Yield: 12 servings Prep Time: 25 minutes, plus 1 hour to chill Cook Time: 35 minutes

This delicious coffee cake is the dairy-free version of a popular recipe on my blog, *All Day I Dream About Food*. At the advice of a longtime reader, I also cut back the cake part so it has a better cake-to-filling ratio. Now it's lighter and less filling but just as delicious.

Blueberry Filling:

1 cup frozen blueberries

¼ cup water

¼ teaspoon glucomannan or xanthan gum

Cream Cheese Filling:

1 (8-ounce) package dairy-free cream cheese, softened

1 large egg

¼ cup powdered erythritol sweetener

2 teaspoons grated lemon zest

Cake:

1½ cups (150g) blanched almond flour

⅓ cup granulated erythritol sweetener

¼ cup unflavored egg white protein powder

2 teaspoons baking powder

¼ teaspoon salt

2 large eggs, room temperature

¼ cup melted (but not hot) coconut oil or ghee

¼ cup unsweetened almond milk

½ teaspoon vanilla extract

COCONUT-FREE OPTION:

Use ghee in the cake.

TO MAKE THE BLUEBERRY FILLING:

1. In a small saucepan over medium heat, bring the blueberries and water to a boil, then reduce the heat to medium-low and simmer for 5 minutes.

2. Remove the pan from the heat and sprinkle the glucomannan over the berries, whisking vigorously to combine. Let cool.

TO MAKE THE CREAM CHEESE FILLING:

3. In a medium bowl, beat the dairy-free cream cheese with an electric mixer until smooth. Beat in the egg until well combined, then beat in the sweetener and lemon zest.

TO MAKE THE CAKE:

4. Preheat the oven to 325°F and grease a 9-inch springform pan.

5. In a medium bowl, whisk together the almond flour, sweetener, protein powder, baking powder, and salt.

6. Add the eggs, coconut oil, almond milk, and vanilla and mix until well combined. Spread the batter in the prepared pan, pushing it slightly up the sides to create a well for the fillings.

7. Spread the cream cheese mixture evenly in the center of the cake, then spread the blueberry mixture over the top of the cream cheese.

8. Bake for 25 to 30 minutes, until the sides of the cake are golden brown and firm to the touch. The center will still jiggle somewhat. Remove from the oven and let cool in the pan.

9. Once cool, run a sharp knife around the edge of the cake to loosen it, then remove the sides of the pan. Cover the cake tightly with plastic wrap and refrigerate for at least 1 hour.

NUTRITIONAL INFORMATION

CALORIES: 210 | FAT: 17.6g | CARBS: 6.5g | FIBER: 2g | PROTEIN: 8g

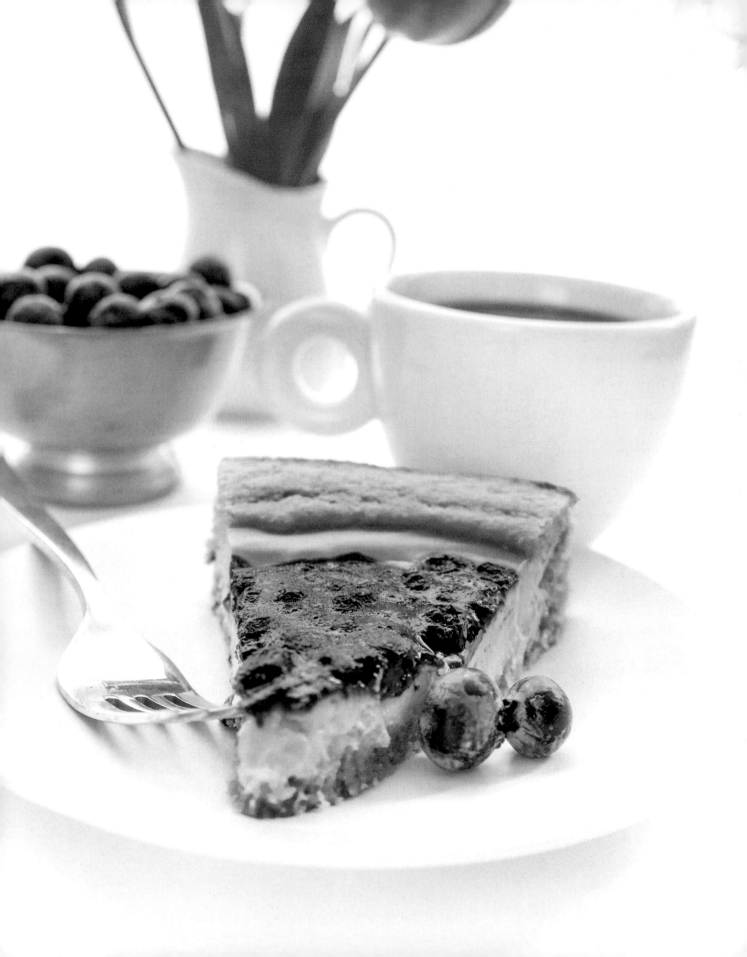

RHUBARB ALMOND SKILLET CAKE

OPTION

Yield: 12 servings Prep Time: 20 minutes Cook Time: 50 minutes

Baking a cake in a skillet gives it a unique texture, with an almost crispy edge. It also makes for a lovely presentation. This cake needs no more than a dusting of powdered sweetener or a dollop of sweetened whipped cream.

3 medium stalks fresh rhubarb, divided

2 cups (200g) blanched almond flour

¼ cup unflavored whey protein powder

2 teaspoons baking powder

¼ teaspoon salt

6 tablespoons unsalted butter, softened

½ cup granulated erythritol sweetener

2 large eggs, room temperature

½ teaspoon almond extract

½ teaspoon vanilla extract

⅓ cup unsweetened almond milk

2 tablespoons sliced almonds

Powdered erythritol sweetener, for garnish

1. Preheat the oven to 325°F and grease a 10-inch ovenproof skillet well.

2. Chop two of the rhubarb stalks and set aside.

3. In a medium bowl, whisk together the almond flour, protein powder, baking powder, and salt.

4. In a large bowl, beat the butter and sweetener with an electric mixer until fluffy and well combined. Beat in the eggs and extracts, then beat in the almond flour mixture in two additions, alternating with the almond milk.

5. Stir in the chopped rhubarb until well mixed, then spread the batter in the prepared skillet and smooth the top.

6. Cut the remaining rhubarb stalk into 3-inch pieces, then cut each piece lengthwise into 3 pieces. Lay the pieces in a starburst pattern on the top of the cake, pressing gently into the batter. Sprinkle with the sliced almonds, pressing lightly to adhere.

7. Bake for 45 to 50 minutes, until the edges are golden and a tester inserted in the center comes out clean. Remove from the oven and let cool in the pan for at least 20 minutes. Dust with powdered sweetener before serving.

DAIRY-FREE OPTION:

Use egg white protein powder in place of the whey protein powder and softened ghee or coconut oil in place of the butter.

TIPS: *When cakes have toppings like this, it can be hard to tell if they are cooked through in the center simply by touching the top. I often use a metal or wooden skewer to test the center of the cake without disturbing the toppings.*

A cast-iron skillet is by no means required here, but it does make the edges even more crispy and gives the cake a rustic look. If you do bake it in cast iron, I suggest removing the leftovers relatively soon after serving. The edges can take on a metallic taste if you leave the cake in the pan too long.

NUTRITIONAL INFORMATION

CALORIES: 229 | FAT: 19.3g | CARBS: 6.9g | FIBER: 3.1g | PROTEIN: 8.4g

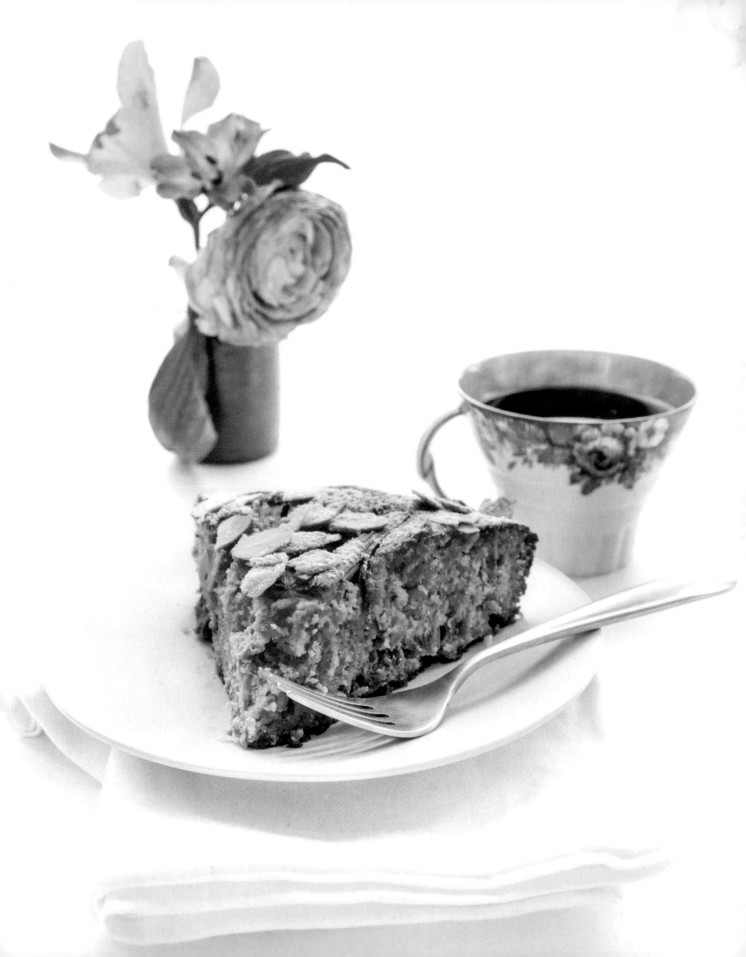

KEY LIME POUND CAKE

Yield: 16 servings   Prep Time: 15 minutes   Cook Time: 1 hour

I originally created this recipe for the Swerve Sweetener website, and from the get-go, it was a reader favorite. Squeezing those tiny Key limes is a lot of work, though, so I won't blame you if you use regular limes instead.

Cake:

3½ cups (350g) blanched almond flour

¼ cup (28g) coconut flour

1 tablespoon baking powder

½ teaspoon salt

½ cup (1 stick) unsalted butter, softened

¾ cup granulated erythritol sweetener

4 large eggs, room temperature

2 teaspoons grated Key lime zest

½ cup fresh Key lime juice

⅓ cup water

Glaze:

3 tablespoons powdered erythritol sweetener

2 to 3 teaspoons Key lime juice

TO MAKE THE CAKE:

1. Preheat the oven to 325°F and grease a 9 by 5-inch loaf pan very well.

2. In a medium bowl, whisk together the almond flour, coconut flour, baking powder, and salt.

3. In a large bowl, beat the butter and sweetener with an electric mixer until lightened and fluffy. Beat in the eggs until well combined, then beat in half of the almond flour mixture. Beat in the lime zest, lime juice, and water, then beat in the remaining almond flour mixture.

4. Transfer the batter to the prepared loaf pan and bake for 50 to 60 minutes, until the edges are golden brown and the top is firm to the touch. Remove from the oven and let cool in the pan for 15 minutes, then flip out onto a wire rack to cool completely.

TO MAKE THE GLAZE:

5. Whisk the powdered sweetener and lime juice together until smooth. The glaze should be somewhat runny. Drizzle over the cooled cake.

DAIRY-FREE OPTION:

Substitute softened coconut oil for the butter.

TIP: This is a large cake, and it really needs to be baked in a 9 by 5-inch loaf pan to cook through properly. So do be careful not to mistake the size and bake it in an 8 by 4-inch pan instead. A 10- to 12-cup Bundt pan would also work well.

NUTRITIONAL INFORMATION

CALORIES: 222 | FAT: 19g | CARBS: 7g | FIBER: 3.3g | PROTEIN: 7.2g

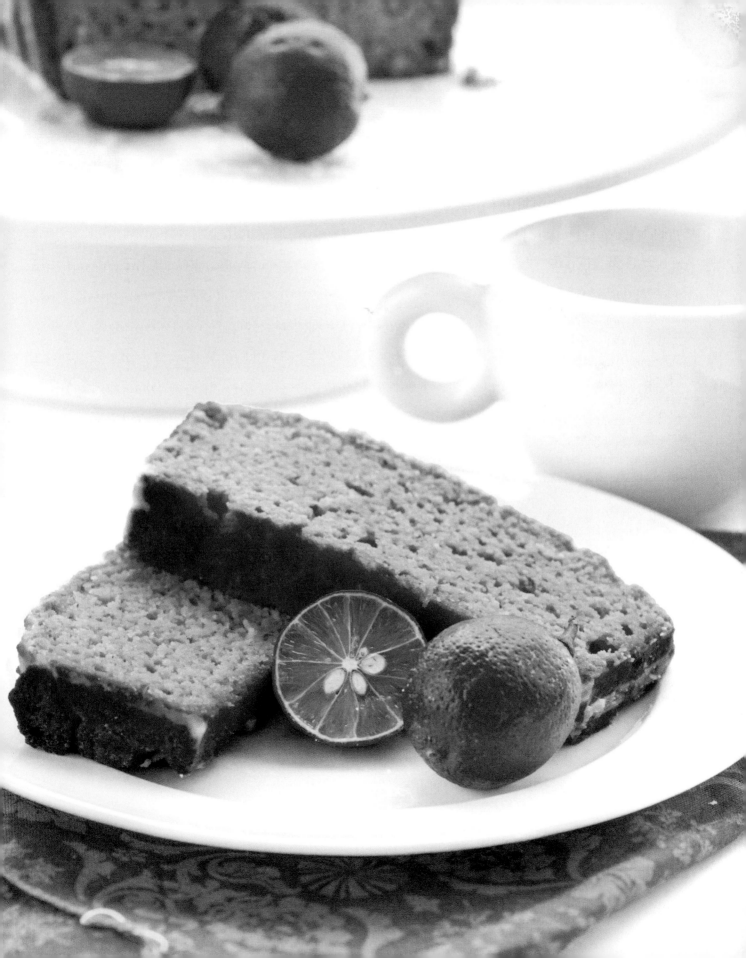

CHOCOLATE CUPCAKES

OPTION

Yield: 12 cupcakes (1 per serving) Prep Time: 15 minutes Cook Time: 25 minutes

The famous coconut flour chocolate cupcakes from my website! I created this recipe way back in 2010, and, amazingly, it has stood the test of time and remains a fan favorite.

½ cup (1 stick) unsalted butter, melted

¼ cup plus 3 tablespoons cocoa powder

1 teaspoon espresso powder

7 large eggs, room temperature

1 teaspoon vanilla extract

⅔ cup (73g) coconut flour

⅔ cup granulated sweetener of choice

2 teaspoons baking powder

½ teaspoon salt

½ cup water, plus additional water if needed

1. Preheat the oven to 350°F and line a standard muffin pan with 12 silicone or parchment paper liners.

2. In a large bowl, whisk together the melted butter, cocoa powder, and espresso powder.

3. Add the eggs and vanilla and stir until well combined. Then add the coconut flour, sweetener, baking powder, and salt and stir until smooth.

4. Stir in the water to thin the batter. If it is still very thick, stir in more water 1 tablespoon at a time until it thins out a bit. The batter should be thick but of scoopable consistency. It will not be pourable.

5. Divide the batter among the prepared muffin cups, filling each about three-quarters full. Bake for 20 to 25 minutes, until the tops are set and a tester inserted in the center of a cupcake comes out clean. Let cool in the pan for 5 to 10 minutes, then transfer to a wire rack to cool completely. Frost if desired (see the suggestions below).

DAIRY-FREE OPTION:

Replace the melted butter with melted coconut oil or ghee.

FROSTING SUGGESTIONS: *So many possibilities! Pair with the Chocolate Buttercream Frosting (page 382) or the Swiss Meringue Buttercream (page 378) for a classic cupcake.*

NUTRITIONAL INFORMATION (DOES NOT INCLUDE ANY FROSTING)
CALORIES: 147 | FAT: 11g | CARBS: 5.9g | FIBER: 3.4g | PROTEIN: 5.3g

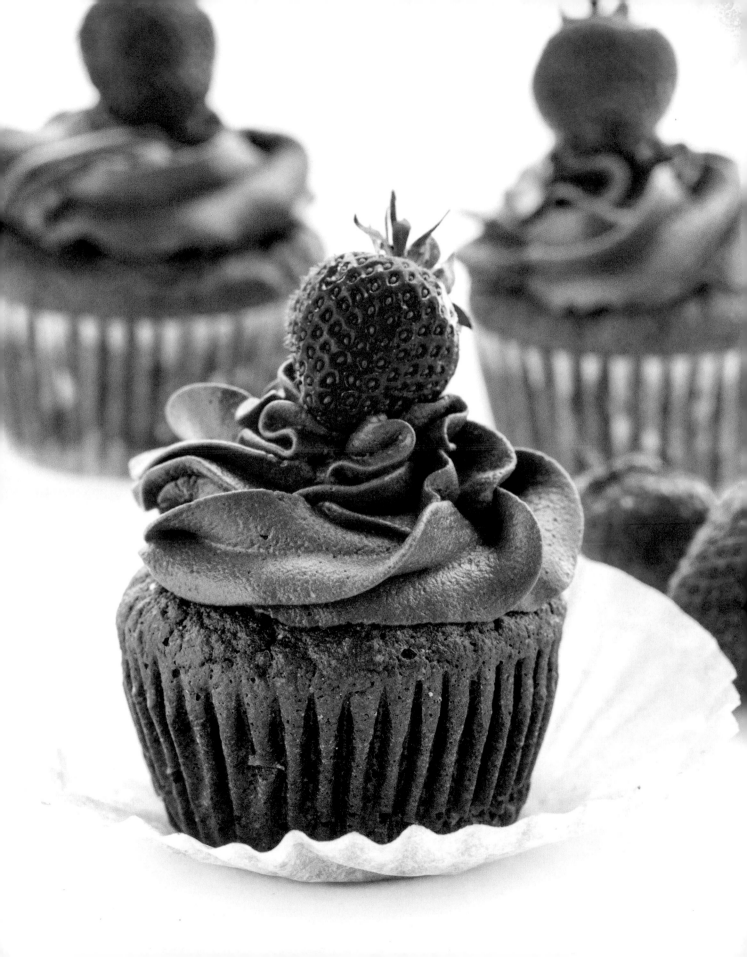

CREAM-FILLED CHOCOLATE CUPCAKES

Yield: 12 cupcakes (1 per serving) Prep Time: 20 minutes (not including time to make cupcakes and glaze) Cook Time: —

This is my keto take on Hostess Cupcakes. You'll feel like a kid again when you bite into one of these!

1 recipe Chocolate Cupcakes (page 78)

3 ounces cream cheese, softened

¾ cup heavy whipping cream, room temperature, divided

⅓ cup powdered erythritol sweetener

½ teaspoon vanilla extract

1 recipe Easy Chocolate Glaze (page 390)

1. Core the cupcakes following Steps 1 and 2 in the visual guide on pages 82 and 83.

2. In a large bowl, use an electric mixer to beat the cream cheese with 6 tablespoons of the cream and the sweetener until well combined.

3. In a medium bowl, beat the remaining 6 tablespoons of cream with the vanilla until it holds stiff peaks. Fold the whipped cream gently into the cream cheese mixture. Reserve about ½ cup of this mixture for decorating the cupcakes.

4. Following Steps 3 through 5 in the visual guide, fill the cored cupcakes with the cream cheese mixture, then plug the cream-filled holes with the tops of the reserved cores, as directed.

5. After making the glaze, allow it to cool and thicken for 10 minutes, then spread the glaze over the tops of the cupcakes.

6. Use the reserved cream mixture to pipe little swirls down the center of each cupcake.

NUTRITIONAL INFORMATION

CALORIES: 292 | FAT: 24.6g | CARBS: 8.5g | FIBER: 4.4g | PROTEIN: 7g

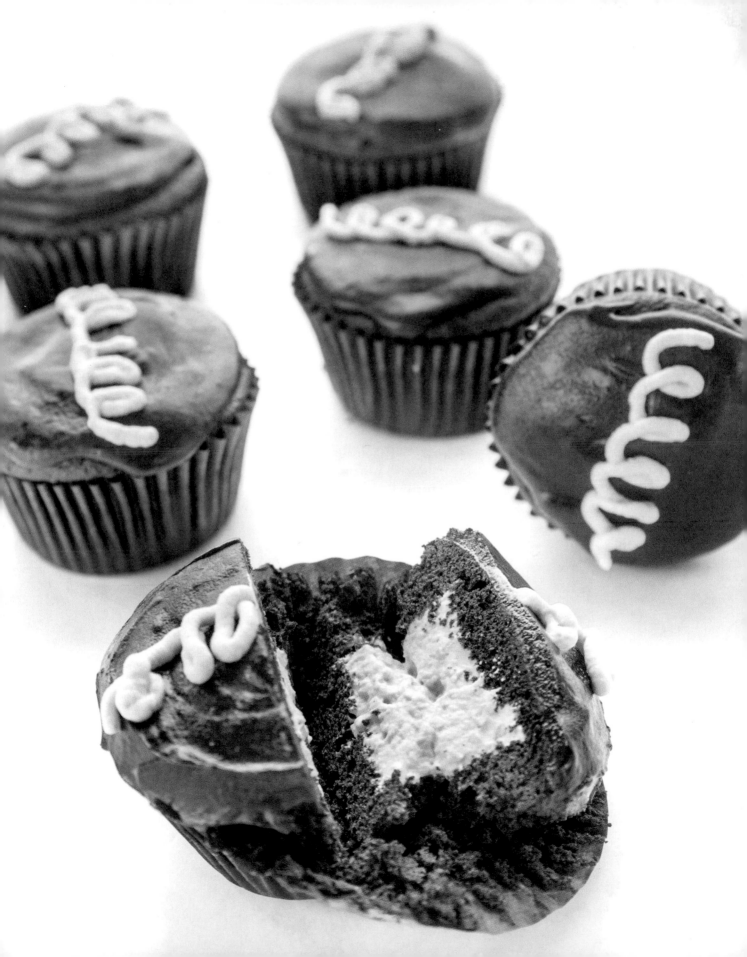

How to Core and Fill Cupcakes

1

Insert a 1-inch cookie cutter into the top of the cupcake and press down about 1 inch. (See note, opposite.)

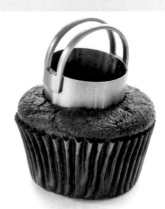

2

Twist a few times and pull the cookie cutter straight up. The core should come out inside the cookie cutter. Reserve the core.

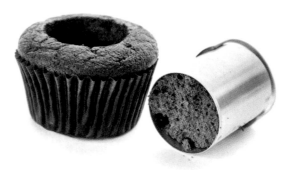

3

Pipe or spoon the filling into the cupcake. Cut off the top ¼ inch of the core.

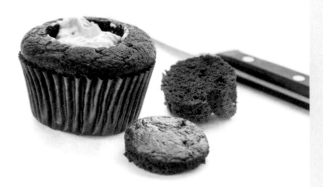

4

Insert the top layer of the core into the cream-filled hole.

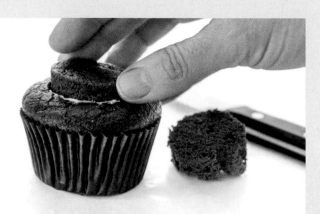

5

Press down firmly to make the top flush with the rest of the cupcake. Frost or glaze as directed.

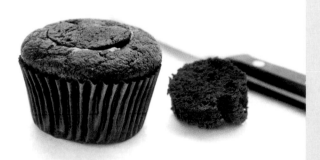

NOTE: *If you do not have a small round cookie cutter, you can use a sharp knife. Cut a cone-shaped piece about 1 inch in diameter and 1 inch deep. Remove and reserve the core. Use a small spoon to scoop out the hole so that it's 1 inch wide all around. Then proceed as directed.*

TIP: *The leftover cores can be eaten on their own or crumbled over ice cream. They freeze well, too, so you can reserve them for another use, such as a parfait, when you have more.*

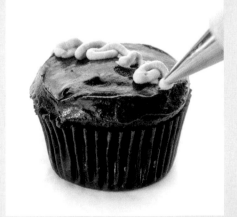

CREAM-FILLED VANILLA CUPCAKES

OPTION

Yield: 12 cupcakes (1 per serving) Prep Time: 30 minutes (not including time to make frosting) Cook Time: 25 minutes

If you loved Twinkies as a kid, you're going to love these Twinkie-inspired cupcakes.

3 cups (300g) blanched almond flour

⅓ cup unflavored whey protein powder

2 teaspoons baking powder

½ teaspoon salt

½ cup (1 stick) unsalted butter, softened

¾ cup granulated erythritol sweetener

3 large eggs

1 large egg yolk

1 teaspoon vanilla extract

¼ cup heavy whipping cream

¼ cup water

½ recipe Whipped Cream Frosting (page 377)

NUT-FREE OPTION:

For a nut-free version, you can make the cupcakes with the batter for the Boston Cream Poke Cake on page 112. Simply complete Steps 2 and 3.

1. Preheat the oven to 325°F and line a standard muffin pan with 12 silicone or parchment paper liners.

2. In a medium bowl, whisk together the almond flour, protein powder, baking powder, and salt.

3. In a large bowl, beat the butter and sweetener with an electric mixer until light and fluffy, about 2 minutes. Beat in the whole eggs one at a time, scraping down the sides of the bowl and the beaters as needed. Beat in the egg yolk and vanilla.

4. Beat in half of the almond flour mixture, then beat in the cream and water. Beat in the remaining almond flour mixture until well combined.

5. Divide the batter among the prepared muffin cups, filling each about three-quarters full.

6. Bake for 20 to 25 minutes, until the edges are just turning golden and the tops are firm to the touch. Remove from the oven and let cool in the pan for at least 10 minutes, then transfer to a wire rack to cool completely.

7. Core the cupcakes following Steps 1 and 2 in the visual guide on pages 82 and 83, setting the cores aside for another use. Pipe or spoon the frosting into the holes, allowing it to mound up and over the tops of the cupcakes.

NUTRITIONAL INFORMATION

CALORIES: 329 | FAT: 29g | CARBS: 7.3g | FIBER: 3g | PROTEIN: 10.4g

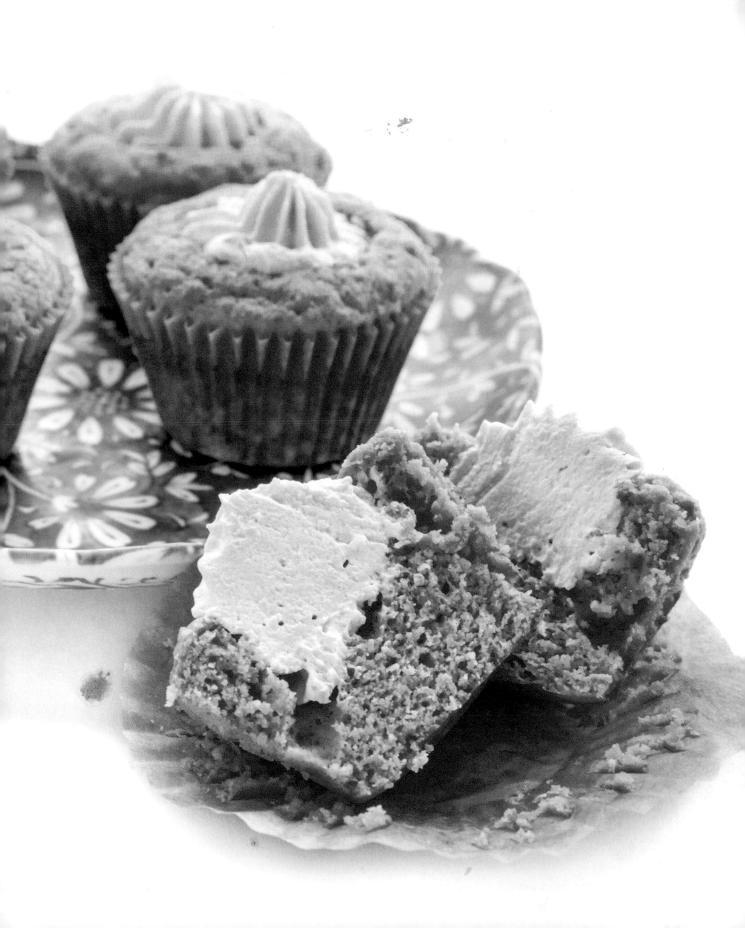

CONFETTI CUPCAKES

Yield: 12 cupcakes (1 per serving)   Prep Time: 20 minutes (not including time to make frosting)   Cook Time: 30 minutes

Sugar-free sprinkles do exist! See page 403 in the Resource Guide to find out where to source them. You can also leave them out, and then these become simple white cupcakes—a great base for any frosting.

2½ cups (250g) blanched almond flour

¾ cup granulated erythritol sweetener

¼ cup unflavored whey protein powder

2 teaspoons baking powder

¼ teaspoon salt

½ cup sour cream or plain Greek yogurt

4 large egg whites

¾ teaspoon vanilla extract

1 tablespoon sugar-free sprinkles, plus more for topping

1 recipe Swiss Meringue Buttercream (page 378)

1. Preheat the oven to 325°F and line a standard muffin pan with 12 silicone or parchment paper liners.

2. In a large bowl, whisk together the almond flour, sweetener, protein powder, baking powder, and salt.

3. Add the sour cream, egg whites, and vanilla and stir until well combined. Gently fold in the sprinkles, trying not to overmix, as they will bleed color a bit.

4. Divide the batter among the prepared muffin cups, filling each about three-quarters full.

5. Bake for 25 to 30 minutes, until the tops are just becoming golden and are firm to the touch. Remove from the oven and let cool completely in the pan before spreading or piping on the buttercream.

6. Top the frosted cupcakes with a few more sprinkles.

TIPS: *Using only egg whites and no butter helps keep the color of the cupcakes whiter. Because almond flour has a bit of a yellowish color naturally, this is about as white as you can get them. You can also use carton egg whites; ¾ cup is the equivalent of 4 large egg whites.*

Can't get your hands on sugar-free sprinkles? I suspect they will become more widely available soon. However, you can also make your own by lightly dyeing unsweetened shredded coconut with a bit of natural food coloring.

NUTRITIONAL INFORMATION
CALORIES: 289 | FAT: 24.4g | CARBS: 5.9g | FIBER: 2.5g | PROTEIN: 8.8g

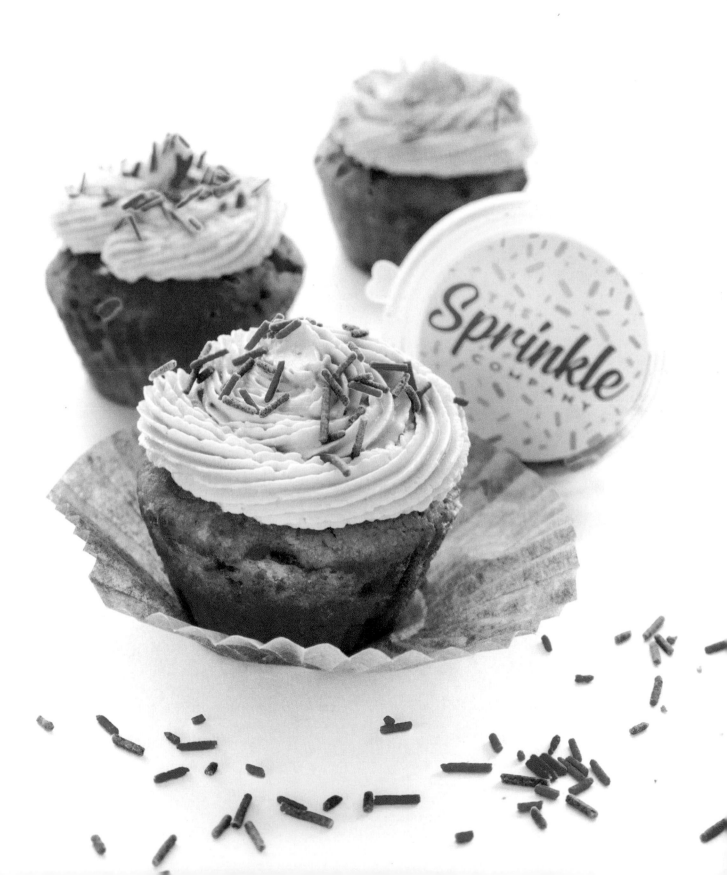

MINI CHOCOLATE PEANUT BUTTER CHEESECAKES

Yield: 6 mini cheesecakes (1 per serving) Prep Time: 20 minutes, plus 2 hours to chill Cook Time: 25 minutes

I love individual treats like these delicious mini cheesecakes. They're easier to make than full-sized cakes, and you have built-in portion control.

Crust:

⅓ cup (33g) blanched almond flour

1½ tablespoons cocoa powder

1½ tablespoons powdered erythritol sweetener

Pinch of salt

1½ tablespoons unsalted butter, melted

Filling:

6 ounces cream cheese, softened

⅓ cup natural peanut butter (creamy or chunky)

⅓ cup powdered erythritol sweetener

½ teaspoon vanilla extract

1 large egg, room temperature

2 tablespoons heavy whipping cream

Topping:

¼ cup heavy whipping cream

1 ounce sugar-free dark chocolate, chopped

2 tablespoons salted peanuts, chopped, for garnish

TO MAKE THE CRUST:

1. Preheat the oven to 350°F and line 6 wells of a standard muffin pan with silicone or parchment paper liners.

2. In a medium bowl, combine the almond flour, cocoa powder, sweetener, and salt. Stir in the melted butter until the mixture begins to clump together.

3. Put about 1 tablespoon of the crust mixture in the bottom of each prepared muffin cup and press down firmly and evenly.

TO MAKE THE FILLING:

4. In a medium bowl, beat the cream cheese, peanut butter, sweetener, and vanilla with an electric mixer until smooth. Beat in the egg and cream until well combined.

5. Spoon the filling mixture into the prepared muffin cups, filling them all the way to the top. Smooth the tops. Bake for 18 to 25 minutes, until just firm to the touch.

6. Remove from the oven and let cool in the pan for 20 minutes, then place in the fridge to chill and firm up, about 2 hours.

TO MAKE THE TOPPING:

7. In a medium microwave-safe bowl, heat the cream on high in 30-second increments until bubbling. Add the chopped chocolate and let sit for a few minutes to melt.

8. Whisk until smooth and spoon over the chilled cheesecakes. Sprinkle with the chopped peanuts.

TIP: *Any nut butter should work here, but be sure to stir it well to mix in any oil from the top of the jar. Too much oil will keep the cheesecakes from setting properly.*

NUTRITIONAL INFORMATION

CALORIES: 311 | FAT: 27.2g | CARBS: 8.1g | FIBER: 2.7g | PROTEIN: 7.3g

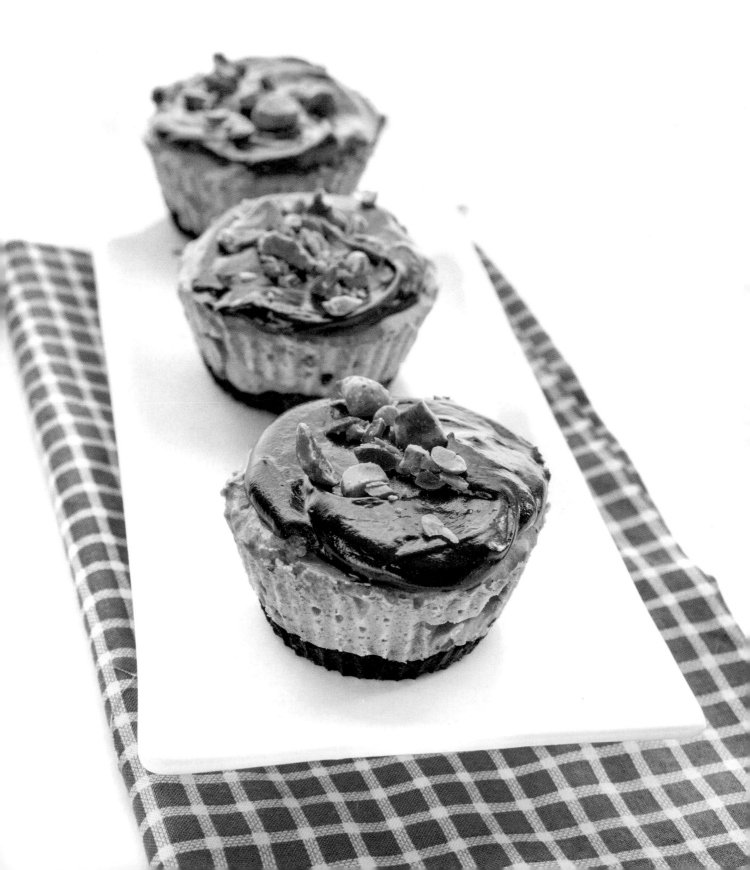

WARM GINGERBREAD CAKE

OPTION

Yield: 12 servings Prep Time: 10 minutes Cook Time: 45 minutes

A cake with an identity crisis! This soft, puddinglike cake is meant to be scooped out by the spoonful rather than cut into slices. Top it with my Sugar-Free Caramel Sauce (page 388) for an amazing gingerbread experience.

2½ cups (250g) blanched almond flour

½ cup brown sugar substitute, packed

⅓ cup granulated sweetener of choice

1 tablespoon cocoa powder

1 tablespoon ginger powder

1½ teaspoons ground cinnamon

½ teaspoon ground cloves

1 teaspoon baking powder

¼ teaspoon salt

2 large eggs

½ cup (1 stick) unsalted butter, melted but not hot

½ teaspoon vanilla extract

⅔ cup hot water (not boiling)

1. Preheat the oven to 325°F and grease a 2-quart glass or ceramic baking dish. (A deep 9-inch pie plate would work as well.)

2. In a large bowl, whisk together the almond flour, sweeteners, cocoa powder, ginger, cinnamon, cloves, baking powder, and salt.

3. Stir in the eggs, melted butter, and vanilla, then slowly add the hot water, stirring as you go, until well combined.

4. Spread the batter in the prepared baking dish and bake for about 45 minutes, until the center is barely set.

5. Remove from the oven and let cool in the baking dish for 10 minutes before scooping out.

TIP: *This cake tends to firm up as it cools, so if you wanted slices, you could let it cool entirely. And if you'd prefer a more cakelike consistency, you can add ¼ cup of whey or egg white protein powder and an additional teaspoon of baking powder to help it rise.*

SERVING SUGGESTION: *Serve warm with Sugar-Free Caramel Sauce (page 388). Also delicious with whipped cream or ice cream.*

DAIRY-FREE OPTION:

Substitute melted coconut oil, melted ghee, or avocado oil for the butter.

NUTRITIONAL INFORMATION

CALORIES: 220 | FAT: 19.6g | CARBS: 6.1g | FIBER: 2.9g | PROTEIN: 6.3g

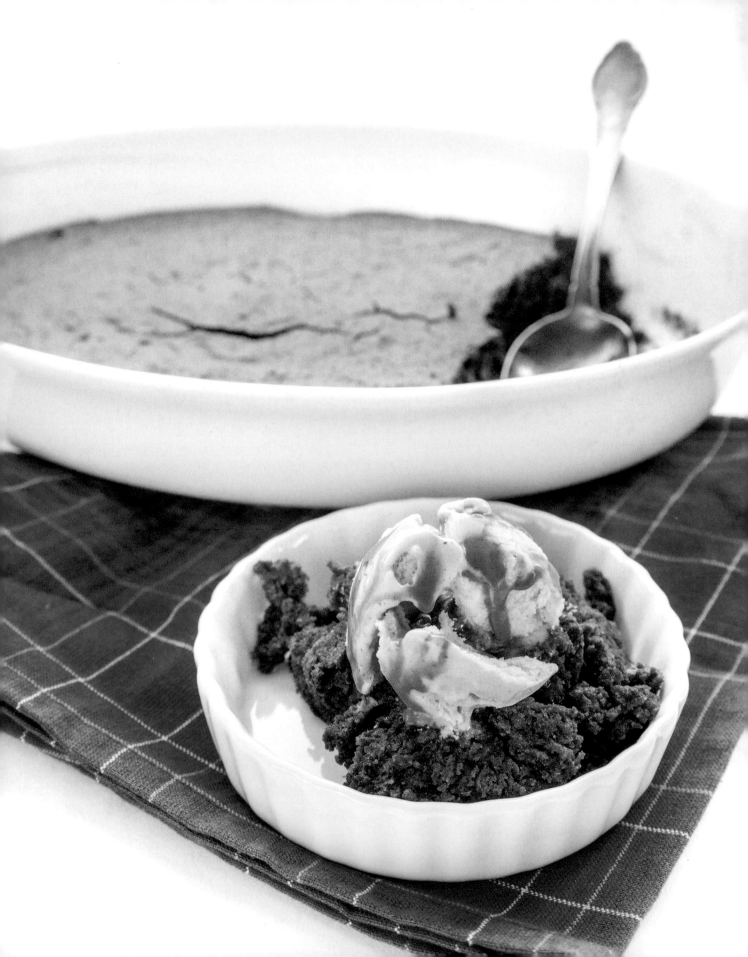

Chapter 5: SPECIAL OCCASION CAKES

Where there is cake, there is hope. And there is always cake. —Dean Koontz

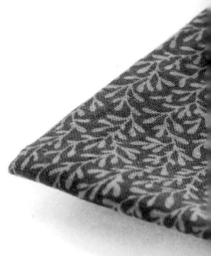

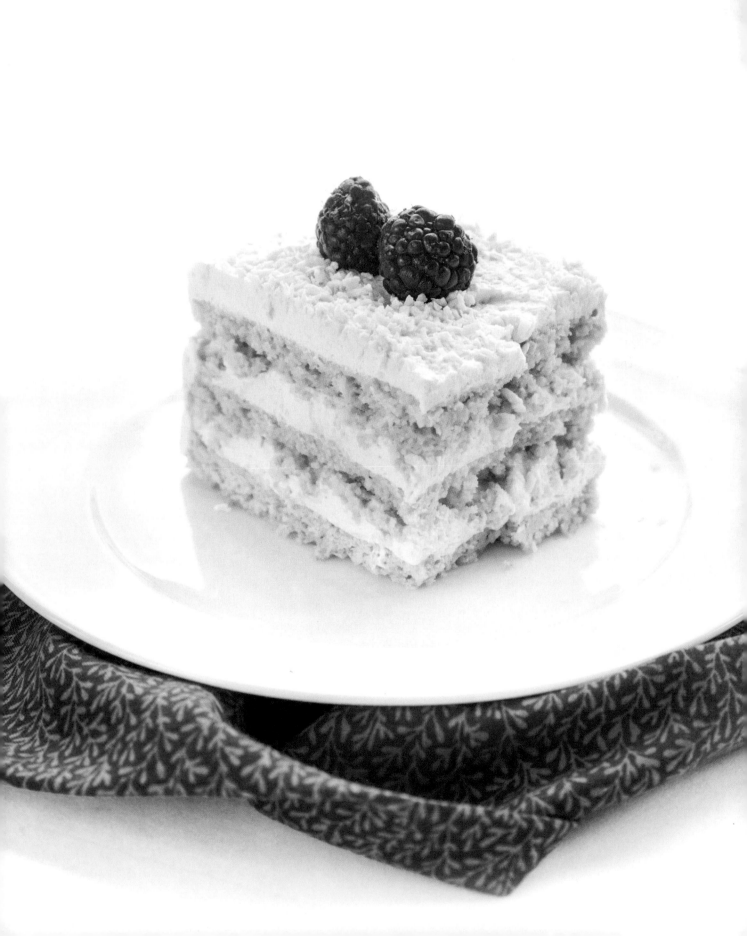

CLASSIC YELLOW BIRTHDAY CAKE

OPTION

Yield: One 2-layer, 8-inch round cake (12 servings) Prep Time: 20 minutes (not including time to make frosting) Cook Time: 25 minutes

The ultimate keto birthday cake! You don't have to pair it with the chocolate buttercream, but it's a classic combination. Sprinkle a little shaved chocolate or perhaps some sugar-free sprinkles (see page 403) on top.

3 cups (300g) blanched almond flour

⅓ cup unflavored whey protein powder

2 teaspoons baking powder

½ teaspoon salt

½ cup (1 stick) unsalted butter, softened

¾ cup granulated erythritol sweetener

3 large eggs

1 large egg yolk

1 teaspoon vanilla extract

½ cup unsweetened almond milk

1 recipe Chocolate Buttercream Frosting (page 382)

DAIRY-FREE OPTION:

Replace the whey protein with egg white protein and the butter with softened coconut oil or ghee. Then use the Dairy-Free Chocolate Frosting (page 384).

1. Preheat the oven to 325°F and grease two 8-inch round cake pans. Line the bottoms of the pans with parchment paper and grease the paper.

2. In a medium bowl, whisk together the almond flour, protein powder, baking powder, and salt.

3. In a large bowl, beat the butter and sweetener with an electric mixer until light and fluffy, about 2 minutes. Beat in the whole eggs one at a time, scraping down the sides of the bowl and the beaters as needed. Beat in the egg yolk and vanilla.

4. Beat in half of the almond flour mixture, then beat in the almond milk. Beat in the remaining almond flour until well combined.

5. Divide the batter between the prepared pans. Spread to the edges and smooth the tops.

6. Bake for 20 to 25 minutes, until the edges are golden brown and the tops are firm to the touch. Remove from the oven and let cool in the pans for at least 20 minutes, then flip out onto a wire rack to cool completely. Peel off the parchment paper.

7. To frost, place one cake layer on a plate or serving platter. Top with one-third of the frosting, spreading it all the way to the edges. Gently place the second layer on top and spread the top with another third of the frosting. Spread the sides with the remaining frosting.

TIP: *In the cake, you could use other sweeteners, such as Bocha Sweet or xylitol. I don't recommend allulose here, as it could make the sides of the cake very dark. For the frosting, you will need a good powdered erythritol sweetener, such as Swerve.*

NUTRITIONAL INFORMATION

CALORIES: 346 | FAT: 31.4g | CARBS: 7.1g | FIBER: 3.3g | PROTEIN: 8.6g

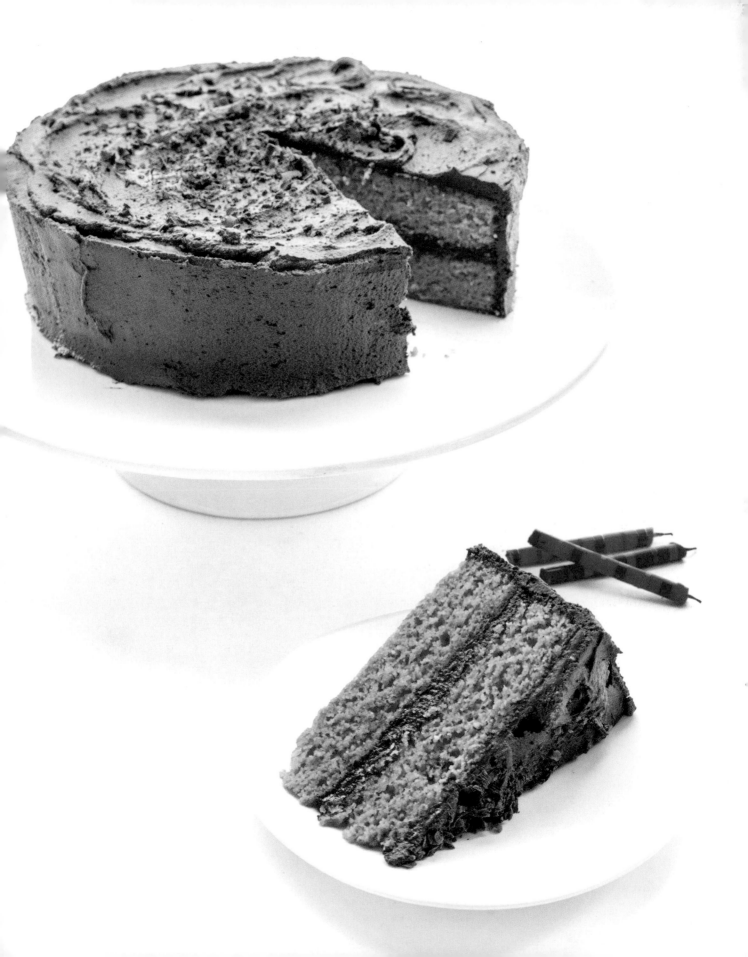

CHOCOLATE MAYONNAISE CAKE

Yield: One 2-layer, 8-inch round cake (16 servings) Prep Time: 15 minutes (not including time to make frosting) Cook Time: 25 minutes

Mayonnaise makes cake extra moist and delicious while being entirely dairy-free. It plays the role of the oil, some of the egg, and some of the liquid. I never knew dairy-free could taste so good!

2 cups (200g) blanched almond flour

¾ cup granulated erythritol sweetener

⅔ cup cocoa powder

1 tablespoon baking powder

1 teaspoon espresso powder (optional)

½ teaspoon salt

1 cup mayonnaise

3 large eggs

⅓ cup water

1 teaspoon vanilla extract

1 recipe Dairy-Free Chocolate Frosting (page 384)

1. Preheat the oven to 350°F and grease two 8-inch round pans. Line the bottoms of the pans with parchment paper and grease the paper.

2. In a large bowl, whisk together the almond flour, sweetener, cocoa powder, baking powder, espresso powder (if using), and salt.

3. Stir in the mayonnaise, eggs, water, and vanilla until well combined. Divide the batter between the prepared pans, then use an offset spatula to spread it to the edges and smooth the tops.

4. Bake for 20 to 25 minutes, until the cakes are just firm to the touch. Remove from the oven and let cool in the pans for at least 20 minutes, then flip out onto a wire rack to cool completely. Peel off the parchment paper.

5. To frost the cake, place one layer on a plate or serving platter. Top with one-third of the frosting, spreading it all the way to the edges. Gently place the second layer on top and spread the top with another third of the frosting. Spread the sides with the remaining frosting.

TIPS: *Adding coffee to a chocolate recipe enhances and deepens the chocolate flavor. In a large cake such as this, it does not make it taste like coffee or mocha at all, but you can skip the coffee if you prefer.*

If you don't need to be dairy-free, pair this gorgeous cake with any frosting you like. It would be fabulous with the Swiss Meringue Buttercream (page 378).

SERVING SUGGESTION: *Top with Chocolate Shards (page 396) for an elegant presentation.*

NUTRITIONAL INFORMATION

CALORIES: 366 | FAT: 35.7g | CARBS: 7.3g | FIBER: 3.4g | PROTEIN: 6.3g

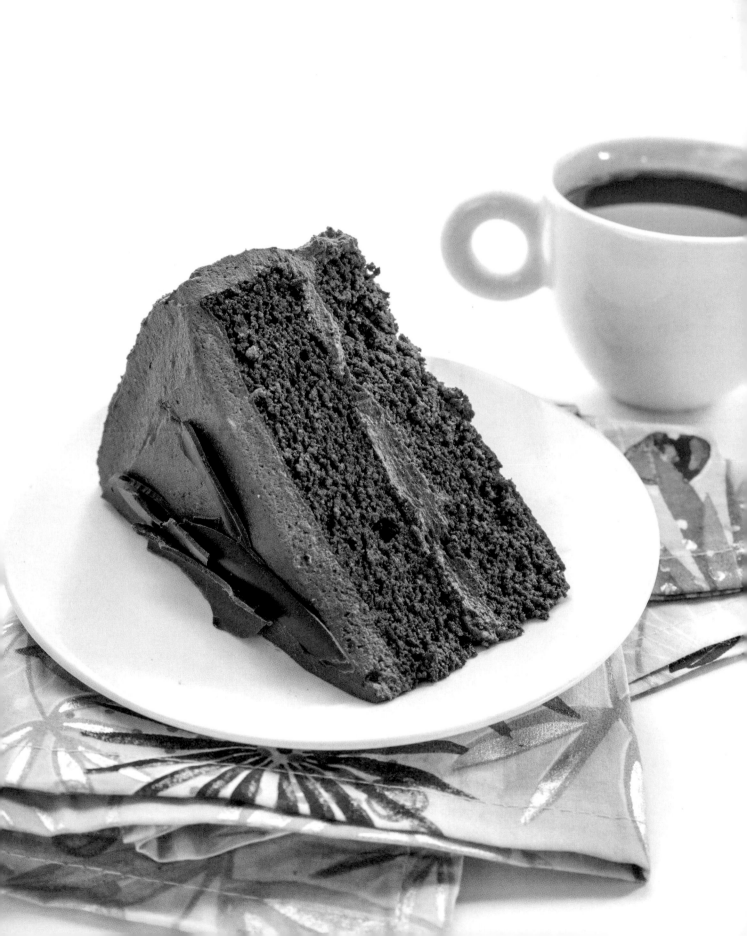

COCONUT LAYER CAKE

Yield: One 3-layer rectangular cake (16 servings) Prep Time: 40 minutes, plus 1 hour to chill Cook Time: 25 minutes

It's like eating a creamy coconut-flavored cloud! If you're a coconut lover, this cake is worth every second of the effort. Garnish it with a few fresh raspberries for a pretty pop of color.

Cake:

2½ cups (250g) blanched almond flour

⅔ cup granulated erythritol sweetener

⅓ cup unsweetened shredded coconut

⅓ cup unflavored whey protein powder

1 tablespoon baking powder

½ teaspoon xanthan gum

½ teaspoon salt

5 large egg whites, room temperature

⅓ cup coconut oil, melted but not hot

1 teaspoon coconut extract

¾ cup unsweetened almond milk, room temperature

Frosting:

1 recipe Whipped Cream Frosting (page 377)

1 teaspoon coconut extract

Garnish:

½ cup unsweetened shredded coconut

TO MAKE THE CAKE:

1. Preheat the oven to 325°F and grease an 11 by 17-inch rimmed baking sheet. Line the bottom with parchment paper and grease the paper.

2. In a large bowl, whisk together the almond flour, sweetener, shredded coconut, protein powder, baking powder, xanthan gum, and salt. Whisk in the egg whites, melted coconut oil, coconut extract, and almond milk until well combined.

3. Spread the batter in the prepared baking sheet and bake for about 25 minutes, until the edges are just golden and the center is set to the touch. Remove from the oven and let cool completely in the pan.

TO MAKE THE FROSTING:

4. Follow the instructions for the whipped cream frosting, but add the coconut extract along with the vanilla.

TO ASSEMBLE:

5. Gently loosen the edges of the cake with a sharp knife, then cover the whole pan with a large cookie sheet or cutting board and flip it upside down. Remove the baking sheet and carefully peel off the parchment paper. Cut the cake crosswise into 3 even pieces to create 3 layers.

6. Gently place one cake layer on a plate or serving platter and spread about 1 cup of the frosting on the top. Repeat with the remaining layers. Spread the remaining 1 cup of frosting over the sides of the cake.

7. Sprinkle the top with the shredded coconut. Refrigerate for at least 1 hour before serving.

TIPS: *The cake layers are very fragile and may break or crack a bit as you lift and try to stack them, but it's easy to piece them back together. The cracks won't show in the final product!*

To slice this lovely but fragile cake, use a very sharp knife to cut the cake in half lengthwise down the center and then cut slices off each side.

NUTRITIONAL INFORMATION

CALORIES: 288 | FAT: 26.6g | CARBS: 6.2g | FIBER: 2.4g | PROTEIN: 7.5g

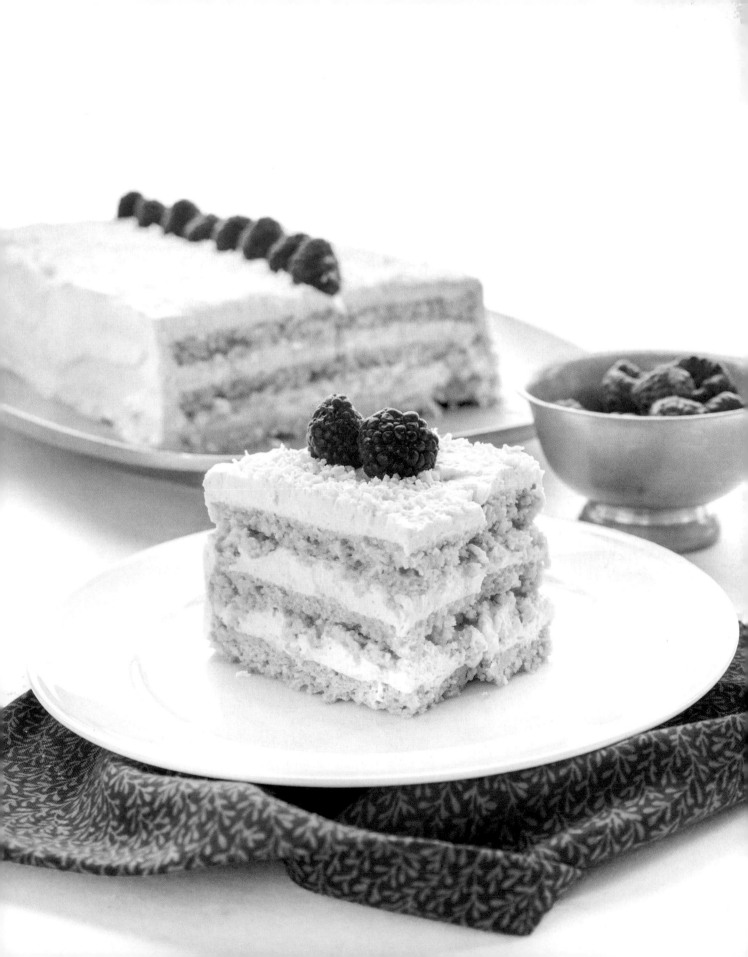

FLOURLESS SWISS ROLL

Yield: 12 servings   Prep Time: 45 minutes, plus 1 hour to chill   Cook Time: 15 minutes

A cake roll is labor-intensive, but the results are worth the trouble. It looks spectacular and tastes like heaven. And it will impress your friends and family!

6 tablespoons cocoa powder, divided

¼ cup plus 2 tablespoons powdered erythritol sweetener

1 tablespoon grass-fed gelatin

6 large eggs, separated

2 tablespoons allulose or Bocha Sweet (see tips)

2 tablespoons coffee or water, room temperature

½ teaspoon vanilla extract

¼ teaspoon cream of tartar

Pinch of salt

1 recipe Cream Cheese Frosting (page 380), for the filling

1 recipe Easy Chocolate Glaze (page 390)

SERVING SUGGESTION: *Top with a few fresh berries or Chocolate Shards (page 396).*

1. Preheat the oven to 350°F and line an 11 by 17-inch rimmed baking sheet with parchment paper. Grease the paper and pan sides very well. Dust thoroughly with 1 tablespoon of the cocoa powder.

2. In a medium bowl, whisk together ¼ cup of the cocoa powder, the powdered sweetener, and the gelatin.

3. In another medium bowl, beat the egg yolks and allulose with an electric mixer until lighter yellow and thickened, about 2 minutes. Beat in the coffee and vanilla. Clean the beaters.

4. Using the mixer and a large bowl, beat the egg whites with the cream of tartar and salt until they hold stiff peaks. Gently fold the egg yolk mixture into the beaten egg whites. Then fold in the cocoa powder mixture until no streaks remain.

5. Spread the batter evenly in the prepared baking sheet and bake for 10 to 15 minutes, until the top springs back when touched. Remove from the oven and let cool in the pan for a few minutes, then run a knife around the edges to loosen.

6. Sprinkle with the remaining 1 tablespoon of cocoa powder. Cover with another large piece of parchment paper, then a kitchen towel. Place another large cookie sheet on top and flip the whole thing over. Keep it covered to help keep the cake warm as you prepare the cream cheese frosting.

7. When ready to fill the cake, uncover it and gently peel off the parchment from what is now the top of the cake. Spread the frosting evenly on top, leaving a ½-inch border.

8. Starting at a short end, gently and carefully roll up the cake. The inner, tighter rolls may crack a little, but the cracks will be hidden inside the cake. Place the cake roll seam side down on a platter.

9. Prepare the chocolate glaze and let cool for 10 to 20 minutes to thicken. Pour the glaze over the top of the cake roll. You can either let it drip down the sides or use an offset spatula to spread it over the cake roll, including the ends. Refrigerate for 1 hour, until set.

NUTRITIONAL INFORMATION

CALORIES: 276 | FAT: 23.9g | CARBS: 4.6g | FIBER: 1.8g | PROTEIN: 6.5g

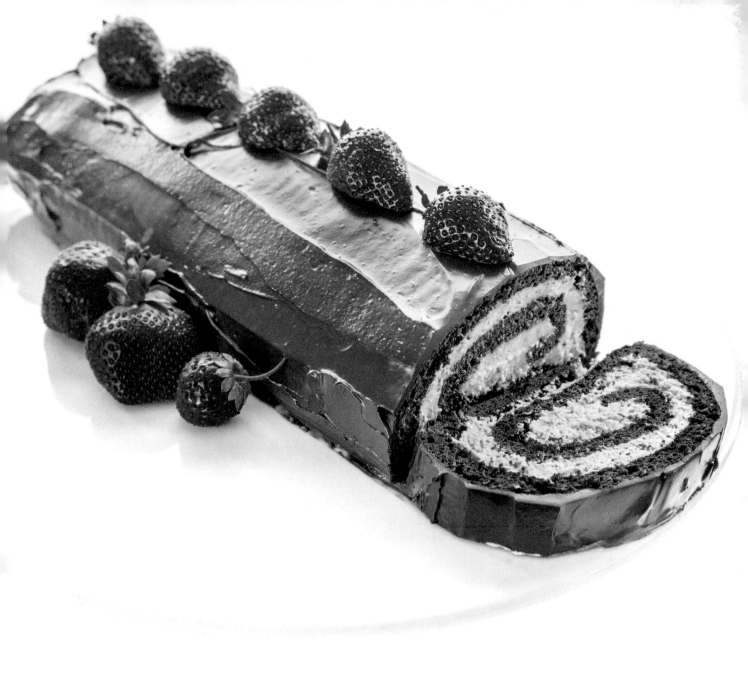

TIPS: *Conventional cake rolls call for rolling the warm cake in a towel, then unrolling it again to spread the filling. I find that for keto cakes, this process makes the cake crack even more. So I simply keep the cake covered warm in the pan as I prepare the filling.*

The gelatin in this recipe helps keep the cake more flexible and less prone to cracking as you roll it.

Using allulose or Bocha Sweet also keeps the cake softer for rolling. If you just want to use an erythritol-based sweetener, that's fine, but the cake may crack a bit more as you roll it.

CREAM CHEESE-FILLED CARROT CAKE

Yield: 16 servings   Prep Time: 25 minutes   Cook Time: 55 minutes

Putting the cream cheese on the inside is a fun twist on classic carrot cake! You can serve this cake as is or top it with a beautiful cream cheese glaze. It's perfect for Easter or any holiday celebration.

Filling:

1 (8-ounce) package cream cheese, softened

⅓ cup powdered erythritol sweetener

1 large egg, room temperature

½ teaspoon vanilla extract

Cake:

3 cups (300g) blanched almond flour

¾ cup granulated erythritol sweetener

½ cup chopped pecans

¼ cup unflavored whey protein powder

1 tablespoon baking powder

1½ teaspoons ground cinnamon

¼ teaspoon ground cloves

¼ teaspoon salt

1 cup peeled and grated carrots

3 large eggs

½ cup (1 stick) unsalted butter, melted but not hot

½ cup unsweetened almond milk

1 teaspoon vanilla extract

Glaze (Optional):

3 ounces cream cheese, softened

1 tablespoon unsalted butter, softened

3 tablespoons powdered erythritol sweetener

½ teaspoon vanilla extract

2 to 4 tablespoons water, to thin

TO MAKE THE FILLING:

1. In a medium bowl, beat the cream cheese and sweetener with an electric mixer until well combined. Beat in the egg and vanilla until the mixture is smooth and creamy. Set aside.

TO MAKE THE CAKE:

2. Preheat the oven to 325°F and grease a 10- to 12-cup Bundt pan very well.

3. In a large bowl, whisk together the almond flour, sweetener, pecans, protein powder, baking powder, cinnamon, cloves, and salt. Stir in the grated carrots.

4. Add the eggs, melted butter, almond milk, and vanilla and stir until well combined.

5. Spread about two-thirds of the batter in the prepared pan, then use a spoon to create a trench in the middle of the batter, about 1 inch deep and 2 inches wide, all the way around the pan.

6. Spoon the filling into the trench and cover with the remaining batter. Smooth the top.

7. Bake for 45 to 55 minutes, until the top is firm to the touch. The cake shouldn't jiggle at all when you shake the pan.

8. Remove from the oven and let cool completely in the pan, then loosen the edge with a knife before carefully flipping the cake out onto a serving plate.

TO MAKE THE GLAZE (OPTIONAL):

9. In a medium bowl, beat the cream cheese and butter with an electric mixer until smooth. Beat in the sweetener and vanilla.

10. Add 2 tablespoons of water and beat until well combined. If the glaze is too thick, add 1 to 2 tablespoons more water to thin it to a drizzling consistency. Drizzle over the cooled cake.

NUTRITIONAL INFORMATION (WITHOUT GLAZE)

CALORIES: 274 | FAT: 23.4g | CARBS: 6.9g | FIBER: 2.9g | PROTEIN: 8.4g

NUTRITIONAL INFORMATION (WITH GLAZE)

CALORIES: 301 | FAT: 25.8g | CARBS: 7.2g | FIBER: 2.9g | PROTEIN: 8.8g

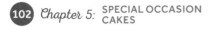

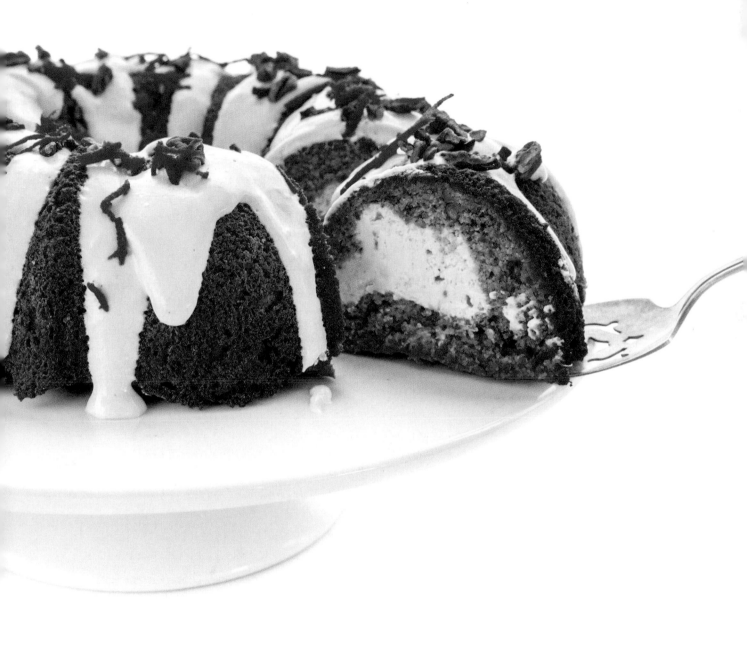

TIPS: *A Bundt pan makes for an elegant presentation, but getting the cake out of the pan can be tricky. I suggest avoiding the pans that have all sorts of peaks and valleys and sticking with a regular fluted pan. Also, grease it very, very well before adding the batter.*

Be sure to let the cake cool completely before trying to flip it out, or you may find it breaking and the filling oozing out.

SERVING SUGGESTION: *Garnish with a few chopped pecans and some shredded carrots.*

RUM CAKE

OPTION

Yield: 16 servings Prep Time: 20 minutes Cook Time: 1 hour

When I was developing and testing this recipe, my home was undergoing renovations. I had to use a friend's kitchen up the street and then rush home with my cake to take photos. Thankfully, it was worth all the trouble!

Cake:

⅓ cup chopped pecans, toasted

2½ cups (250g) blanched almond flour

¼ cup (28g) coconut flour

¼ cup unflavored whey protein powder

1 tablespoon baking powder

½ teaspoon salt

½ cup (1 stick) plus 2 tablespoons unsalted butter, softened

⅓ cup brown sugar substitute

⅓ cup granulated erythritol sweetener (see tips)

4 large eggs, room temperature

2 large egg yolks, room temperature

1 teaspoon vanilla extract

½ cup white rum

Rum Syrup:

6 tablespoons unsalted butter

⅓ cup granulated sweetener of choice (see tips)

¼ cup water

¼ cup white rum

DAIRY-FREE OPTION:

Replace the whey protein with egg white protein and the butter with coconut oil or ghee.

TO MAKE THE CAKE:

1. Preheat the oven to 325°F and grease a 10- to 12-cup Bundt pan very well. Sprinkle the bottom with the chopped pecans.

2. In a large bowl, whisk together the almond flour, coconut flour, protein powder, baking powder, and salt.

3. In another large bowl, beat the butter and sweeteners with an electric mixer until well combined. Beat in the whole eggs one at a time, scraping down the sides of the bowl and the beaters as needed. Beat in the egg yolks and vanilla.

4. Add the almond flour mixture all at once and beat until combined. Beat in the rum until the batter is uniform.

5. Spread the batter in the prepared pan and bake for 45 to 55 minutes, until the top is golden brown and firm to the touch. Remove from the oven and let cool completely in the pan.

TO MAKE THE SYRUP:

6. In a medium saucepan over medium heat, melt the butter with the sweetener. Add the water and bring to a boil, stirring until the sweetener is dissolved. Boil for 2 minutes.

7. Stir in the rum and boil for another 2 minutes.

TO ASSEMBLE:

8. While it's still in the pan, poke the cake all over with a skewer. Pour about half of the hot rum syrup over the cake and let it soak in for 10 minutes.

9. Loosen the edge of the cake with a knife, then flip the cake out onto a serving platter. Drizzle with the remaining rum syrup.

NUTRITIONAL INFORMATION
CALORIES: 275 | FAT: 22.3g | CARBS: 5.5g | FIBER: 2.7g | PROTEIN: 6.9g

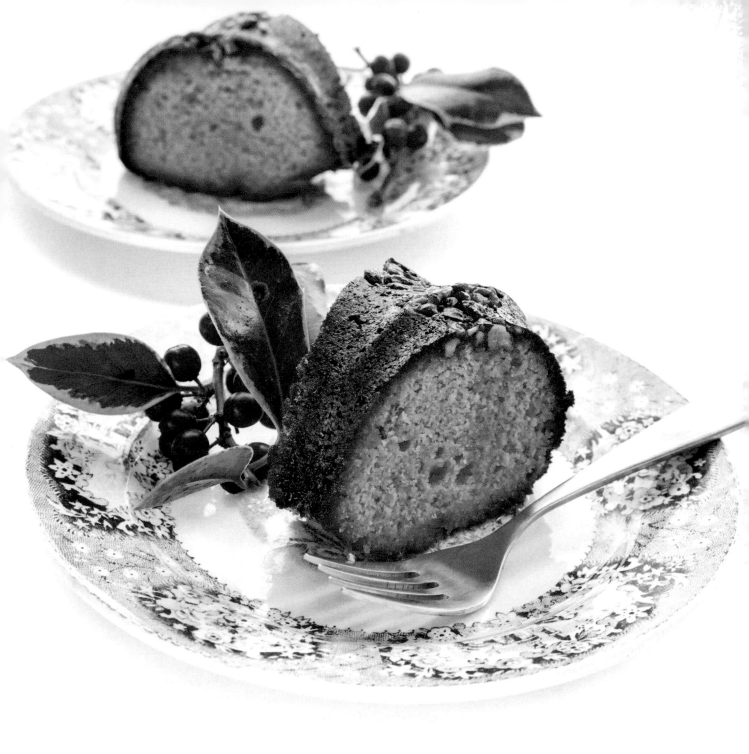

TIPS: *You will notice the surprisingly dark color on the outside of this cake in the photo. I was experimenting with allulose as part of the sweetener, and it appears to have made the portion of the cake that was touching the pan very dark. My recipe testers all used Swerve or Bocha Sweet, and their cakes were much lighter in color.*

The syrup will be fine with any granulated sweetener you prefer, although it may recrystallize some if you use an erythritol-based sweetener.

PECAN PIE POUND CAKE

Yield: 16 servings **Prep Time:** 20 minutes **Cook Time:** 65 minutes

Pecan pie in cake form! This is a divine cake to serve around the holidays.

Cake:

3 cups (300g) blanched almond flour

⅓ cup (37g) coconut flour

¼ cup unflavored whey protein powder

1 tablespoon baking powder

½ teaspoon salt

¾ cup (1½ sticks) unsalted butter, softened

½ cup granulated erythritol sweetener

½ cup brown sugar substitute

6 large eggs, room temperature

1 teaspoon caramel extract

1 cup unsweetened almond milk

¾ cup chopped pecans, toasted

Glaze:

3 tablespoons unsalted butter

3 tablespoons brown sugar substitute

3 tablespoons Bocha Sweet or allulose

1 tablespoon heavy whipping cream

¼ teaspoon caramel extract

¼ cup toasted pecan halves, for garnish

TO MAKE THE CAKE:

1. Preheat the oven to 325°F and grease a 10- to 12-cup Bundt pan very well.

2. In a medium bowl, whisk together the almond flour, coconut flour, protein powder, baking powder, and salt.

3. In a large bowl, beat the butter and sweeteners with an electric mixer until lightened and fluffy, about 3 minutes. Beat in the eggs one at a time, scraping down the sides of the bowl and the beaters as needed. Beat in the caramel extract.

4. Beat in the almond flour mixture in two additions, alternating with the almond milk. Stir in the chopped pecans.

5. Dollop the batter into the prepared pan and smooth the top. Bake for 50 to 60 minutes, until the cake is golden brown and the top is firm to the touch. A tester inserted in the center should come out clean.

6. Remove from the oven and let cool in the pan for 20 minutes, then transfer to a wire rack to cool completely.

TO MAKE THE GLAZE:

7. In a small saucepan over medium heat, melt the butter with the sweeteners until the sweeteners are completely dissolved, 3 to 4 minutes.

8. Remove the pan from the heat and stir in the cream and caramel extract. Drizzle over the cooled cake. Arrange the pecan halves on top.

TIP: *The combination of brown sugar erythritol sweetener and Bocha Sweet gives the glaze a lovely caramel color and keeps it softer. You can use just regular granulated erythritol and, if you want to give the glaze a caramel color, add a teaspoon of molasses.*

NUTRITIONAL INFORMATION

CALORIES: 315 | FAT: 27.7g | CARBS: 7.4g | FIBER: 3.8g | PROTEIN: 9.1g

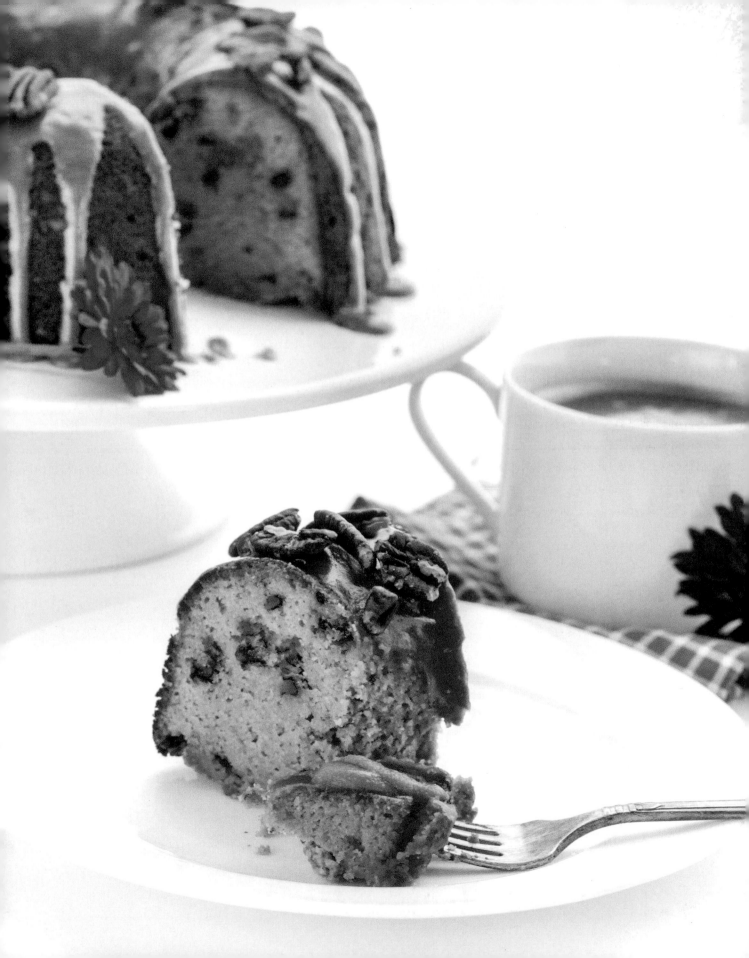

CHIFFON CAKE

Yield: 16 servings   Prep Time: 25 minutes   Cook Time: 1 hour

Chiffon cake is similar in method and texture to angel food cake, but it uses whole eggs rather than just the whites. So you don't have to find uses for 12 leftover yolks, and you still end up with a light, airy sponge cake that pairs perfectly with berries, whipped cream, ice cream, or anything that strikes your fancy.

1½ cups (150g) blanched almond flour

½ cup unflavored egg white protein powder

½ cup granulated erythritol sweetener

½ cup powdered erythritol sweetener

1 tablespoon baking powder

¼ teaspoon salt

4 large eggs, separated, room temperature

2 large whole eggs, room temperature

¼ cup water

¼ cup avocado oil

1 teaspoon vanilla extract

½ teaspoon almond extract

½ teaspoon cream of tartar

Powdered erythritol sweetener, for garnish

VARIATION: ORANGE CHIFFON CAKE.

Add 1 tablespoon freshly grated orange zest to the eggs, water, and oil mixture. Replace the almond extract with ¾ teaspoon orange extract.

1. Place an oven rack in the second-lowest position and preheat the oven to 325°F.

2. Line the bottom of a 16-cup nonstick tube pan with parchment paper but leave the pan ungreased (see tips).

3. In a large bowl, whisk together the almond flour, protein powder, sweeteners, baking powder, and salt. In a medium bowl, whisk together the egg yolks, whole eggs, water, oil, and extracts. Whisk the yolk mixture into the dry ingredients until smooth and well combined.

4. In another large bowl, whip the egg whites with the cream of tartar until they hold very stiff peaks. They should look dry and be very firm.

5. With a large rubber spatula, fold the egg whites into the batter until well combined and no streaks of egg white remain (see tips). Spread the batter in the prepared pan and smooth the top. Wipe off any drops of batter from the sides of the pan and tap the whole thing on the counter a few times to release any air bubbles.

6. Bake for 50 to 60 minutes, rotating the pan halfway through baking, until the top is uniformly golden brown and springs back when pressed. Remove from the oven and let cool completely in the pan.

7. If your tube pan has a removable bottom, you should be able to simply push the bottom up to release the cake. Otherwise, run a small knife around the inside of the pan to loosen the cake. Invert the pan over a cake plate and gently tap to release the cake.

8. Peel off the parchment paper from what is now the top of the cake and dust with powdered sweetener.

NUTRITIONAL INFORMATION

CALORIES: 119 | FAT: 10.5g | CARBS: 3g | FIBER: 1.1g | PROTEIN: 6.7g

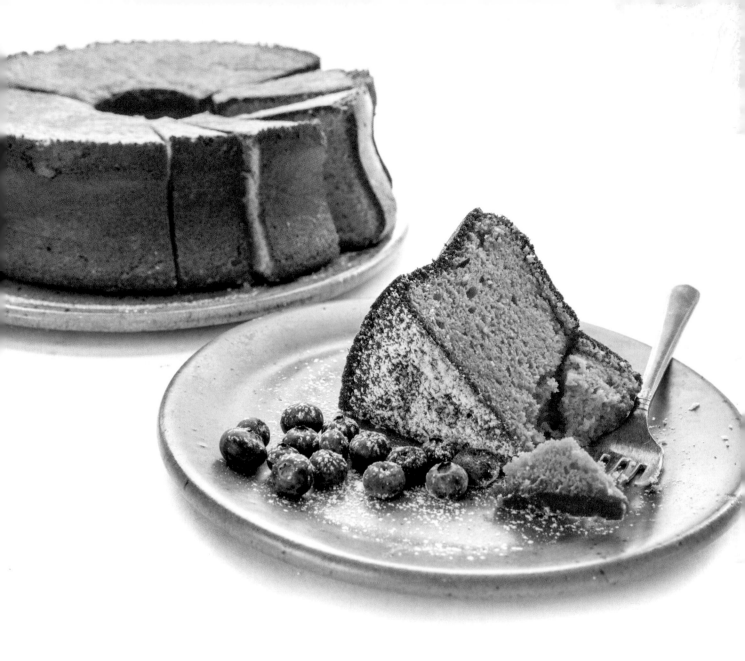

TIPS: *To line the cake pan, you will need a 9-inch circle of parchment paper. Fold the paper in half and then in half again to create a cone shape. Cut enough out of the very tip of the cone so that, when it is opened up, it fits over the center of the tube pan. It doesn't need to be perfect.*

The beaten egg whites need to be very stiff to give the cake the proper structure. You almost want to overbeat them. You can tell when they are done when they not only hold stiff peaks, but a lot of the whites stick to the beaters as you lift them out.

Folding such stiffly beaten egg whites into the batter can be tricky. If you find that there are clumps of egg white that won't combine easily, you can rub them up against the side of the bowl with a rubber spatula to break them up.

TRES LECHES CAKE

Yield: 15 servings   Prep Time: 30 minutes, plus 1½ hours to soak and chill cake (not including time to make condensed milk)
Cook Time: 25 minutes

Tres leches cake is the original poke cake recipe. The name means "three milks," and the traditional version involves pouring sweetened condensed milk, evaporated milk, and heavy cream over a cake poked with small holes. I had a lot of fun keto-fying this Latin American classic.

Cake:

1 cup (100g) blanched almond flour

⅓ cup (37g) coconut flour

2 teaspoons baking powder

5 large eggs, separated, room temperature

½ teaspoon salt

¾ cup granulated erythritol sweetener

1 teaspoon vanilla extract

Filling:

1 cup Keto Sweetened Condensed Milk (page 386)

¼ cup heavy whipping cream

¼ cup unsweetened vanilla-flavored almond milk

Topping:

1¼ cups heavy whipping cream

3 tablespoons powdered erythritol sweetener

SERVING SUGGESTION: *Top with a few fresh raspberries.*

TO MAKE THE CAKE:

1. Preheat the oven to 350°F and grease a 9 by 13-inch baking pan.

2. Using a sieve, sift the almond flour and coconut flour into a medium bowl to break up any clumps. Whisk in the baking powder.

3. In a large bowl, beat the egg whites and salt with an electric mixer until the whites hold medium peaks (the tip of the peak should fall over as you lift the beaters away from it).

4. In another large bowl, beat the egg yolks with the sweetener until thickened and pale yellow in color, about 2 minutes. Beat in the vanilla.

5. Gently fold the egg whites into the yolks until well combined. Then fold in the almond flour mixture in 3 additions. The egg whites will deflate some.

6. Spread the batter in the prepared pan and bake for 25 minutes, or until golden brown and firm to the touch.

7. Remove from the oven and let cool for 10 minutes, then use a skewer to poke holes all over the cake in ½-inch increments or even closer together. The more holes you poke, the better the filling will soak into the cake.

TO MAKE THE FILLING:

8. In a large bowl, whisk together the condensed milk, cream, and almond milk until well combined. Pour all over the warm cake and let it soak in for about 1 hour.

TO MAKE THE TOPPING:

9. In a large bowl, beat the cream with the sweetener until it holds stiff peaks. Spread all over the cooled cake. Refrigerate for at least 30 minutes to set.

NUTRITIONAL INFORMATION

CALORIES: 233 | FAT: 20.9g | CARBS: 4.6g | FIBER: 1.7g | PROTEIN: 5g

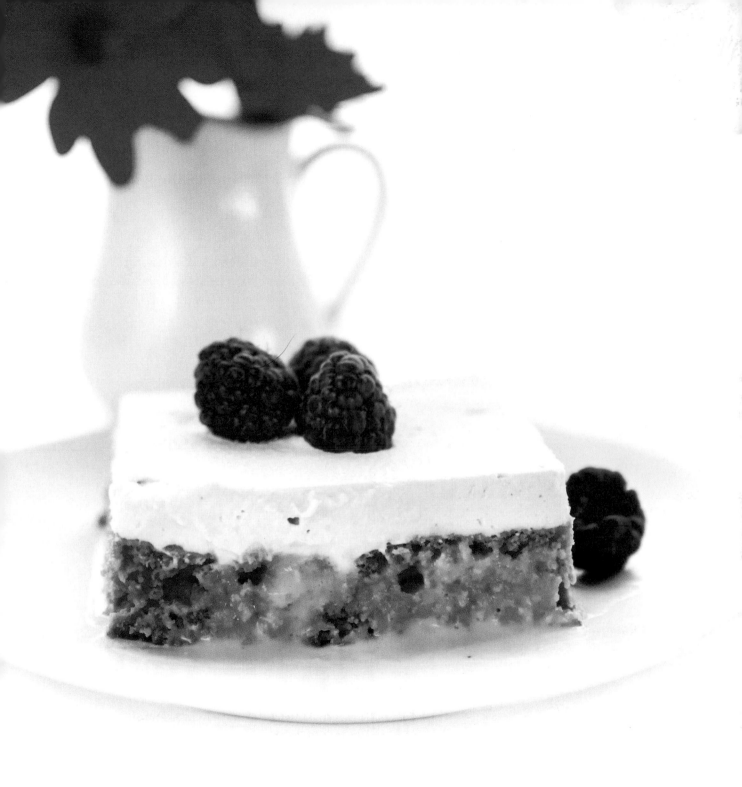

TIPS: *The cake itself is quite dry, and it's supposed to be. This allows the filling to soak in and create an incredibly moist dessert.*

When beating egg whites, you want to stop and check the consistency fairly often. Stiff peaks means that they should stand absolutely upright as you pull the beaters away. Medium peaks will have tips that curl over.

BOSTON CREAM POKE CAKE

Yield: 16 servings **Prep Time:** 30 minutes, plus 2½ to 4 hours to chill **Cook Time:** 45 minutes

I lived in the Boston area for 11 years, and the only time I ever tasted Boston cream pie was when I made my own keto version. This poke cake is deliciously gooey and as fun to make as it is to eat.

⅔ cup (73g) coconut flour

½ cup granulated erythritol sweetener

2 teaspoons baking powder

¼ teaspoon salt

3 large eggs

2 large egg whites

6 tablespoons unsalted butter, melted but not hot

¼ cup heavy whipping cream

¼ cup water

½ teaspoon vanilla extract

1 recipe Pastry Cream (page 392)

1 recipe Easy Chocolate Glaze (page 390)

1. Preheat the oven to 350°F and grease an 8-inch square baking pan.

2. In a large bowl, whisk together the coconut flour, sweetener, baking powder, and salt.

3. Add the whole eggs, egg whites, melted butter, cream, water, and vanilla and stir until well combined.

4. Pour the batter into the prepared baking pan and bake for 30 minutes, or until the edges are golden and the top is firm to the touch. Remove from the oven and let cool completely in the pan.

5. Using the handle of a wooden spoon, poke large holes all over the cake.

6. Prepare the pastry cream as directed. Let cool for about 10 minutes, then pour all over the cake. Refrigerate for 2 to 3 hours, until the pastry cream is mostly set.

7. Prepare the chocolate glaze as directed and let cool for 10 to 15 minutes, until slightly thickened. Pour over the pastry cream and spread to the edges of the cake. Refrigerate for another 30 to 60 minutes, until set.

TIPS: *Unlike the Tres Leches Cake (page 110), you want bigger holes here, and a skewer won't cut it. The pastry cream doesn't sink willingly into small holes, so using a wooden spoon handle to poke bigger holes ensures delicious cream all the way down.*

Let the pastry cream set properly before adding the chocolate glaze. It shouldn't feel wet to the touch, but it's okay if it's still a little tacky.

NUTRITIONAL INFORMATION

CALORIES: 223 | FAT: 19.5g | CARBS: 4.9g | FIBER: 2.3g | PROTEIN: 4.1g

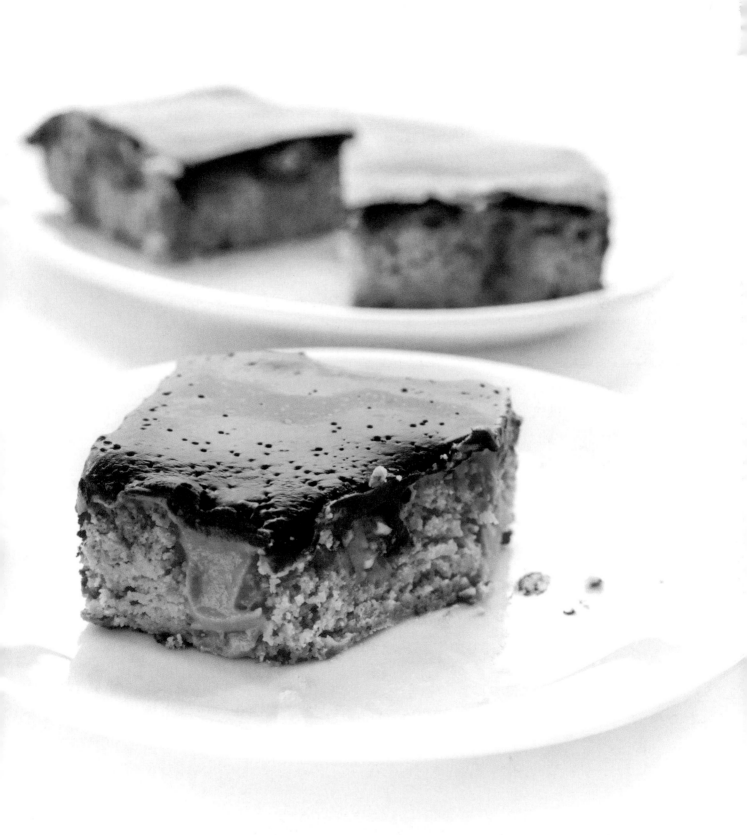

MARBLE CHEESECAKE

OPTION

Yield: 16 servings Prep Time: 35 minutes, plus 4 hours to chill Cook Time: 90 minutes

Creamy vanilla and chocolate cheesecake, swirled together over a chocolate "cookie" crust. Pure keto heaven!

1 recipe Keto Chocolate Pie Crust (page 370)

2 ounces unsweetened chocolate, chopped

1 tablespoon unsalted butter

3 (8-ounce) packages cream cheese, softened

½ cup granulated sweetener of choice

½ cup powdered erythritol sweetener

½ cup heavy whipping cream, room temperature, divided

1 teaspoon vanilla extract

3 large eggs, room temperature

SERVING SUGGESTION: *Top with a fresh strawberry.*

NUT-FREE OPTION:

Use the nut-free version of the crust.

1. Preheat the oven to 325°F and grease the bottom of a 9-inch springform pan.

2. Prepare the crust according to the directions and press firmly and evenly into the bottom of the prepared pan. Par-bake for 10 minutes, then remove from the oven and let cool while you prepare the filling.

3. Reduce the oven temperature to 300°F.

4. Place the chopped chocolate and butter in a small saucepan over low heat. Whisk until melted and smooth, then immediately remove the pan from the heat. Set aside to cool.

5. In a large bowl, beat the cream cheese and sweeteners with an electric mixer on medium speed until well combined. Beat in ¼ cup of the cream and the vanilla until smooth. With the mixer on medium-low, beat in the eggs one at a time until just incorporated.

6. Transfer about one-third of the cream cheese mixture to a separate bowl and set aside. Add the melted chocolate and stir together. The mixture will be quite thick. Stir in the remaining ¼ cup of cream to thin it.

7. Brush the sides of the pan lightly with oil, taking care not to disturb the crust. Pour about one-third of the vanilla cheesecake mixture over the crust. Alternately dollop the remaining vanilla and chocolate mixtures on top. Use a knife or an offset spatula to swirl the two together.

8. Gently shake the pan to even out the top of the filling. Place the pan on the middle rack in the oven. Fill another pan, such as a 9 by 13-inch, with water and place it on the rack below. Bake for 65 to 75 minutes, until the cheesecake is mostly set but still has a little jiggle in the middle.

9. Remove the pan from the oven and let cool for only 5 minutes before carefully running a sharp knife around the edge of the pan. Let cool to room temperature, then loosen the sides of the pan (see tips). Refrigerate until firm, at least 4 hours. Remove the sides of the pan before serving.

NUTRITIONAL INFORMATION

CALORIES: 288 | FAT: 24.7g | CARBS: 5.6g | FIBER: 2g | PROTEIN: 6.5g

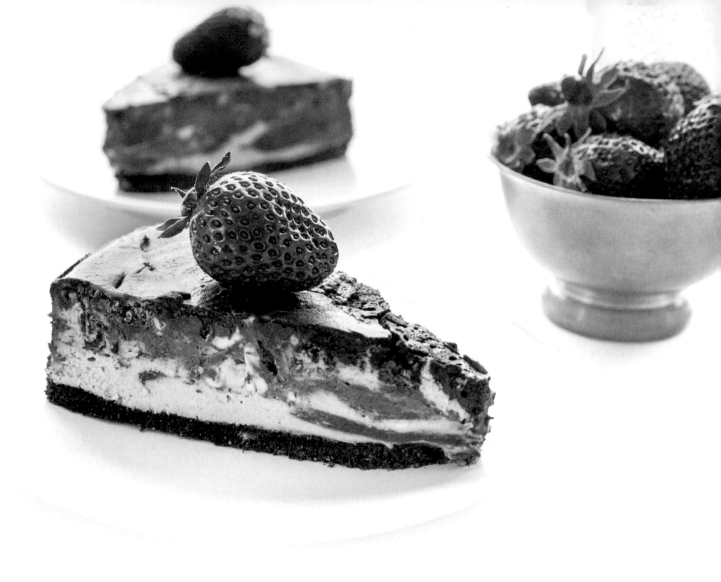

TIPS: *Cheesecakes can be finicky, especially ones made with chocolate. They are prone to cracking, and a number of the steps in this recipe are designed to minimize that.*

It's important to have the chocolate mixture be about the same consistency as the vanilla mixture. This makes it easier to swirl them together and prevents cracks from forming between them. Depending on the brand of unsweetened chocolate you use, the chocolate filling may be too thick. Add more cream, 1 tablespoon at a time, until it's about the same consistency as the vanilla mixture.

Putting a pan of water in the oven creates a moist heat that helps bake the cake more gently and minimizes cracking. It also catches any drips of oil that may leak out during baking.

Finally, the cheesecake shrinks a bit as it cools. If the sides of the cake are stuck to the pan, the top can crack. I have found that for this recipe, to keep the cake from sticking to the pan, I need to run a sharp knife around the edge of the pan early in the cooling process and then, once cool, loosen the sides of the pan before chilling the cheesecake.

RICOTTA CHEESECAKE WITH FRESH BERRIES

Yield: 12 servings Prep Time: 20 minutes, plus 3 hours to chill Cook Time: 90 minutes

This was my first time ever making a cheesecake with ricotta, and I was blown away by the results. This cake is creamy and smooth, and quite a bit easier to make than regular cheesecake.

1 recipe Easy Almond Flour Pie Crust (page 366)

1 pound whole-milk ricotta cheese, room temperature

12 ounces cream cheese, softened

½ cup powdered erythritol sweetener

¼ cup granulated sweetener of choice

2 teaspoons grated lemon zest

1 teaspoon vanilla extract

3 large eggs, room temperature

1 tablespoon coconut flour

For Garnish:

1 cup chopped strawberries or other berries of choice

Powdered erythritol sweetener

1. Preheat the oven to 325°F and grease the bottom of a 9-inch springform pan.

2. Prepare the crust according to the directions and press firmly and evenly into the bottom of the prepared pan. Prick the crust all over with a fork. Par-bake for 12 minutes, then remove from the oven and let cool while you prepare the filling.

3. Reduce the oven temperature to 300°F.

4. Place the ricotta, cream cheese, sweeteners, lemon zest, and vanilla in a food processor. Blend on high until smooth. Add the eggs and coconut flour and blend until fully combined.

5. Brush the sides of the pan lightly with oil, taking care not to disturb the crust. Pour the filling over the crust and tap the pan lightly on the counter to remove any air bubbles.

6. Place the pan on a rimmed baking sheet to catch any oil that might leach out. Bake for 65 to 75 minutes, until the cheesecake is mostly set but still has a little jiggle in the middle.

7. Remove from the oven and let cool in the pan for 20 minutes, then run a sharp knife around the edge of the pan and loosen and remove the sides. Refrigerate the cake until firm, at least 3 hours.

8. Top with the berries and dust with sweetener before serving.

TIP: *Depending on the brand, ricotta can be kind of grainy. So it's imperative to use a food processor to mix the batter, as it works out all the clumps and creates an incredibly smooth mixture. It also makes the filling very easy to whip together, unlike traditional cheesecake.*

NUTRITIONAL INFORMATION (BASED ON AN ALMOND FLOUR CRUST)
CALORIES: 285 | FAT: 22.9g | CARBS: 5.9g | FIBER: 1.8g | PROTEIN: 10.6g

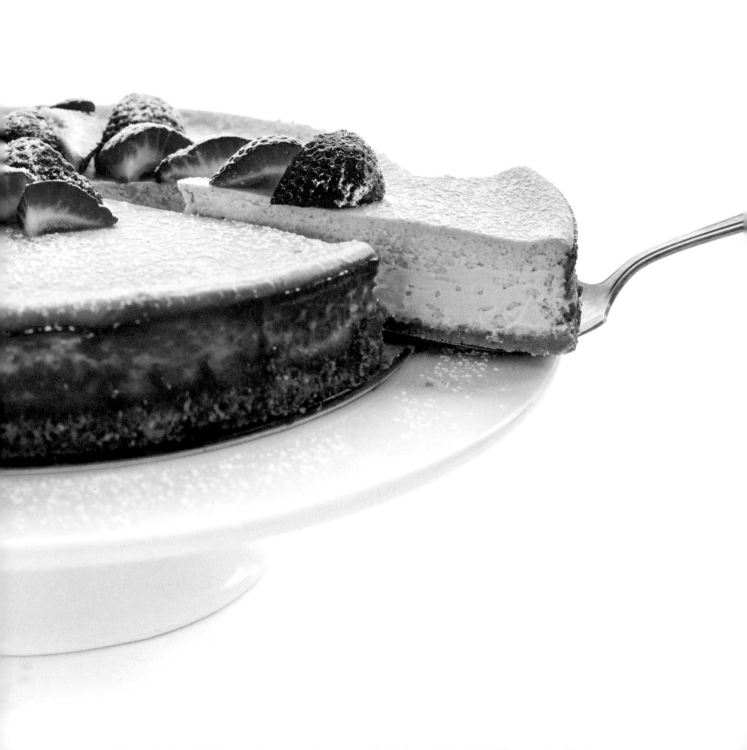

CANNOLI ICEBOX CAKE

Yield: 16 servings   Prep Time: 20 minutes, plus 3 hours to chill (not including time to make graham crackers)   Cook Time: —

If this were a conventional cookbook, a cake like this would be considered a no-bake recipe. But in the keto world, you have to make your own graham crackers from scratch. So, while this is an icebox cake, you still need to do some baking!

1 cup whole-milk ricotta cheese

6 ounces cream cheese, softened

¾ cup powdered erythritol sweetener, plus more for garnish

½ teaspoon vanilla extract

1 cup heavy whipping cream

1 recipe Graham Crackers (page 300)

⅓ cup sugar-free chocolate chips

1. Place the ricotta, cream cheese, sweetener, and vanilla in a food processor. Blend on high until smooth and creamy.

2. In a large bowl, beat the cream with an electric mixer until it holds stiff peaks. Gently fold in the ricotta mixture until well combined.

3. Place a layer of graham crackers in an 8-inch square baking dish, breaking or cutting to fit as needed. Spread one-third of the whipped cream evenly on top. Repeat two more times.

4. Sprinkle the top with the chocolate chips. Refrigerate for at least 3 hours to soften the graham crackers. Dust lightly with powdered sweetener just before serving.

TIP: *You want the graham crackers soften properly, so don't skimp on the chilling time. If they are too crisp, the graham crackers will move as you try to cut the cake, and the slices won't come out nicely.*

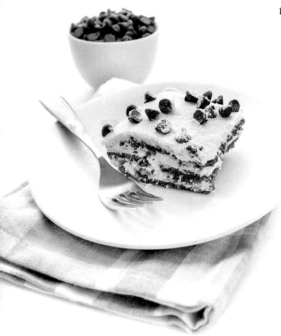

NUTRITIONAL INFORMATION

CALORIES: 235 | FAT: 20.2g | CARBS: 6.4g | FIBER: 3g | PROTEIN: 6.4g

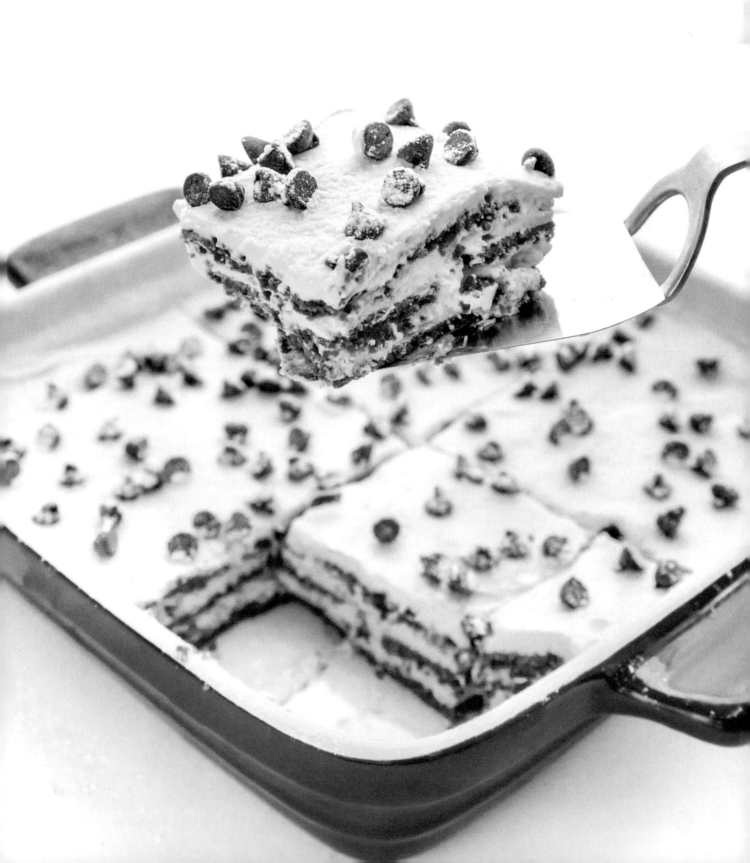

CHOCOLATE HAZELNUT TORTE

Yield: 12 servings **Prep Time:** 25 minutes **Cook Time:** 1 hour

Want a cake that tastes like you're biting into a Ferrero Rocher chocolate? Done! Toasting the hazelnut meal and using hazelnut oil really brings that flavor to the forefront in this delicious torte.

1¼ cups hazelnut meal

¾ cup granulated erythritol sweetener, divided

5 large eggs, separated, room temperature

¼ teaspoon cream of tartar

¼ teaspoon salt

4 ounces unsweetened chocolate, chopped

⅓ cup toasted hazelnut oil

¼ cup warm water

1 teaspoon hazelnut or vanilla extract

Powdered erythritol sweetener, for garnish

SERVING SUGGESTION: *Top with lightly sweetened whipped cream and a few chopped hazelnuts for garnish.*

1. Spread the hazelnut meal in a large skillet. Toast over medium heat, stirring continuously, until lightly colored and fragrant, about 5 minutes. Let cool for a few minutes, then whisk in ½ cup of the granulated sweetener and set aside.

2. Preheat the oven to 325°F and grease a 9-inch springform pan. Line the bottom of the pan with parchment paper and grease the paper.

3. In a large bowl, use an electric mixer to whip the egg whites with the cream of tartar and salt until frothy. Slowly add the remaining ¼ cup of sweetener and continue to beat until the whites hold stiff peaks.

4. Set a large heatproof bowl over a pan of barely simmering water. Place the chopped chocolate and hazelnut oil in the bowl and stir until melted and smooth. Remove the bowl from the heat and stir in the hazelnut meal mixture, then whisk in the egg yolks until well combined. The mixture may thicken and seize a bit; this is normal. Slowly whisk in the water until it smooths out. Stir in the extract.

5. Add about one-third of the whipped egg whites and fold in to lighten the chocolate mixture. Then fold the chocolate mixture carefully back into the remaining egg whites.

6. Spread the mixture in the prepared pan and bake for 45 to 50 minutes, until the top is just firm to the touch and a tester inserted in the center comes out clean.

7. Remove from the oven and let cool completely in the pan, then run a sharp knife around the inside of the pan and loosen and remove the pan sides. Sprinkle the torte with powdered sweetener.

TIP: *Don't panic if the chocolate mixture thickens and seizes when you add the egg yolks. Unsweetened chocolate tends to do this. Adding the warm liquid slowly as you continue to whisk will help it become smooth again.*

NUTRITIONAL INFORMATION

CALORIES: 223 | FAT: 19.4g | CARBS: 5g | FIBER: 2.8g | PROTEIN: 5.6g

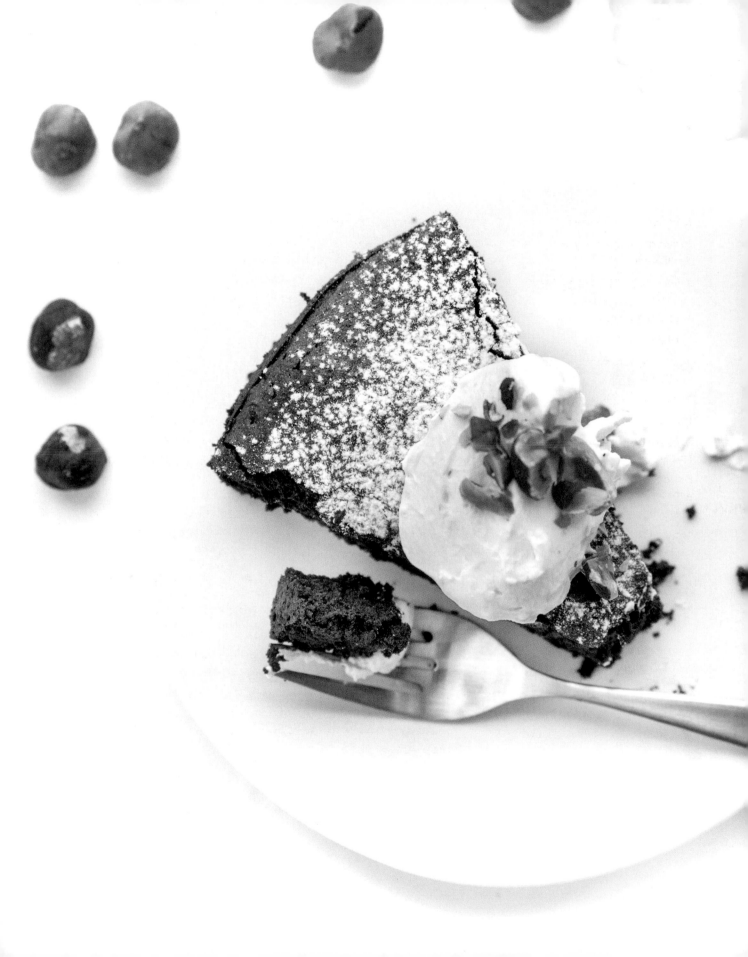

Chapter 6:
EVERYDAY COOKIES

C is for cookie; that's good enough for me.
—Cookie Monster

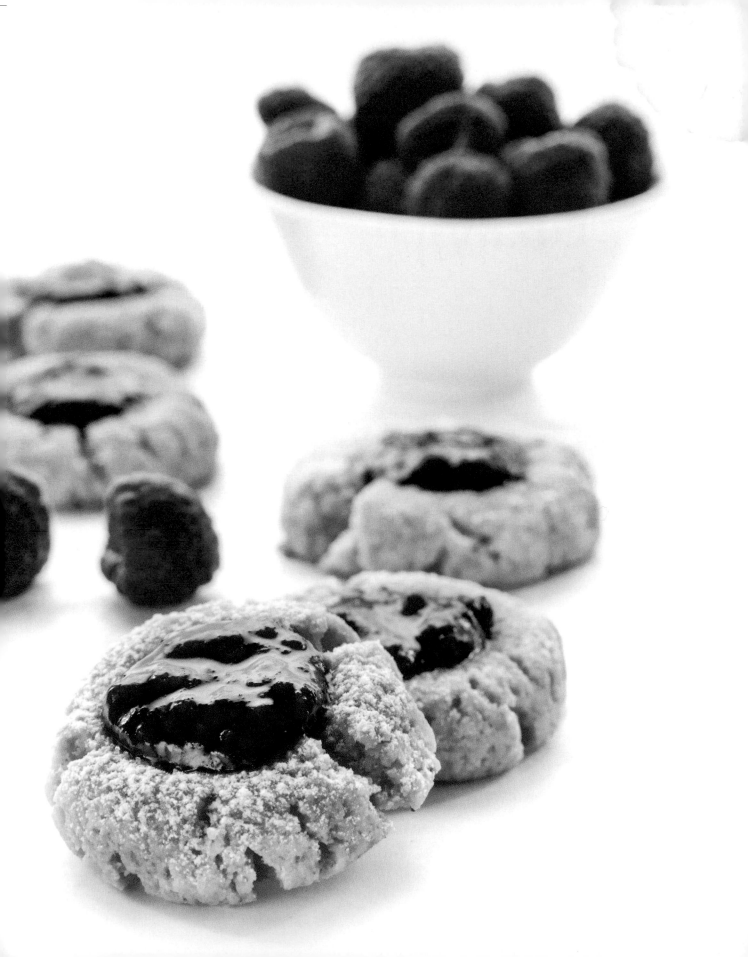

SOFT AND CHEWY CHOCOLATE CHIP COOKIES

Yield: 18 cookies (2 per serving) Prep Time: 25 minutes Cook Time: 15 minutes

I typically don't like cookies made with coconut flour, as you can't get that crispy-chewy quality. But these are delicious soft batch–style cookies. I kept sneaking bites of the batter as I made them, which is always a good sign.

4 ounces cream cheese, softened

¼ cup (½ stick) unsalted butter, softened

¼ cup granulated erythritol sweetener

¼ cup brown sugar substitute

2 large eggs, room temperature

½ teaspoon vanilla extract

½ cup (55g) coconut flour

1 tablespoon grass-fed gelatin (optional; see tips)

1 teaspoon baking powder

¼ teaspoon salt

⅓ cup sugar-free chocolate chips

1. Preheat the oven to 350°F and line a cookie sheet with a silicone baking mat or parchment paper.

2. In a large bowl, beat the cream cheese and butter with an electric mixer until smooth. Beat in the sweeteners until well combined. Add the eggs and vanilla and beat until smooth.

3. All at once, add the coconut flour, gelatin (if using), baking powder, and salt and beat until the dough comes together. It will be a bit sticky and thin at this point. Stir in the chocolate chips and let the dough rest for about 10 minutes to thicken.

4. Roll the dough into 1½-inch balls and place on the prepared cookie sheet, at least 2 inches apart. If the dough is too sticky to roll, work in another tablespoon or two of coconut flour.

5. Press the balls down with the palm of your hand to about ¾ inch thick. They will spread a little. Bake for about 15 minutes, until the cookies are just firm to the touch on top. Remove from the oven and let cool completely on the pan.

TIPS: *Gelatin adds chewiness to many keto cookie recipes. It's not required, but it will improve the overall texture.*

In conventional baking, you can just drop chocolate chip cookie dough right off the spoon onto the cookie sheet and they will spread into perfect cookies. But this doesn't always work in keto baking. I find that rolling the dough into balls first and then pressing them down with my hands gets me the perfect cookie shape.

NUTRITIONAL INFORMATION

CALORIES: 169 | FAT: 12.7g | CARBS: 7.3g | FIBER: 4.6g | PROTEIN: 4.3g

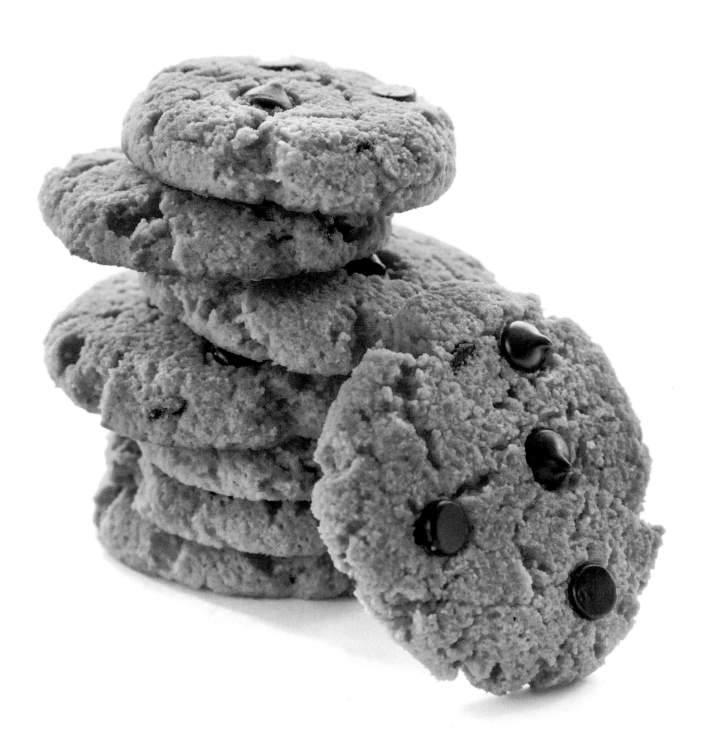

SOFT AND CHEWY SNICKERDOODLES

Yield: 18 cookies (2 per serving) Prep Time: 25 minutes Cook Time: 18 minutes

When I was creating the chocolate chip cookies on page 124, it struck me that the dough would also make fabulous snickerdoodles. It needed a bit of tweaking to get a true snickerdoodle flavor, but it's the same basic idea.

4 ounces cream cheese, softened

¼ cup (½ stick) unsalted butter, softened

¼ cup granulated erythritol sweetener

¼ cup brown sugar substitute

2 large eggs, room temperature

½ teaspoon vanilla extract

½ cup (55g) coconut flour

1 tablespoon grass-fed gelatin (optional; see tip)

1 teaspoon cream of tartar

½ teaspoon baking soda

¼ teaspoon salt

Topping:

2 tablespoons granulated sweetener of choice

2 teaspoons ground cinnamon

1. Preheat the oven to 350°F and line a cookie sheet with a silicone baking mat or parchment paper.

2. In a large bowl, beat the cream cheese and butter with an electric mixer until smooth. Beat in the sweeteners until well combined. Add the eggs and vanilla and beat until smooth.

3. All at once, add the coconut flour, gelatin (if using), cream of tartar, baking soda, and salt and beat until the dough comes together. It will be a bit sticky and thin at this point. Let the dough rest for about 10 minutes to thicken.

4. In a shallow bowl, combine the 2 tablespoons of granulated sweetener with the cinnamon. Roll the dough into 1½-inch balls, then roll the balls in the cinnamon mixture to coat. If the dough is too sticky to roll, work in another tablespoon or two of coconut flour.

5. Place the balls on the prepared cookie sheet, at least 2 inches apart. Press the balls down with the palm of your hand to about ¾ inch thick. They will spread a little.

6. Bake for 15 to 18 minutes, until the cookies are just firm to the touch on top. Remove from the oven and let cool completely on the pan.

TIP: *Gelatin is featured in a lot of the cookie recipes in this chapter and the next. In this recipe, it is optional, but it really does make the cookies much chewier. I know it can seem like yet another ingredient to purchase, but I recommend it. A single bag can last for months and months.*

NUTRITIONAL INFORMATION

CALORIES: 139 | FAT: 10.3g | CARBS: 4.9g | FIBER: 2.5g | PROTEIN: 3.8g

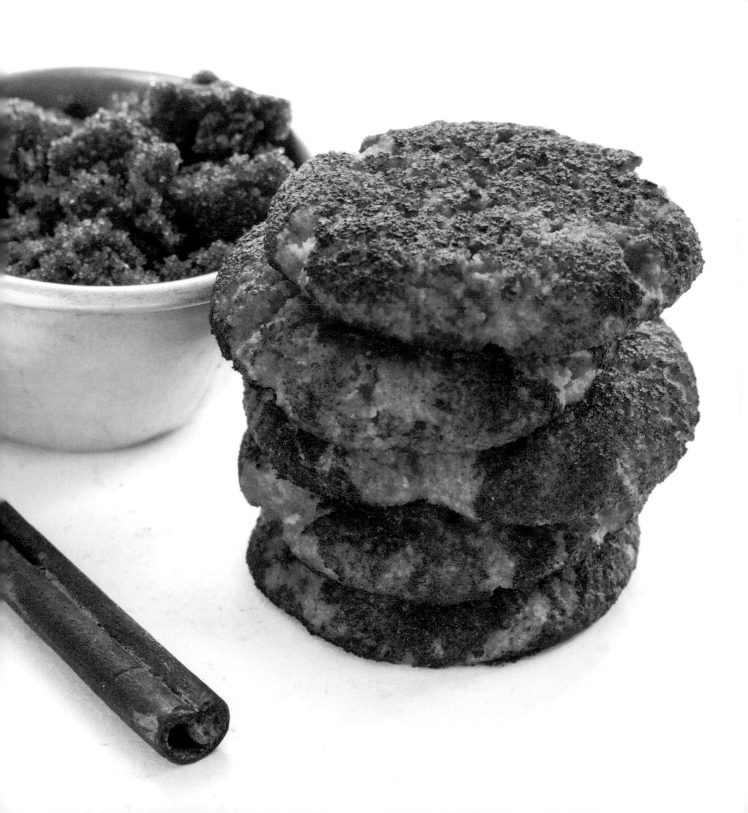

CLASSIC PEANUT BUTTER COOKIES

Yield: 24 cookies (2 per serving) **Prep Time:** 15 minutes **Cook Time:** 15 minutes

Can't have a baking book without a recipe for peanut butter cookies!

½ cup creamy natural peanut butter

¼ cup (½ stick) unsalted butter, softened

¼ cup granulated sweetener of choice

¼ cup brown sugar substitute

1 large egg, room temperature

½ teaspoon vanilla extract

1 cup (100g) blanched almond flour

¼ cup roasted, defatted peanut flour (see tip)

½ teaspoon baking soda

¼ teaspoon salt

1. Preheat the oven to 325°F and line a cookie sheet with a silicone baking mat or parchment paper.

2. In a large bowl, beat the peanut butter and butter with an electric mixer until smooth. Beat in the sweeteners until lightened and fluffy, about 2 minutes, then beat in the egg and vanilla.

3. Add the almond flour, peanut flour, baking soda, and salt and beat until well combined.

4. Roll the dough into 1-inch balls and place on the prepared cookie sheet, about 2 inches apart. Press the balls down with the palm of your hand to about ½ inch thick. Use a wet fork to create hatchmarks.

5. Bake for 12 to 15 minutes, until just starting to brown around the edges. Let cool completely on the pan. The cookies will be very soft coming out of the oven but will firm up as they cool.

VARIATION: CHOCOLATE PEANUT BUTTER SANDWICH COOKIES.

Use a half recipe of Chocolate Buttercream Frosting (page 382) as a filling to make tasty sandwich cookies. You can also use a half recipe of Easy Chocolate Glaze (page 390) if you let it sit and thicken up a bit before spreading.

TIP: *Be sure to use peanut flour that has been roasted and defatted, such as Protein Plus, to get the right consistency and flavor. Peanut butter powders like PBFit can be used, but they sometimes contain sugar, so be sure to read the labels.*

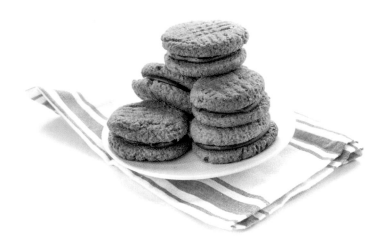

NUTRITIONAL INFORMATION

CALORIES: 178 | FAT: 15.1g | CARBS: 5.6g | FIBER: 2.2g | PROTEIN: 5.6g

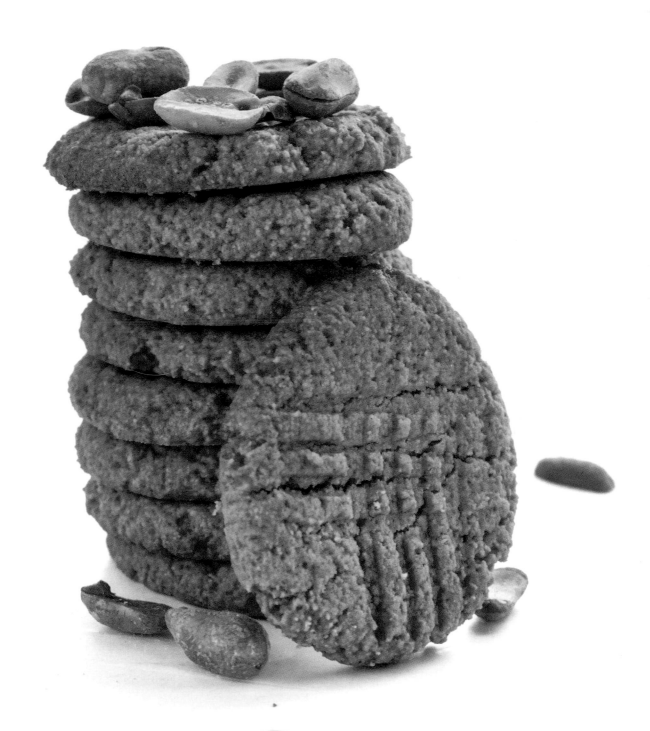

COWBOY COOKIES

Yield: 24 large cookies (1 per serving) Prep Time: 25 minutes Cook Time: 20 minutes

These big chocolate chip cookies with coconut and pecans have an amazing crispy-chewy texture. The recipe makes a big batch, so feel free to halve the ingredients.

¾ cup (1½ sticks) butter, softened

½ cup plus 2 tablespoons brown sugar substitute (see tip)

½ cup plus 2 tablespoons granulated erythritol sweetener

2 large eggs, room temperature

1½ teaspoons vanilla extract

2 cups (200g) blanched almond flour

2 tablespoons grass-fed gelatin (optional)

1½ teaspoons baking powder

1 teaspoon baking soda

½ teaspoon salt

1 cup unsweetened flaked coconut

1 cup chopped pecans

⅔ cup sugar-free chocolate chips

1. Set the oven racks to the second highest and second lowest positions and preheat the oven to 325°F. Line two cookie sheets with silicone baking mats or parchment paper.

2. In a large bowl, beat the butter and sweeteners with an electric mixer until lightened and fluffy, about 2 minutes. Beat in the eggs and vanilla until well combined.

3. Add the almond flour, gelatin (if using), baking powder, baking soda, and salt. Beat until just mixed together. Stir in the coconut, pecans, and chocolate chips.

4. Form the dough into 2-inch balls place on the prepared cookie sheets, at least 3 inches apart, 12 balls per sheet. Press the balls down with the palm of your hand to about ½ inch thick.

5. Bake for 15 to 20 minutes, switching and rotating the pans halfway through baking, until the edges of the cookies are golden brown. Remove from the oven and let cool completely on the pans.

TIP: *If you want the crispy texture of a classic cookie, use Swerve Sweetener. Don't use Bocha Sweet or allulose, as it will make the cookies cakey and soft. My recipe testers liked them best made with half Swerve Brown and half Swerve Granular.*

NUTRITIONAL INFORMATION
CALORIES: 187 | FAT: 16.9g | CARBS: 5.7g | FIBER: 3.6g | PROTEIN: 4.1g

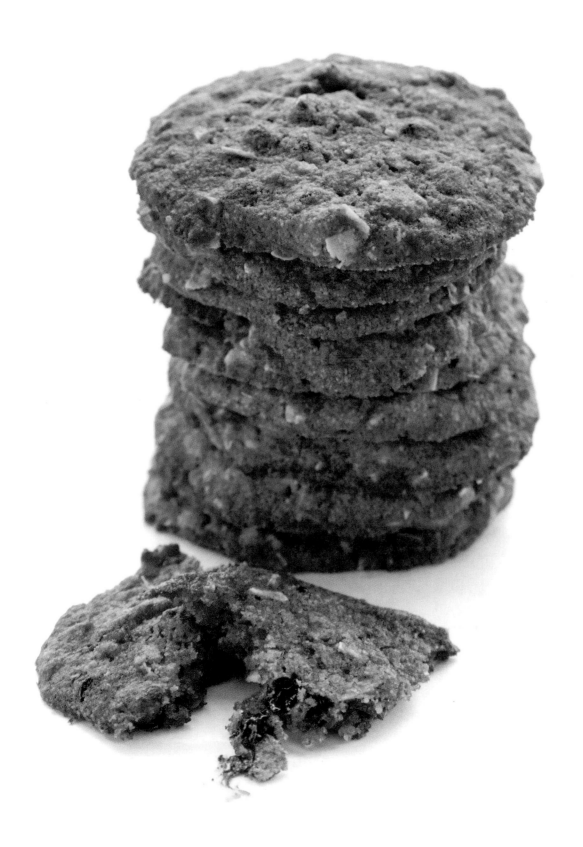

BROWNIE COOKIES

OPTION OPTION

Yield: About 36 cookies (2 per serving) Prep Time: 20 minutes, plus 30 minutes to chill dough Cook Time: 17 minutes

Cookies or brownies? Brownies or cookies? Now you don't need to choose.

6 ounces sugar-free chocolate chips

6 tablespoons unsalted butter

1 cup (100g) blanched almond flour

¼ cup cocoa powder

2 tablespoons grass-fed gelatin (optional; adds chewiness)

½ teaspoon baking powder

3 large eggs

½ cup granulated erythritol sweetener

½ cup Bocha Sweet or allulose (see tip)

2 teaspoons vanilla extract

¼ teaspoon salt

½ cup chopped pecans

DAIRY-FREE OPTION:

Use coconut oil or ghee in place of the butter.

NUT-FREE OPTION:

Use sunflower seed or pumpkin seed meal in place of the almond flour, and leave out the pecans. Add a few additional chocolate chips on top if desired.

1. In a medium saucepan over low heat, melt the chocolate chips and butter until smooth. Remove the pan from the heat and set aside.

2. In a medium bowl, whisk together the almond flour, cocoa powder, gelatin (if using), and baking powder.

3. In a large bowl, beat the eggs, sweeteners, vanilla, and salt with an electric mixer on high until thickened, about 5 minutes. Reduce the speed to low and beat in the melted chocolate mixture until well combined. Stir in the pecans.

4. Add the almond flour mixture and beat until just combined. Cover with plastic wrap and refrigerate for 30 minutes.

5. Preheat the oven to 350°F and line two cookie sheets with silicone baking mats or parchment paper.

6. Using about 1½ tablespoons at a time, scoop the dough onto the prepared cookie sheets, about 2 inches apart. Use a flat-bottomed glass covered in plastic wrap or parchment paper to flatten the mounds to ½ inch thick.

7. Bake for 10 to 12 minutes, until set around the edges but still a bit wet-looking on top. Remove from the oven and let cool completely on the pan.

TIP: Using both Swerve and Bocha Sweet gives these cookies a softer, brownielike consistency. You can make them with all Swerve if you prefer, but they may dry out a little faster.

NUTRITIONAL INFORMATION

CALORIES: 148 | FAT: 12.3g | CARBS: 6g | FIBER: 4.1g | PROTEIN: 4.3g

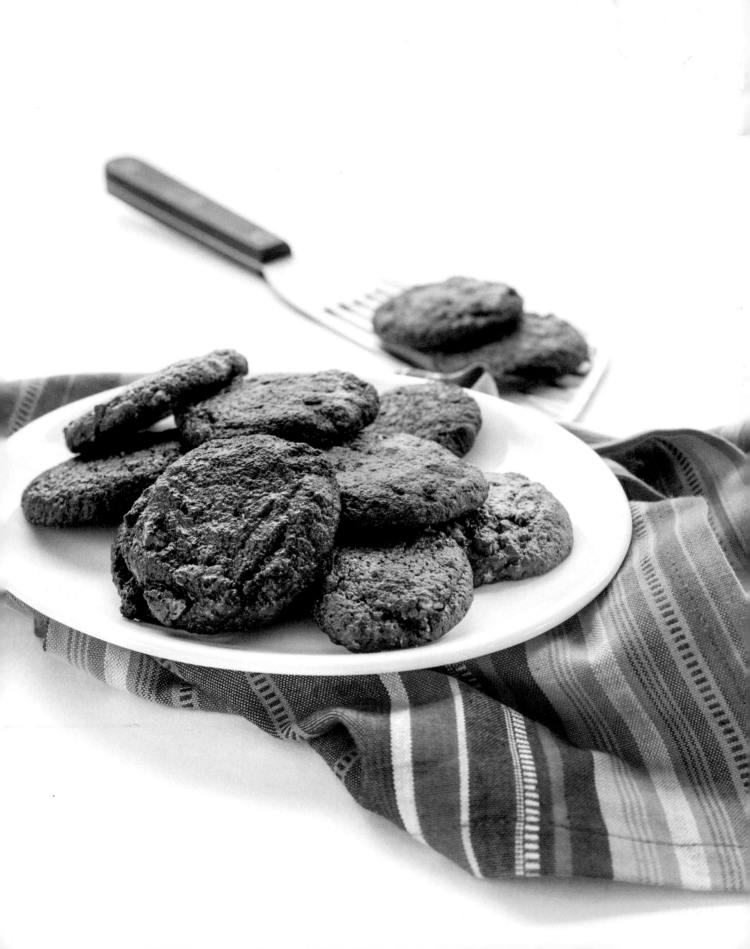

CHEWY GINGER "MOLASSES" COOKIES

Yield: 40 cookies (2 per serving) Prep Time: 20 minutes Cook Time: 12 minutes

A truly chewy, delicious ginger cookie with a hint of "molasses" flavor. This was the first recipe to which I tried adding gelatin, and I was blown away by the results.

2 cups (200g) almond flour

2 tablespoons grass-fed gelatin (optional; adds chewiness)

1 tablespoon ginger powder

1 teaspoon ground cinnamon

¼ teaspoon ground cloves

½ teaspoon baking soda

½ teaspoon salt

½ cup (1 stick) unsalted butter, softened

½ cup creamy unsalted almond butter

1 cup brown sugar substitute (see tips)

2 large eggs, room temperature

½ teaspoon vanilla extract

1. Preheat the oven to 325°F and line two cookie sheets with silicone baking mats or parchment paper.

2. In a medium bowl, whisk together the almond flour, gelatin (if using), ginger, cinnamon, cloves, baking soda, and salt.

3. In a large bowl, beat the butter, almond butter, and sweetener with an electric mixer until smooth. Beat in the eggs and vanilla until well combined.

4. Add the almond flour mixture and continue to beat until the dough comes together.

5. Roll the dough into 1-inch balls and place on the prepared cookie sheets, a few inches apart.

6. Bake for 5 minutes, then remove from the oven and gently press down a bit (to encourage the cookies to spread). Return to the oven and bake for another 7 minutes or so, until just barely golden brown. They will still be very soft.

7. Remove from the oven and let cool completely on the pan. The cookies will firm up as they cool.

DAIRY-FREE OPTION:

Replace the softened butter with softened coconut oil or ghee.

TIPS: *Swerve Brown has the best molasses flavor of all the brown sugar substitutes, so I highly recommend using it here.*

This recipe makes a lot of cookies! You can easily halve the ingredients, but you can also roll the balls, freeze them on a cookie sheet, and then place them in a resealable bag. They will last for up to 2 months in the freezer. Thaw the balls before baking as directed above.

NUTRITIONAL INFORMATION

CALORIES: 157 | FAT: 12.5g | CARBS: 4.3g | FIBER: 2g | PROTEIN: 5g

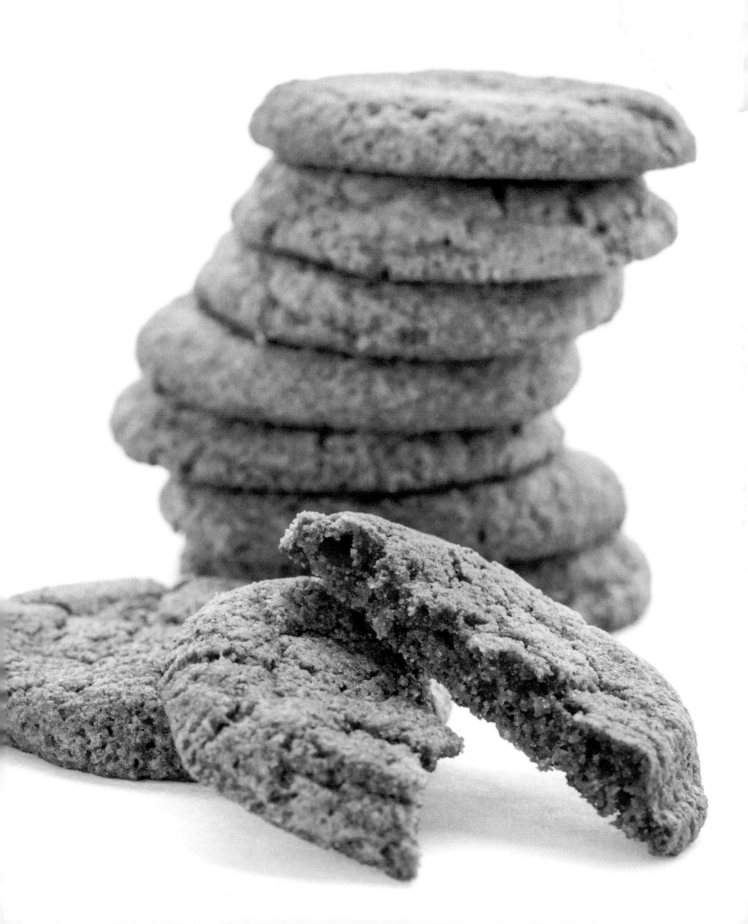

DAIRY-FREE JAM THUMBPRINTS

Yield: 24 cookies (2 per serving) Prep Time: 20 minutes, plus 1 hour for filling to set Cook Time: 20 minutes

Thumbprint cookies are so much fun to make and look so pretty. These cookies are incredibly tender, and the raspberry filling is an easy shortcut for jam.

Cookies:

2 cups (200g) blanched almond flour

½ cup granulated erythritol sweetener

½ teaspoon baking powder

¼ teaspoon salt

1 large egg

⅓ cup coconut oil, melted but not hot

½ teaspoon almond extract

Powdered erythritol sweetener, for garnish (optional)

Filling:

1 cup fresh raspberries

2 tablespoons water

2 tablespoons powdered erythritol sweetener

1½ teaspoons grass-fed gelatin

TO MAKE THE COOKIES:

1. Preheat the oven to 325°F and line a cookie sheet with a silicone baking mat or parchment paper.

2. In a large bowl, whisk together the almond flour, sweetener, baking powder, and salt. Add the egg, melted coconut oil, and almond extract and stir until the dough comes together.

3. Roll the dough into 1-inch balls and place on the prepared cookie sheet, 2 inches apart. Press the balls down with the palm of your hand to about ½ inch thick, then use your thumb to create an indentation in the center of each cookie.

4. Bake for 12 to 15 minutes, until the edges are just golden. Remove from the oven and use the end of a wooden spoon to gently redefine the well in the center of each cookie, as they will have puffed up a bit. Let cool completely on the cookie sheet.

5. Dust the cooled cookies lightly with powdered sweetener, if desired.

TO MAKE THE FILLING:

6. Place the raspberries and water in a medium saucepan over medium heat. Bring to a boil, then reduce the heat to a simmer and cook for 5 minutes, until the berries are soft enough to mash with a wooden spoon.

7. Stir in the sweetener and gelatin and let cool until thickened but not entirely gelled. Spoon about ½ teaspoon of the raspberry filling into the well in each cookie and let set until firm, about 1 hour.

TIP: *If you prefer, you can substitute vanilla extract for the almond extract and any type of fresh berry for the raspberries. You can also use store-bought sugar-free jam for the filling. See page 403 for healthy options.*

NUTRITIONAL INFORMATION
CALORIES: 175 | FAT: 16g | CARBS: 5.3g | FIBER: 2.7g | PROTEIN: 4.9g

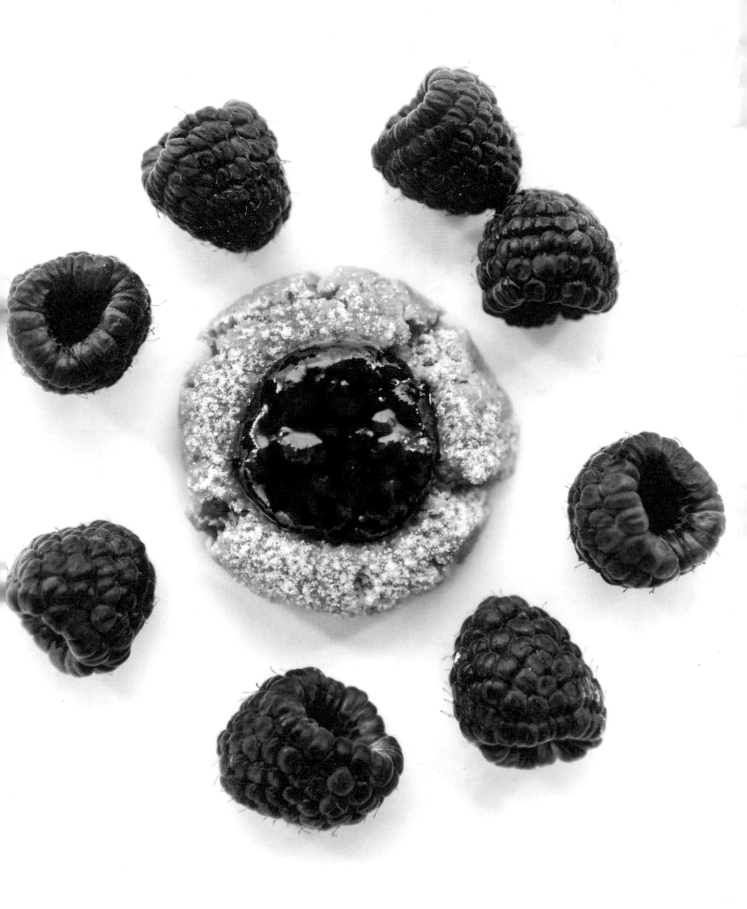

PECAN SNOWBALLS

OPTION

Yield: 36 cookies (2 per serving) Prep Time: 15 minutes Cook Time: 18 minutes

Pecan snowballs were my late father's favorite holiday cookie, so creating a keto-friendly version was of the utmost importance to me. Every time I bite into one, I think of him. Here's to you, Dad!

2 cups (200g) blanched almond flour

1 cup finely chopped pecans

2 tablespoons coconut flour

½ teaspoon baking powder

½ teaspoon salt

½ cup (1 stick) unsalted butter, softened

⅔ cup brown sugar substitute

1 large egg, room temperature

½ teaspoon vanilla extract

½ cup powdered erythritol sweetener, for coating

1. Preheat the oven to 325°F and line a cookie sheet with a silicone baking mat or parchment paper.

2. In a medium bowl, whisk together the almond flour, pecans, coconut flour, baking powder, and salt.

3. In a large bowl, beat the butter and brown sugar substitute with an electric mixer until well combined. Beat in the egg and vanilla.

4. Beat in the almond flour mixture until the dough comes together. Form into 1-inch balls and place on the prepared cookie sheet.

5. Bake for 15 to 18 minutes, until just lightly golden brown. They will not be firm to the touch coming out of the oven but will firm up as they cool. Let cool completely on the pan.

6. Place the powdered sweetener in a shallow bowl and roll the cooled cookies in the sweetener to coat.

DAIRY-FREE OPTION:

Softened ghee would be the best replacement for butter in this recipe so that you don't lose the wonderful buttery flavor.

TIP: These ball-shaped cookies don't spread much, so you can place them pretty close together on the cookie sheet.

NUTRITIONAL INFORMATION

CALORIES: 165 | FAT: 15.1g | CARBS: 4g | FIBER: 2.1g | PROTEIN: 3.7g

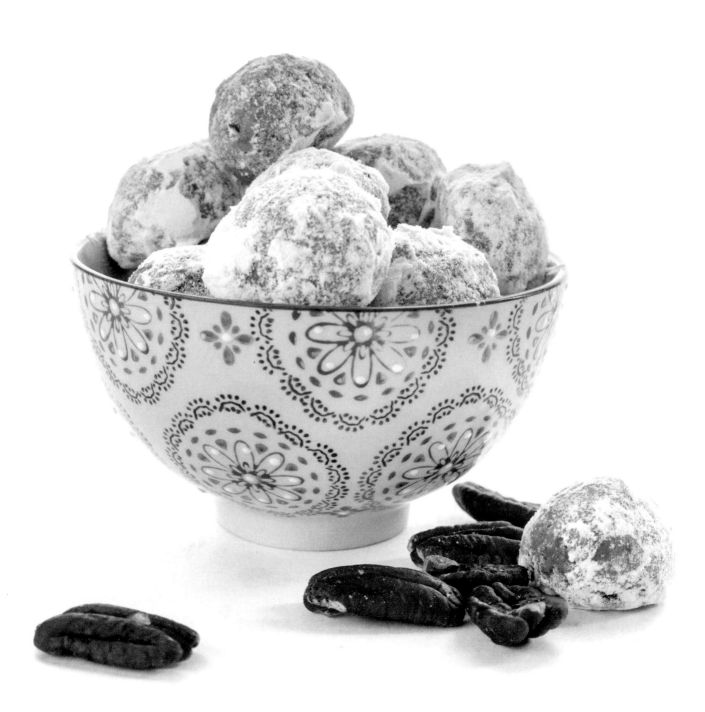

ITALIAN SESAME SEED COOKIES

Yield: 24 cookies (2 per serving) Prep Time: 25 minutes Cook Time: 22 minutes

These cookies are deceptively simple. They look rather unassuming, but the taste and texture are out of this world—light and puffy, with a unique flavor from the toasted sesame seeds.

½ cup sesame seeds

½ cup (1 stick) unsalted butter, softened

⅔ cup granulated erythritol sweetener

1 large egg, room temperature

1 teaspoon vanilla extract

1 teaspoon grated lemon zest

2 cups (200g) blanched almond flour

1½ teaspoons baking powder

¼ teaspoon salt

2 tablespoons heavy whipping cream

2 tablespoons water

1. Preheat the oven to 325°F and line two cookie sheets with silicone baking mats or parchment paper.

2. Spread the sesame seeds in a medium skillet. Toast over medium heat, stirring continuously, until most of the seeds are golden, about 5 minutes. Spread the seeds in a shallow dish.

3. In a large bowl, beat the butter and sweetener with an electric mixer until well combined and fluffy. Add the egg, vanilla, and lemon zest and beat until well combined.

4. Add the almond flour, baking powder, and salt and beat until the dough comes together.

5. In a shallow bowl, whisk together the cream and water. Roll the dough into 1-inch balls, then roll the balls into 2-inch logs. Dunk lightly in the cream and water mixture, then roll in the toasted sesame seeds.

6. Place the coated logs on the prepared cookie sheets, at least 2 inches apart. Bake for 18 to 22 minutes, switching and rotating the pans halfway through baking, until golden brown and just firm to the touch. Remove from the oven and let cool completely on the pans.

TIP: *You can toast sesame seeds on a rimmed baking sheet in the oven, but they are so small that they burn easily. I recommend the skillet method, but you do need to stand there stirring and watching constantly to get them evenly toasted.*

NUTRITIONAL INFORMATION

CALORIES: 247 | FAT: 22.1g | CARBS: 6.8g | FIBER: 3.4g | PROTEIN: 6.3g

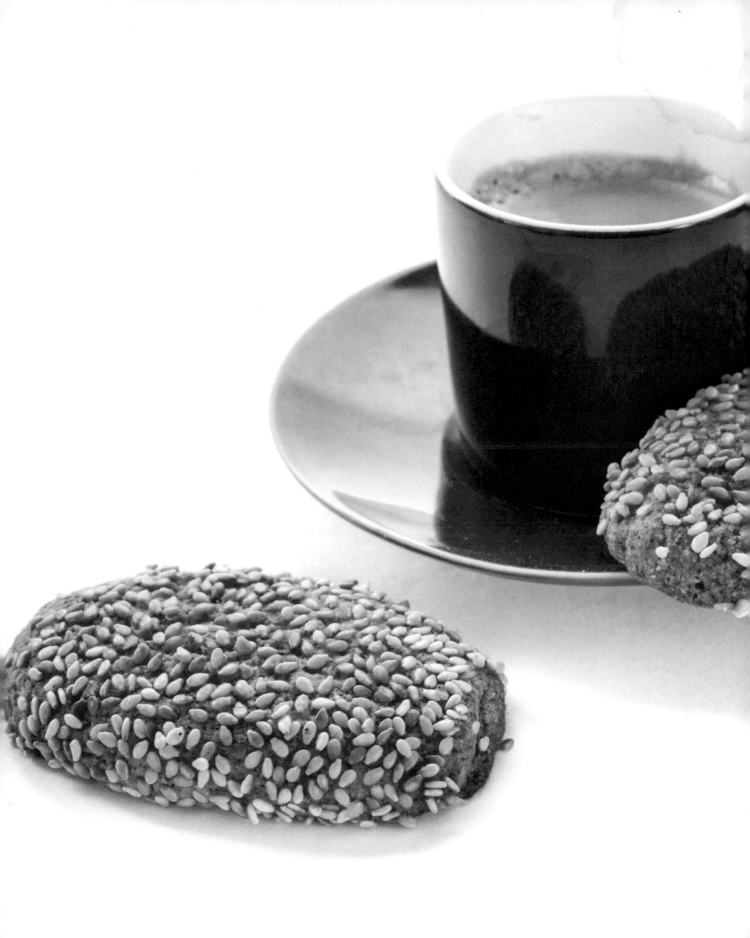

DAIRY-FREE CHOCOLATE CHIP SKILLET COOKIE

OPTION

Yield: One 10-inch cookie (10 servings) Prep Time: 10 minutes Cook Time: 25 minutes

What's easier than making a batch of chocolate chip cookies? Making one big cookie in a skillet. So easy, so deliciously gooey, and everyone loves digging right in with their spoons.

1¼ cups (125g) blanched almond flour

¾ cup unsweetened shredded coconut

⅓ cup brown sugar substitute

⅓ cup granulated sweetener of choice (see tip)

½ teaspoon baking soda

½ teaspoon salt

½ cup melted (but not hot) coconut oil

1 large egg, room temperature

½ teaspoon vanilla extract

⅓ cup sugar-free chocolate chips

1. Preheat the oven to 325°F and grease a 10-inch cast-iron or other ovenproof skillet well.

2. In a large bowl, whisk together the almond flour, shredded coconut, sweeteners, baking soda, and salt.

3. Stir in the melted coconut oil, egg, and vanilla until the dough comes together, then stir in the chocolate chips.

4. Spread the dough evenly in the prepared skillet and bake for 20 to 25 minutes, until light golden brown. The cookie will be very soft and puffed when removed from the oven, and it won't seem cooked through.

5. Let cool for at least 15 minutes before serving. When warm, it will not come out of the pan in proper slices, so you will need scoop it out onto plates to serve it. It will continue to firm up as it cools, so if you want to serve it in slices, let it cool completely before cutting.

COCONUT-FREE OPTION:

You can replace the shredded coconut with more almond flour if you wish, but the coconut provides an absolutely delightful chewiness. Replace the coconut oil with ghee or any nut oil.

TIP: *You can use your favorite sweetener here, but be forewarned that allulose may make the edges of the cookie overly dark.*

SERVING SUGGESTION: *If you don't need to be dairy-free, try topping the warm skillet cookie with a scoop of Keto Vanilla Ice Cream (page 394) and a drizzle of Easy Chocolate Glaze (page 390).*

NUTRITIONAL INFORMATION
CALORIES: 257 | FAT: 24.8g | CARBS: 7.3g | FIBER: 4.4g | PROTEIN: 4.6g

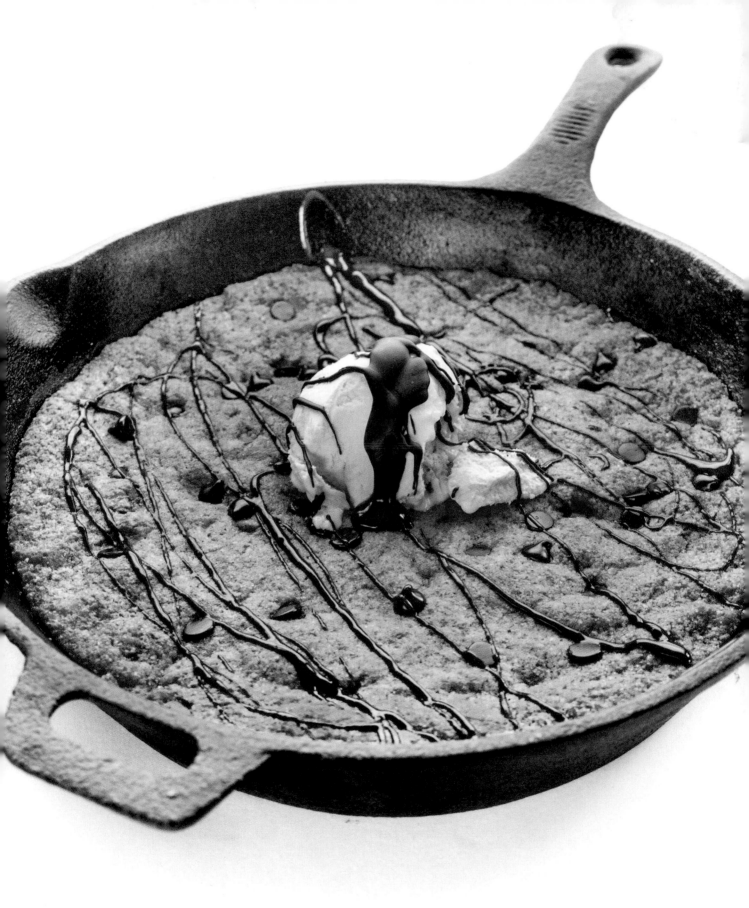

Chapter 7:
FANCY COOKIES

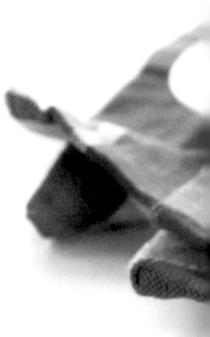

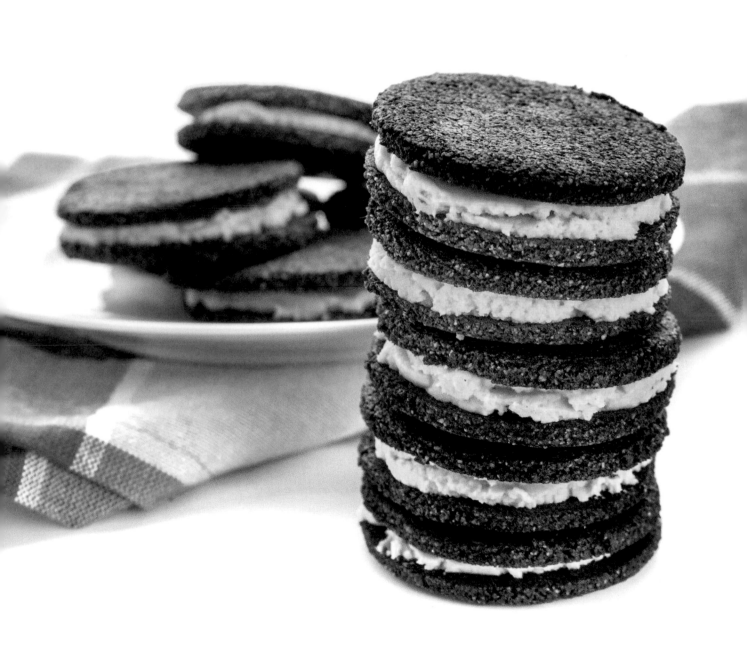

CHOCOLATE WAFERS

OPTION OPTION

Yield: 36 cookies (2 per serving)   **Prep Time:** 25 minutes   **Cook Time:** 30 minutes

These chocolate wafers are actually quite simple to make, and they are delicious on their own. But they are also the basis for some fancier cookies, like my keto "thin mints" (page 148) and "no-reos" (page 150).

1¾ cups (175g) blanched almond flour

½ cup granulated erythritol sweetener

⅓ cup cocoa powder

1 teaspoon baking powder

¼ teaspoon salt

1 large egg, room temperature

2 tablespoons unsalted butter, melted but not hot

½ teaspoon vanilla extract

DAIRY-FREE OPTION:

Use melted ghee or avocado oil in place of the butter. Coconut oil tends to make things very tender and isn't the best choice here.

NUT-FREE OPTION:

Coconut flour won't work in this recipe, but the cookies do turn out well when made with a seed flour like sunflower or pumpkin. If the dough is too sticky to handle, you may need to add a little more flour.

1. Place the oven racks in the second lowest and second highest positions and preheat the oven to 300°F. Line two cookie sheets with silicone baking mats or parchment paper.

2. In a large bowl, combine the almond flour, sweetener, cocoa powder, baking powder, and salt. Add the egg, melted butter, and vanilla and stir well until the dough comes together.

3. Roll out the dough between two pieces of parchment paper to about ¼ inch thick. Remove the top piece of parchment.

4. Using a 2-inch round cookie cutter, cut out circles of dough. Then, using an offset spatula, gently lift and place the cookies on the prepared cookie sheets. Gather up the scraps of dough, reroll, and cut into circles. Repeat until too few dough scraps are left to roll out.

5. Bake the cookies until firm to the touch, 20 to 30 minutes, switching and rotating the pans halfway through baking. Remove from the oven and let cool completely on the pans. The cookies will continue to crisp up as they cool.

TIP: *These cookies are meant to be crisp, so you really need an erythritol-based sweetener such as Swerve.*

NUTRITIONAL INFORMATION

CALORIES: 82 | FAT: 7.1g | CARBS: 3.4g | FIBER: 1.8g | PROTEIN: 3g

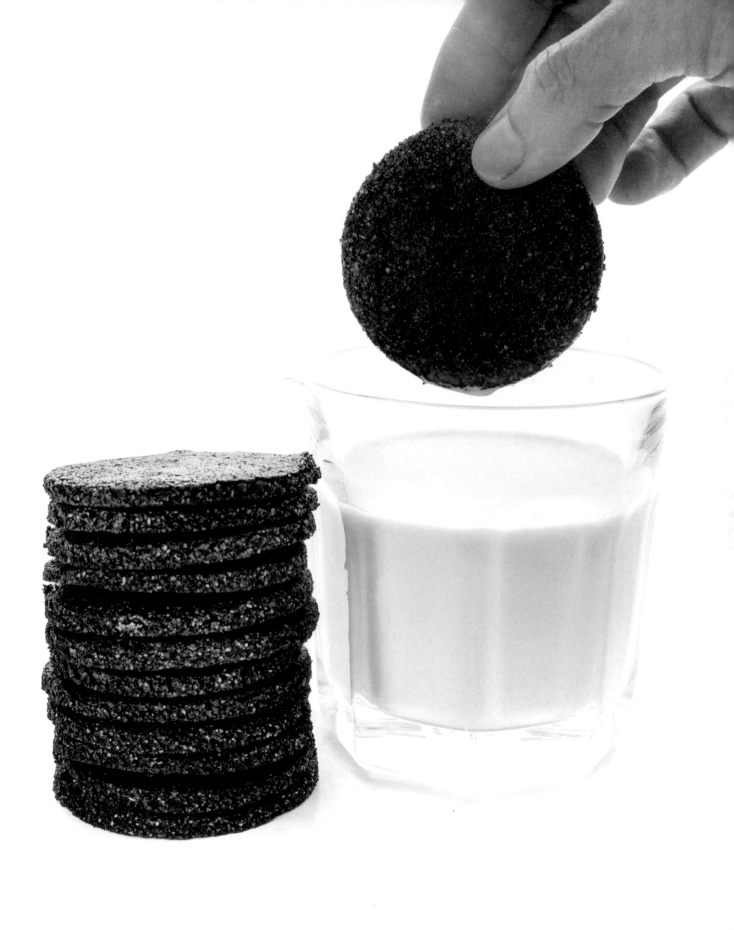

MINT CHOCOLATE THINS

OPTION OPTION

Yield: 36 cookies (2 per serving) Prep Time: 20 minutes (not including time to make chocolate wafers) Cook Time: 5 minutes

Keep the temptations of the Girl Scout cookies at bay with this healthy homemade version of Thin Mints! My family can't get enough of them.

6 ounces sugar-free dark chocolate, chopped

¾ ounce cocoa butter, or
1 tablespoon coconut oil

1 teaspoon peppermint extract

1 recipe Chocolate Wafers (page 146)

DAIRY-FREE OPTION:

Use the dairy-free version of the chocolate wafers.

NUT-FREE OPTION:

Use the nut-free version of the chocolate wafers.

1. Line a cookie sheet with waxed paper.

2. Set a heatproof bowl over a pot of gently simmering water, not allowing the bottom of the bowl to touch the water. Melt the chocolate and cocoa butter in the bowl, stirring until smooth. Remove from the heat and stir in the peppermint extract.

3. Dip the wafers one at a time into the chocolate, using two forks to turn over and fully coat each cookie. Lift out the cookie and gently tap the fork on the side of the bowl to remove the excess chocolate, then place the cookie on the prepared cookie sheet.

4. Refrigerate until fully set, at least 20 minutes.

TIP: *Melting the dark chocolate coating with cocoa butter helps thin it out so that it coats the cookies more easily. Coconut oil works, too, but don't use butter, which tends to make the coating thicker.*

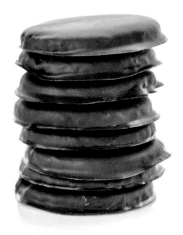

NUTRITIONAL INFORMATION

CALORIES: 127 | FAT: 11.5g | CARBS: 7.1g | FIBER: 3.6g | PROTEIN: 3.3g

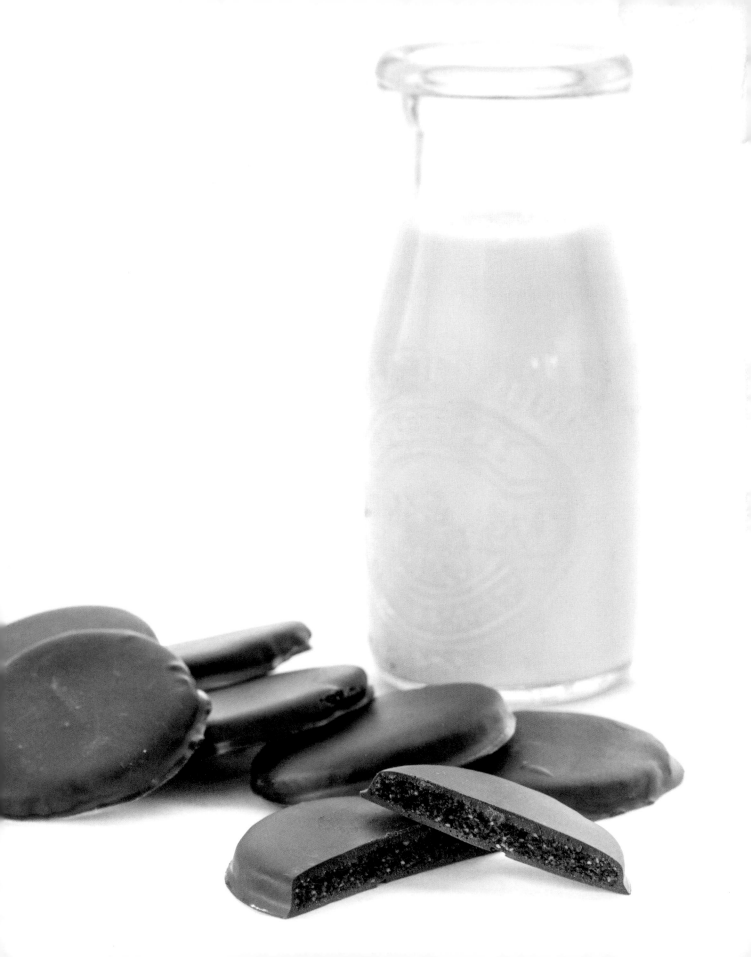

CHOCOLATE SANDWICH COOKIES (AKA NO-REOS)

OPTION

Yield: 18 cookies (1 per serving) Prep Time: 15 minutes (not including time to make chocolate wafers) Cook Time: —

Classic and timeless! My son, who is perhaps my biggest critic, said these cookies taste just like Oreos.

6 tablespoons unsalted butter, softened

2 ounces cream cheese, softened

⅔ cup powdered erythritol sweetener

2 tablespoons heavy whipping cream, room temperature

½ teaspoon vanilla extract

1 recipe Chocolate Wafers (page 146)

1. In a medium bowl, beat the butter and cream cheese with an electric mixer until smooth. Beat in the sweetener until well combined, then beat in the cream and vanilla. The filling mixture should be like a thick frosting.

2. Take a chocolate wafer and spread it with about 1 tablespoon of filling, then top with another wafer. Repeat until all the wafers and filling are used up.

NUT-FREE OPTION:

Use the nut-free version of the chocolate wafers.

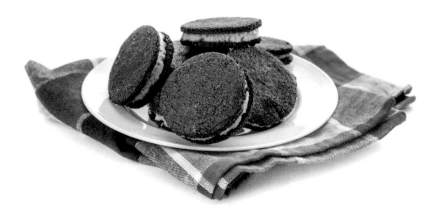

NUTRITIONAL INFORMATION
CALORIES: 134 | FAT: 12.2g | CARBS: 3.6g | FIBER: 1.8g | PROTEIN: 3.3g

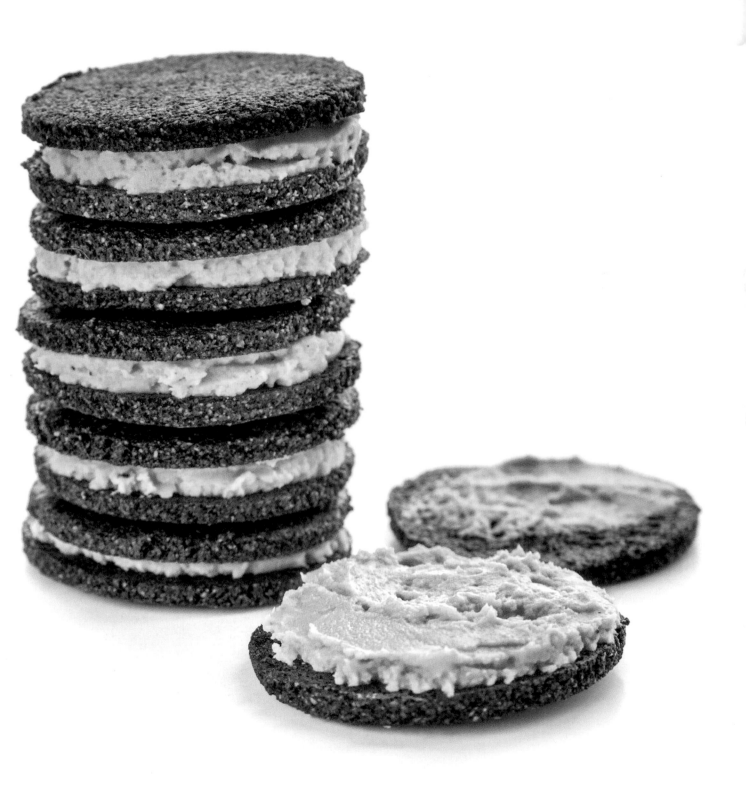

CREAM CHEESE CUTOUT COOKIES

OPTION

Yield: About 48 cookies (2 per serving) Prep Time: 40 minutes, plus 30 minutes to chill (not including time to make frosting)
Cook Time: 15 minutes

Egg-free sugar cookies! The cream cheese helps these delicious cookies hold together. This recipe makes a lot of cookies, perfect for decorating and giving away during the holidays.

3½ cups (350g) almond flour, plus more for the work surface

1 teaspoon baking powder

½ teaspoon xanthan gum

¼ teaspoon salt

4 ounces cream cheese, softened

6 tablespoons unsalted butter, softened

¾ cup powdered erythritol sweetener

1 teaspoon vanilla extract

½ recipe Cream Cheese Frosting (page 380), colored with natural food coloring as desired

DAIRY-FREE OPTION:

One of my recipe testers had great success making these with Kite Hill almond milk cream cheese and ghee. You can make a dairy-free version of the cream cheese frosting (page 380) using the Kite Hill product as well.

1. Line two or three cookie sheets with silicone baking mats or parchment paper, depending on how big your sheets are. You can also work in batches with one or two cookie sheets.

2. In a medium bowl, whisk together the almond flour, baking powder, xanthan gum, and salt.

3. In a large bowl, beat the cream cheese and butter with an electric mixer until well combined. Beat in the powdered sweetener and vanilla, then beat in the almond flour mixture until the dough comes together. Divide the dough in half and form each half into a disc.

4. Dust a silicone baking mat with almond flour and place a disc on the mat. Cover with parchment paper and roll out to ¼ inch thick. Remove the top piece of parchment.

5. Use 2- to 3-inch cookie cutters to cut out desired shapes. Very gently loosen the shapes from the mat with an offset spatula and place on the prepared cookie sheets. They are very soft, so if they tear, simply patch them back together gently. Repeat with the remaining disc of dough. Refrigerate for 30 minutes.

6. Preheat the oven to 325°F. Bake for 12 to 15 minutes, switching and rotating the pans halfway through baking, until just barely browned around the edges. Remove from the oven and let cool completely on the pans.

7. Frost the cooled cookies as desired.

TIPS: *Choose cookie cutters that don't have too many thin points. This dough is delicate, and you may find that it rips and tears as you try to lift the cookie cutters.*

The unfrosted cookies freeze really well, but you could easily cut the recipe in half if you wanted fewer cookies.

NUTRITIONAL INFORMATION (UNFROSTED)

CALORIES: 137 | FAT: 12.2g | CARBS: 3.8g | FIBER: 1.8g | PROTEIN: 3.8g

NUTRITIONAL INFORMATION (FROSTED)

CALORIES: 184 | FAT: 16.8g | CARBS: 4g | FIBER: 1.8g | PROTEIN: 4.2g

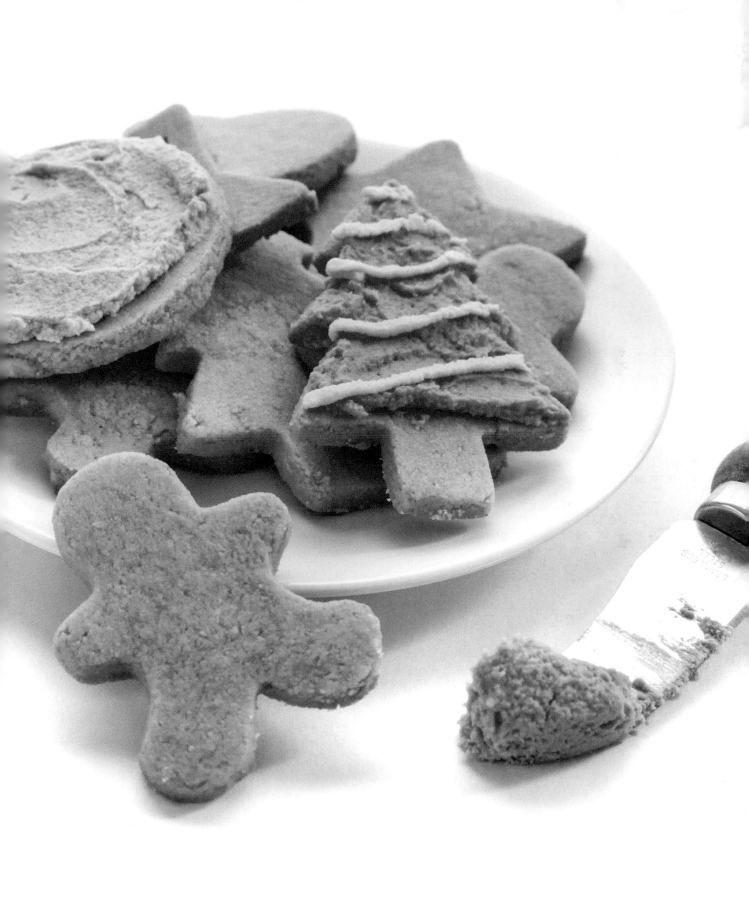

CINNAMON ROLL COOKIES

Yield: About 60 cookies (2 per serving) Prep Time: 35 minutes, plus 30 to 60 minutes to freeze dough logs Cook Time: 21 minutes

Another large-batch cookie recipe that's perfect for holidays and other special occasions. The dough logs can be made ahead and frozen for up to two months. Just be sure to let them soften for 15 minutes or so before attempting to slice them.

Cookie Dough:

2¼ cups (225g) blanched almond flour

3 tablespoons coconut flour

1 tablespoon grass-fed gelatin

1 teaspoon baking powder

¼ teaspoon salt

½ cup (1 stick) unsalted butter, softened

¾ cup granulated sweetener of choice (see tips)

1 large egg, room temperature

½ teaspoon vanilla extract

Cinnamon Filling:

2 tablespoons unsalted butter, melted, divided

¼ cup brown sugar substitute, divided

1 teaspoon ground cinnamon, divided

Drizzle:

6 tablespoons powdered erythritol sweetener

2½ tablespoons water

¼ teaspoon vanilla extract

1. Lay a piece of parchment or waxed paper on a work surface and grease lightly with avocado or coconut oil spray.

2. In a large bowl, whisk together the almond flour, coconut flour, gelatin, baking powder, and salt.

3. In another large bowl, beat the butter and granulated sweetener with an electric mixer until combined. Beat in the egg and vanilla, then beat in the flour mixture until the dough comes together.

4. Divide the dough into two equal portions. Place one portion on the prepared work surface and pat into a rough rectangle. Cover with another piece of parchment and roll out to an 8 by 10-inch rectangle. Remove the top piece of parchment.

5. Brush the dough with 1 tablespoon of the melted butter and sprinkle with 2 tablespoons of the brown sugar substitute and ½ teaspoon of the cinnamon.

6. Use an offset spatula or sharp knife to loosen the dough from the parchment paper. Starting at one of the long sides, gently roll the dough up as tightly as you can, using the parchment to help lift it. If it cracks a bit, simply patch it back together. Once the dough is rolled, wrap it tightly in the paper and place in the freezer for 30 to 60 minutes to firm up.

7. Repeat with the remaining dough, melted butter, brown sugar substitute, and cinnamon.

8. Once the dough logs have chilled, preheat the oven to 325°F and line two cookie sheets with silicone baking mats or parchment paper.

9. Using a sharp knife, cut the dough logs into ¼-inch-thick slices and place on the prepared cookie sheets. Bake for 5 minutes, then remove from the oven and press a little flatter with a flat-bottomed glass. Bake for another 12 to 16 minutes, until just golden around the edges. Remove from the oven and let cool completely on the pans.

NUTRITIONAL INFORMATION

CALORIES: 87 | FAT: 7.7g | CARBS: 2.3g | FIBER: 1.2g | PROTEIN: 2.4g

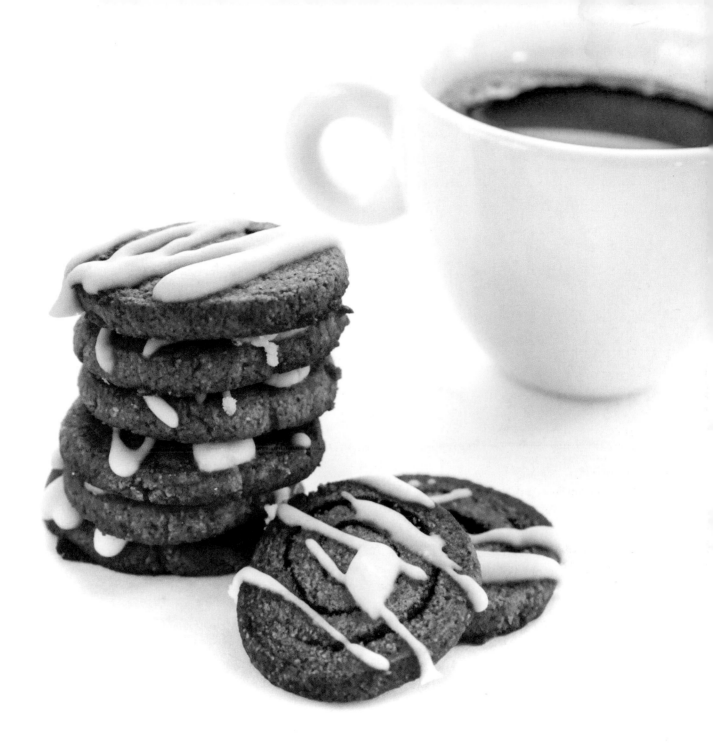

10. In a small bowl, whisk together the powdered sweetener, water, and vanilla. Drizzle over the cooled cookies and let set for 5 minutes.

TIPS: *The gelatin in this recipe is critical, as it gives the dough more flexibility to be rolled. Using half Swerve Sweetener and half allulose for the granulated sweetener also will help, but using all allulose will make them rather cakey.*

You can freeze the baked cookies for up to 2 months, but leave off the drizzle until you are ready to serve them.

SCOTTISH SHORTBREAD

Yield: 16 cookies (1 per serving) Prep Time: 20 minutes Cook Time: 50 minutes

When I was growing up, Scottish shortbread was a staple in our house during the holidays. We could always see the plaid boxes of Walkers sticking out of our stockings as we came down the stairs. It simply wouldn't be Christmas without shortbread!

2¼ cups (225g) blanched almond flour

⅔ cup powdered erythritol sweetener

½ teaspoon salt

6 tablespoons unsalted butter, softened

1 tablespoon water

½ teaspoon vanilla extract

TIPS: *The sides of a springform pan are perfect for helping you press the shortbread dough into a perfect 9-inch circle. You can do it free-form if you prefer.*

Parchment paper will work in place of a silicone baking mat, but the shortbread may brown more on the bottom and sides. A silicone mat will protect it better and keep it the pale color of traditional shortbread.

You can dip the ends in chocolate for a pretty presentation. Follow the same method as in the Slice-and-Bake Mocha Shortbread (page 158), completing Steps 6 and 7. If desired, sprinkle coarse sea salt onto the chocolate-dipped ends, then allow the chocolate to set.

1. Preheat the oven to 300°F and line a cookie sheet with a silicone baking mat or parchment paper. Remove the bottom of a 9-inch springform pan and set aside; you will be using only the sides of the pan for this recipe. Place the sides of the pan on the prepared cookie sheet with the clip closed.

2. Place the almond flour, sweetener, and salt in a food processor. Pulse a few times to combine. Add the butter in chunks and pulse until the mixture resembles coarse crumbs. Add the water and vanilla and process on high until the dough clumps up into one large ball.

3. Press the dough firmly and evenly inside the springform pan sides to create a perfect 9-inch circle, then loosen and remove the sides.

4. Using a large sharp knife, cut the dough into 16 even wedges, but do not separate them yet. Use a fork to prick the wedges decoratively. You can crimp the edges a bit as well.

5. Bake for about 30 minutes, until the edges are becoming golden. Remove from the oven and turn off the oven. Recut along the cut lines. Gently separate the wedges and space them around the cookie sheet.

6. Return the cookie sheet to the warm oven and prop the door open. Let the shortbread sit inside for another 10 to 20 minutes, until just firm to the touch. Watch carefully in case it is browning too quickly. Remove from the oven and let cool completely on the pan.

NUTRITIONAL INFORMATION

CALORIES: 130 | FAT: 11.9g | CARBS: 3.4g | FIBER: 1.7g | PROTEIN: 3.4g

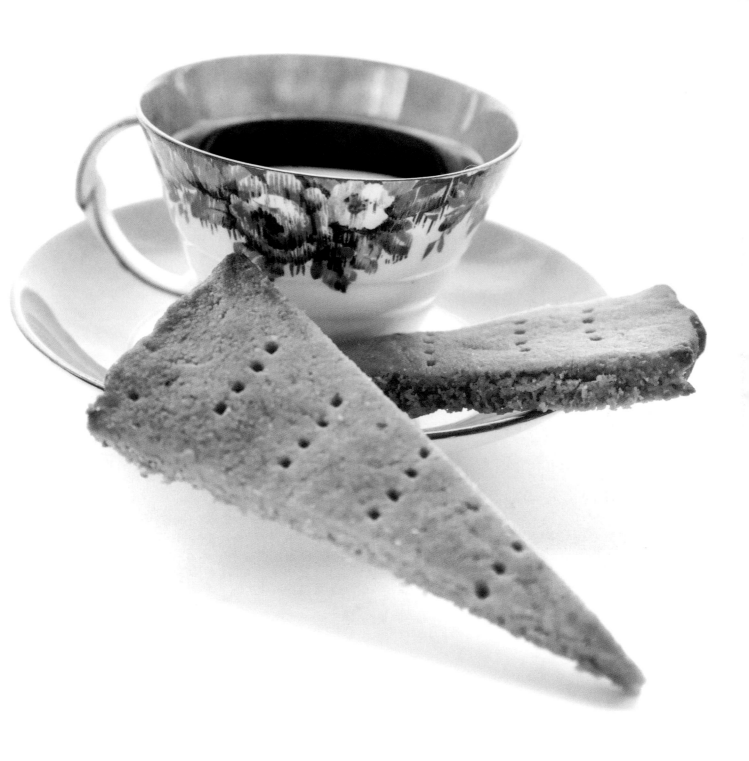

SLICE-AND-BAKE MOCHA SHORTBREAD

Yield: 40 cookies (2 per serving) **Prep Time:** 25 minutes, plus 1 hour to freeze dough **Cook Time:** 17 minutes

Like your favorite Starbucks drink in cookie form. And much, much healthier!

½ cup (1 stick) unsalted butter, softened

½ cup powdered erythritol sweetener

1¾ cups (175g) blanched almond flour

¼ cup cocoa powder

2 teaspoons espresso powder

½ teaspoon vanilla extract

½ teaspoon salt

3 ounces sugar-free dark chocolate, chopped

½ ounce cocoa butter

1. In a large bowl, beat the butter and sweetener with an electric mixer until lightened and fluffy, about 2 minutes. Beat in the almond flour, cocoa powder, espresso powder, vanilla, and salt until well combined.

2. Divide the dough into two equal portions and place each on a sheet of waxed paper. Roll into logs about 1½ inches in diameter and wrap tightly in the waxed paper. Freeze for 1 hour.

3. Preheat the oven to 325°F and line two cookie sheets with silicone baking mats or parchment paper. Using a sharp knife, cut the dough logs into ¼-inch slices. Place the slices on the prepared cookie sheets.

4. Bake for 5 minutes, then remove from the oven and use a flat-bottomed glass to press down slightly to flatten. Bake for another 10 to 12 minutes, until just firm to the touch. Remove from the oven and let cool completely on the pans.

5. Line a cookie sheet with waxed paper.

6. Place the chocolate and cocoa butter in a heatproof bowl set over a pan of barely simmering water. Stir until melted and smooth.

7. Dip the cooled cookies into the chocolate, one at a time, coating them about halfway. Place on the prepared cookie sheet and allow to set for at least 20 minutes.

TIP: *As with the other slice-and-bake cookies in this book, the dough logs can be kept in the freezer for up to two months. Just be sure to let them thaw a bit before slicing and baking. You don't want them fully defrosted, but they shouldn't be rock solid.*

NUTRITIONAL INFORMATION

CALORIES: 124 | FAT: 11.6g | CARBS: 4.5g | FIBER: 2.3g | PROTEIN: 2.6g

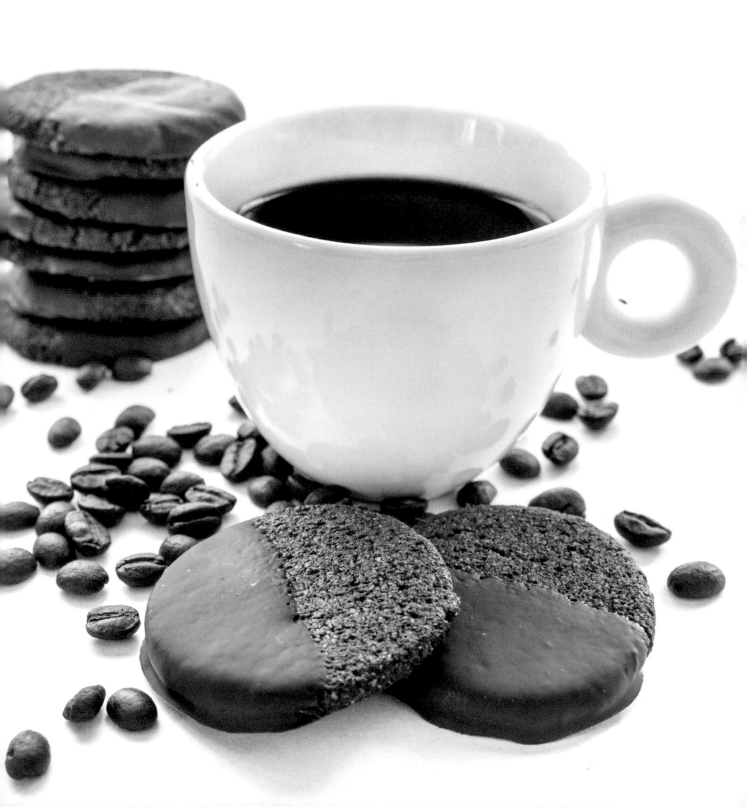

CLASSIC ALMOND BISCOTTI

OPTION

Yield: 14 biscotti (1 per serving)   **Prep Time:** 15 minutes   **Cook Time:** 40+ minutes

Dipping a crunchy biscotto into a cup of coffee might be my favorite morning activity.

2 cups (200g) blanched almond flour

⅓ cup granulated erythritol sweetener

1 teaspoon baking powder

¼ teaspoon salt

¼ cup (½ stick) plus 1 tablespoon butter, melted but not hot, divided

1 large egg

¾ teaspoon almond extract

2 tablespoons sliced almonds

DAIRY-FREE OPTION:

Replace the butter with avocado oil. I don't recommend coconut oil here, as it tends to make the biscotti too tender, and they should be crisp.

1. Preheat the oven to 325°F and line a cookie sheet with a silicone baking mat or parchment paper.

2. In a large bowl, whisk together the almond flour, sweetener, baking powder, and salt. Stir in ¼ cup of the melted butter, the egg, and almond extract until the dough comes together.

3. Turn the dough out onto the prepared cookie sheet and form into a low log, about 4 by 10 inches. Brush with the remaining 1 tablespoon of melted butter and press the sliced almonds into the top.

4. Bake for 22 to 25 minutes, until lightly browned and just firm to the touch. Remove from the oven and let cool for 30 minutes. Reduce the oven temperature to 250°F.

5. Using a sharp knife, cut the log crosswise into about 14 slices. (A straight-up-and-down motion works better than sawing back and forth.) Place the slices back on the cookie sheet cut side down and bake for 15 minutes, then carefully flip them over. Turn off the oven and let the biscotti sit inside until cool.

TIP: *Using an erythritol-based sweetener like Swerve is the key to getting these biscotti to crisp up properly.*

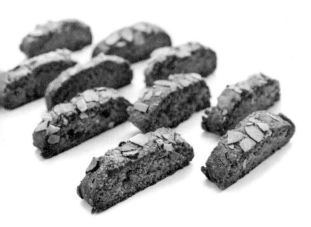

NUTRITIONAL INFORMATION
CALORIES: 123 | FAT: 11.1g | CARBS: 3.9g | FIBER: 1.8g | PROTEIN: 3.8g

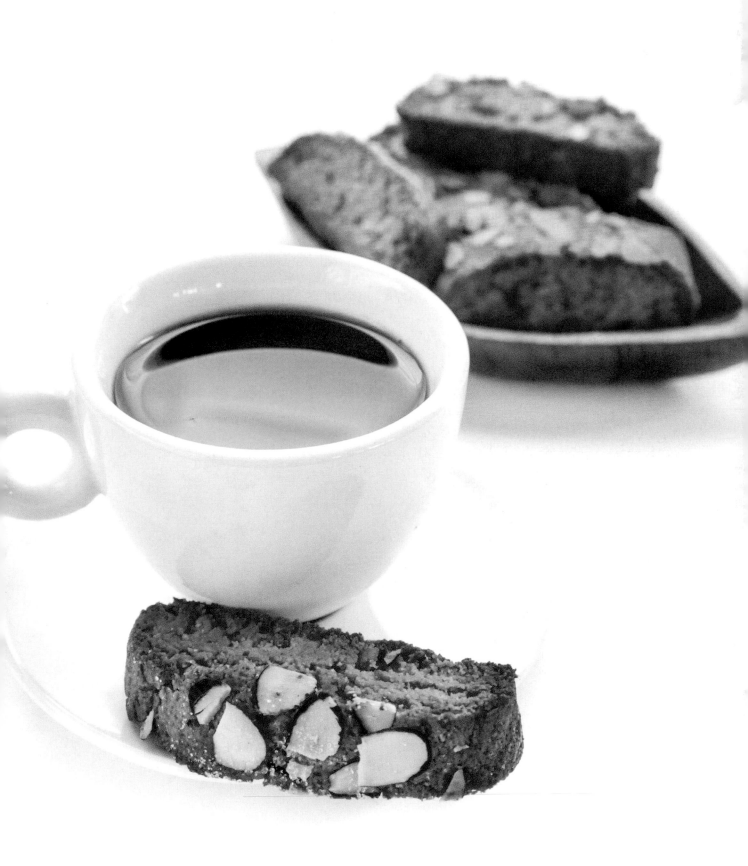

CHOCOLATE HAZELNUT BISCOTTI

Yield: 14 biscotti (1 per serving) **Prep Time:** 15 minutes **Cook Time:** 40+ minutes

I made a version of these cookies back in 2011 when I was still exploring keto baking and how to make it work. I tried to grind the hazelnuts myself to make the meal. I highly recommend using the commercially ground version instead, which makes the biscotti finer and much less crumbly.

1¾ cups hazelnut meal

⅓ cup granulated erythritol sweetener

¼ cup cocoa powder

¼ cup finely chopped hazelnuts

1 teaspoon baking powder

¼ teaspoon salt

¼ cup toasted hazelnut oil or avocado oil

1 large egg

½ teaspoon vanilla extract

1. Preheat the oven to 325°F and line a cookie sheet with a silicone baking mat or parchment paper.

2. In a large bowl, whisk together the hazelnut meal, sweetener, cocoa powder, hazelnuts, baking powder, and salt. Stir in the oil, egg, and vanilla until the dough comes together.

3. Turn the dough out onto the prepared cookie sheet and form into a low log, about 4 by 10 inches.

4. Bake for 22 to 25 minutes, until lightly browned and just firm to the touch. Remove from the oven and let cool for 30 minutes. Reduce the oven temperature to 250°F.

5. Using a sharp knife, cut the log crosswise into 14 slices (a straight-up-and-down motion works better than sawing back and forth). Place the slices back on the cookie sheet cut side down and bake for 15 minutes, then carefully flip them over. Turn off the oven and let the biscotti sit inside until cool.

TIP: *Chop those hazelnuts relatively finely so that it's easier to slice the biscotti for the second baking.*

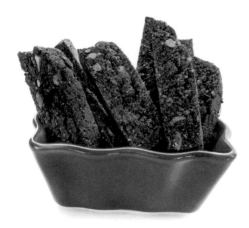

NUTRITIONAL INFORMATION

CALORIES: 149 | FAT: 14.1g | CARBS: 3.9g | FIBER: 2.3g | PROTEIN: 3.1g

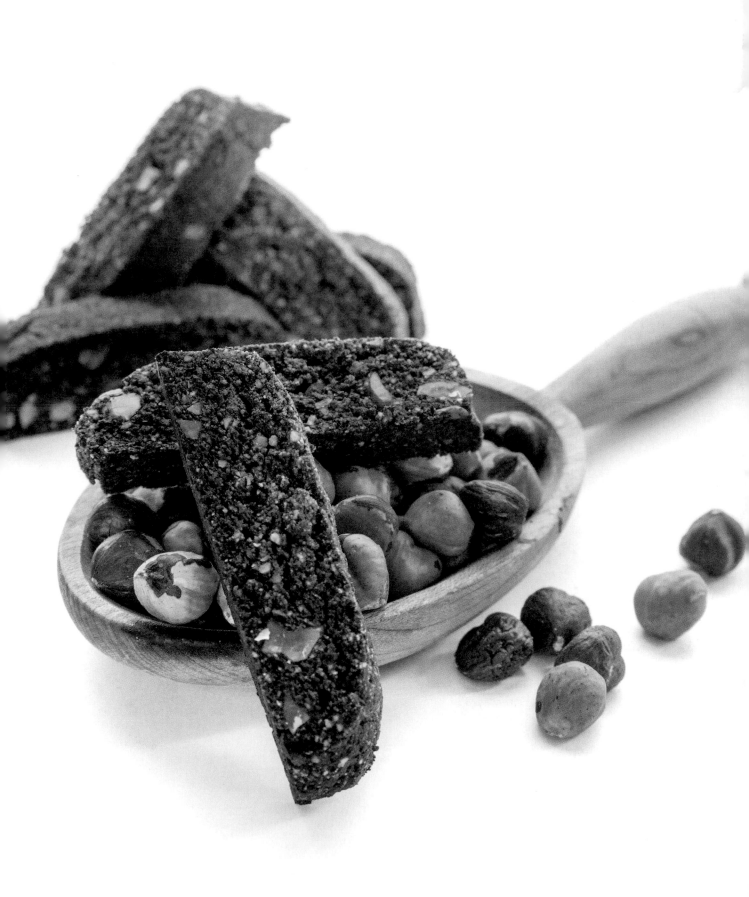

CLASSIC WHOOPIE PIES

Yield: 10 whoopie pies (1 per serving)   Prep Time: 25 minutes (not including time to make frosting)   Cook Time: 20 minutes

Whoopie pies were not something I grew up with in Canada, but I completely understand the appeal now!

½ cup plus 2 tablespoons (69g) coconut flour

½ cup granulated sweetener of choice

¼ cup cocoa powder

¼ cup unflavored whey protein powder

1½ teaspoons baking powder

½ teaspoon salt

4 large eggs, room temperature

½ cup heavy whipping cream

¼ cup (½ stick) unsalted butter, melted

½ teaspoon vanilla extract

½ recipe Swiss Meringue Buttercream (page 378) or Cream Cheese Frosting (page 380)

1. Preheat the oven to 350°F and line a cookie sheet with a silicone baking mat or parchment paper.

2. In a large bowl, whisk together the coconut flour, sweetener, cocoa powder, protein powder, baking powder, and salt. Stir in the eggs, cream, melted butter, and vanilla until well combined. Let sit for 10 minutes to thicken.

3. Wet your hands and roll the batter into balls, using about 2 tablespoons of batter at a time. You should get about 20 balls. You can also use a 2-tablespoon cookie scoop to place the batter on the prepared cookie sheet.

4. Place the balls on the prepared cookie sheet, about 3 inches apart, and press down lightly with the palm of your hand to about ½ inch thick.

5. Bake for 15 to 20 minutes, until the cookies are puffed and set. Remove from the oven and let cool completely on the pan.

6. Once cool, spread the bottom of a cookie with about 1 tablespoon of the frosting and top with another cookie. Repeat with the rest of the cookies and frosting.

TIP: *The protein powder helps give these cookies more of a cakey quality. You can use any sweetener you like.*

NUTRITIONAL INFORMATION (WITH SWISS MERINGUE FROSTING)
CALORIES: 245 | FAT: 20.1g | CARBS: 6.3g | FIBER: 3.3g | PROTEIN: 6.7g

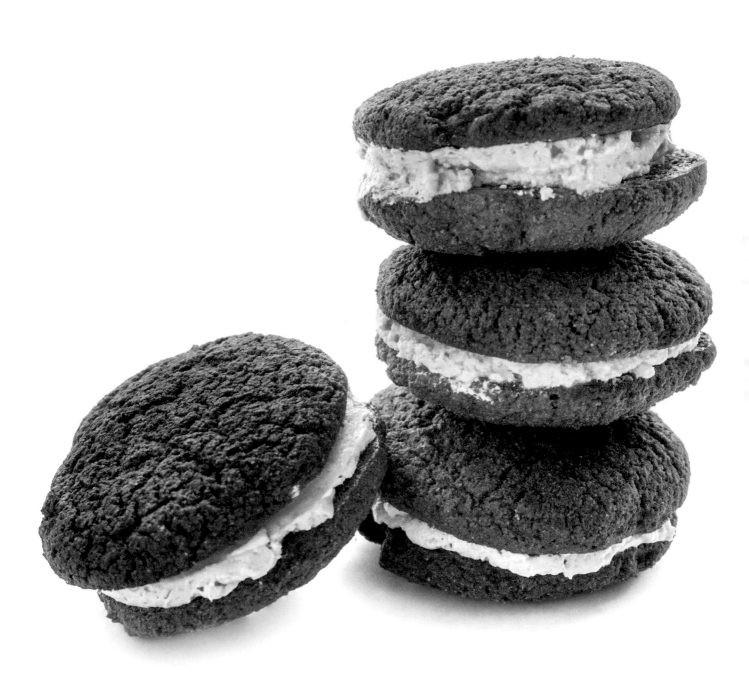

FROSTED LEMON SUGAR COOKIES

Yield: 24 cookies (2 per serving) Prep Time: 30 minutes Cook Time: 18 minutes

Lemon lovers, rejoice! These soft, sweet "sugar" cookies have a delectably tangy lemon flavor. They are great on their own, but add the frosting and they are out of this world!

Cookies:

½ cup (1 stick) unsalted butter, softened

⅔ cup granulated erythritol sweetener

1 large egg, room temperature

1 large egg yolk, room temperature

2 teaspoons grated lemon zest

¾ teaspoon lemon extract

½ teaspoon vanilla extract

2 cups (200g) blanched almond flour

1½ teaspoons baking powder

¼ teaspoon salt

Lemon Frosting:

½ recipe Cream Cheese Frosting (page 380)

1 teaspoon grated lemon zest

2 tablespoons fresh lemon juice

Natural yellow food coloring, as desired

Long strips of lemon zest, for garnish (optional)

1. Preheat the oven to 325°F and line two cookie sheets with silicone baking mats or parchment paper.

2. In a large bowl, beat the butter and sweetener with an electric mixer until well combined and fluffy. Add the whole egg, egg yolk, lemon zest, and extracts and beat until well combined.

3. Add the almond flour, baking powder, and salt and beat until the dough comes together.

4. Roll the dough into 1-inch balls and place on the prepared cookie sheets, at least 2 inches apart. Flatten slightly with the palm of your hand to about ½ inch thick.

5. Bake for 15 to 18 minutes, until just golden around the edges, switching and rotating the pans halfway through baking. The cookies will still be a bit soft. Remove from the oven and let cool completely on the pans. They will continue to firm up as they cool.

6. Prepare the cream cheese frosting according to the directions, beating in the lemon zest and juice after Step 2. Beat in yellow food coloring a little at a time until a light yellow hue is achieved.

7. Spread the frosting over the tops of the cooled cookies and decorate with long strips of lemon zest, if using.

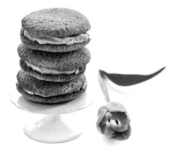

> **VARIATION:** LEMON SANDWICH COOKIES.
>
> *Make lemon sandwich cookies by spreading about 1 tablespoon of the frosting on the bottom of one cookie and topping it with another cookie. Omit the lemon zest.*

NUTRITIONAL INFORMATION (WITH FROSTING)

CALORIES: 262 | FAT: 24g | CARBS: 5.1g | FIBER: 2g | PROTEIN: 5.5g

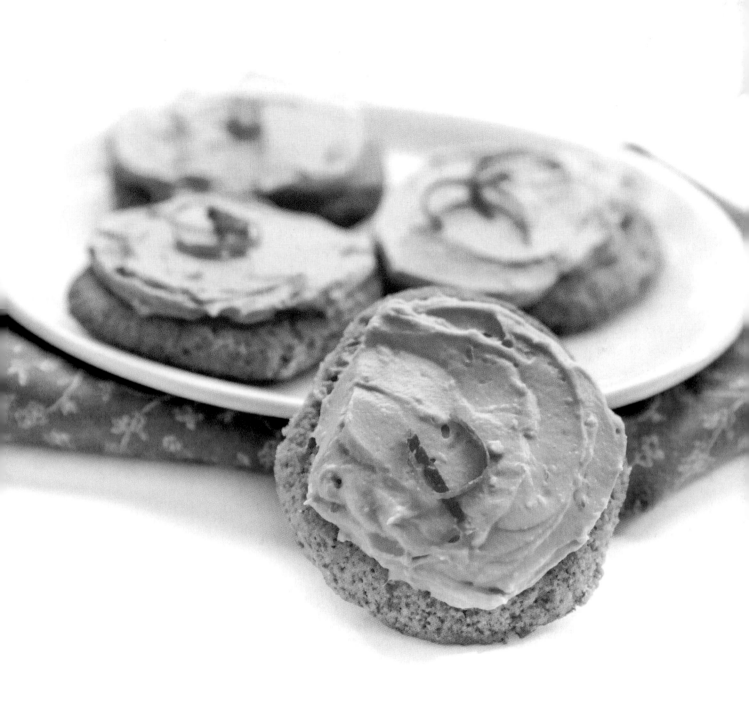

TIP: *For the yellow color, there are several good natural food coloring options. I use Color Kitchen, a vegetable-based powdered food dye. It's potent stuff, though, and it can produce an overly vibrant hue if you use too much. I sprinkle a little in, beat the frosting, and then sprinkle in a bit more until I have the color I want.*

"OATMEAL" LACE COOKIES

Yield: 28 cookies (2 per serving) Prep Time: 20 minutes Cook Time: 12 minutes

These delicate, lacy cookies have a rich caramel flavor and a texture reminiscent of oatmeal.

1 cup unsweetened flaked coconut

1 cup sliced almonds

½ cup (1 stick) unsalted butter, softened

½ cup brown sugar substitute

⅓ cup granulated erythritol sweetener

1 large egg, room temperature

½ teaspoon vanilla extract

2 tablespoons blanched almond flour

¼ teaspoon baking soda

¼ teaspoon salt

1. Preheat the oven to 325°F and line two rimmed baking sheets with silicone baking mats or parchment paper.

2. In a food processor, process the coconut and almonds until they resemble oats.

3. In a large bowl, beat the butter and sweeteners with an electric mixer until light and fluffy, about 2 minutes. Beat in the egg and vanilla.

4. Add the coconut/almond mixture, almond flour, baking soda, and salt. Beat until well combined. Roll the mixture into 1-inch balls and place on the prepared baking sheets, about 3 inches apart.

5. Bake for 5 minutes, then remove from the oven and press down with a flat-bottomed glass to flatten. If the cookies stick to the glass, cover the glass with greased plastic wrap or parchment paper.

6. Return the cookies to the oven and bake for another 5 to 7 minutes, until just brown around the edges. Remove from the oven and let cool completely on the pans.

TIPS: *These very fragile, delicate cookies are best baked on a silicone baking mat. They will leak a lot of butter during baking but will reabsorb it as they cool. Be sure to use rimmed baking sheets so the butter doesn't drip all over your oven!*

This is another cookie that really requires an erythritol-based sweetener to crisp up properly.

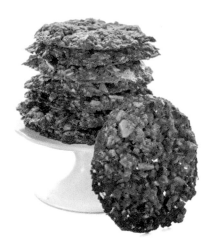

NUTRITIONAL INFORMATION

CALORIES: 138 | FAT: 12.9g | CARBS: 2.8g | FIBER: 1.5g | PROTEIN: 2.4g

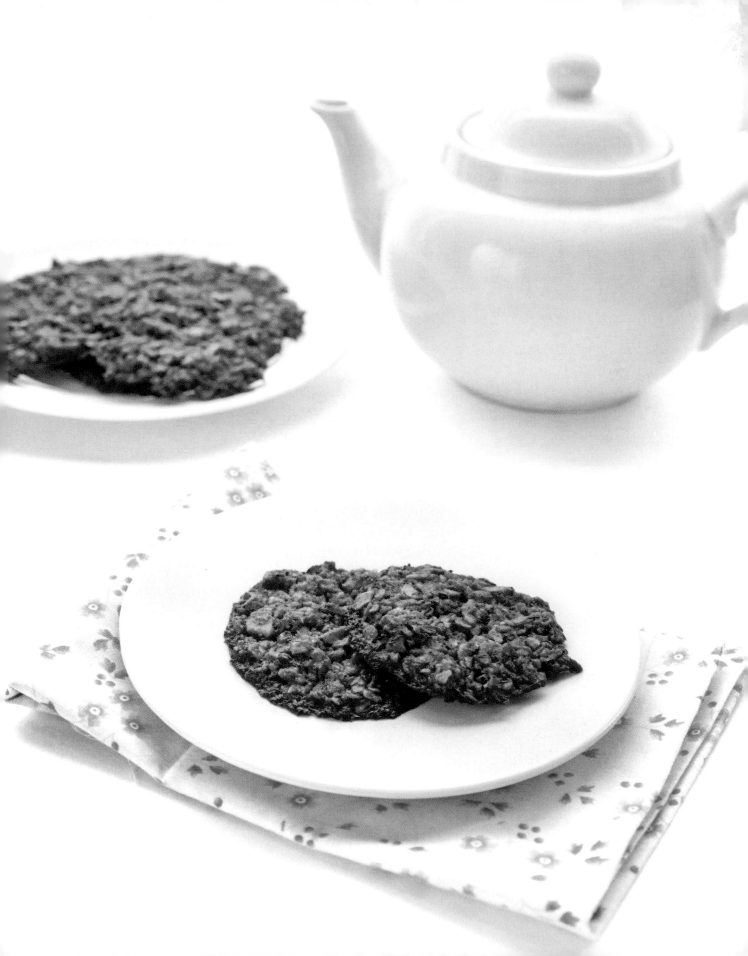

SUGAR-FREE MERINGUES

Yield: 12 servings **Prep Time:** 20 minutes **Cook Time:** 60 to 90 minutes, plus 1 to 2 hours to dry

Crispy light meringues with a pillowy soft inside. The number of meringues you get from this recipe depends on how big you make them.

4 large egg whites, room temperature

¼ teaspoon cream of tartar

⅛ teaspoon salt

½ teaspoon vanilla extract (see tips)

¼ cup granulated erythritol sweetener (see tips)

¼ cup powdered erythritol sweetener

1. Preheat the oven to 200°F and line a cookie sheet with parchment paper.

2. In a large bowl, beat the egg whites, cream of tartar, and salt with an electric mixer until frothy. Beat in the vanilla.

3. Mix the sweeteners together in a small bowl. With the mixer running, add the blended sweeteners to the egg white mixture 1 tablespoon at a time. Beat until the egg whites are glossy and hold medium peaks (the tip of the whites should just fold over as you lift the beaters). Don't beat until completely stiff or the meringues will harden too much.

4. Pipe or dollop the egg white mixture onto the prepared cookie sheet in the desired size. Bake until just barely firm and no longer tacky to the touch, anywhere between 60 and 90 minutes, depending on size.

5. Turn off the oven and let the meringues sit inside for another hour or two. Remove from the oven just as they are beginning to brown. Let cool completely on the pan before gently peeling off the parchment paper.

VARIATION: MERINGUE GANACHE KISSES.

Pipe the meringue into small kisses using a piping bag fitted with a star-shaped tip. Bake as directed. Prepare the Easy Chocolate Glaze (page 390) and let sit for 20 minutes to thicken. Spread the bottom of a meringue with about ½ teaspoon of the glaze and press the bottom of another meringue onto the glaze. Place on a waxed paper–lined cookie sheet to set.

TIPS: *Meringues are finicky, and sugar-free meringues are even more so. Here are my best tips for making them work:*

No sweetener besides erythritol will produce a serviceable meringue. Believe me, I have tried and tried. Allulose, Bocha Sweet, and xylitol all make the meringues so soft and marshmallow-like that you can't get them off the parchment paper. I even tried using mostly Swerve with a single tablespoon of Bocha Sweet, and they never firmed up properly.

The combination of granulated and powdered Swerve helps the overall consistency be soft without residual grittiness.

Do not use an oil-based vanilla extract in this recipe. Even the smallest amount of oil will keep the egg whites from whipping properly.

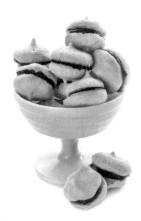

NUTRITIONAL INFORMATION

| CALORIES: | 8 | FAT: | 0g | CARBS: | 0.1g | PROTEIN: | 1.2g |

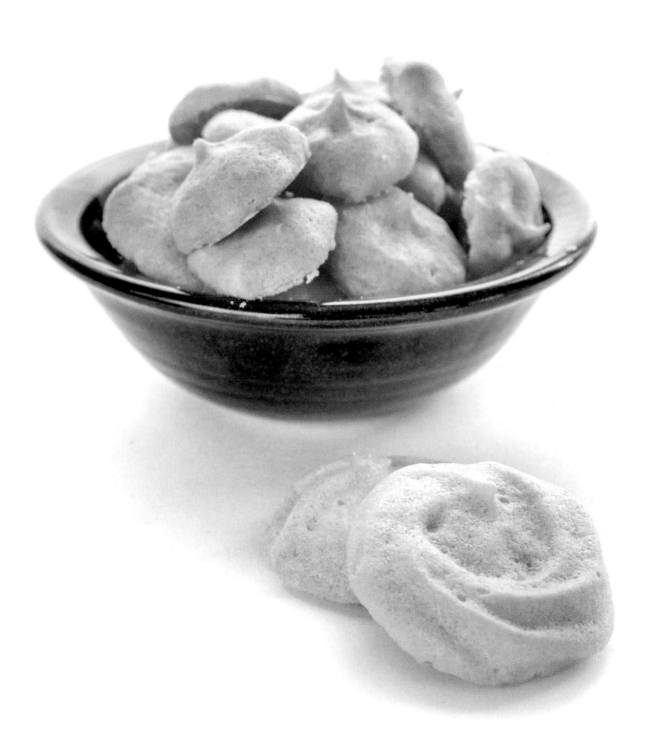

COCONUT MACAROONS

Yield: 16 cookies (1 per serving)   Prep Time: 20 minutes   Cook Time: 35 minutes

These cookies are chewy and coconutty, just like macaroons should be.

¾ cup full-fat coconut milk

½ cup powdered erythritol sweetener

½ teaspoon vanilla extract

¼ teaspoon xanthan gum

2 cups unsweetened shredded coconut

2 large egg whites

¼ teaspoon salt

VARIATION: CHOCOLATE-DIPPED COCONUT MACAROONS.

Place 2 ounces chopped sugar-free dark chocolate and 2 teaspoons coconut oil in a small microwave-safe bowl. Heat on high in 30-second increments, stirring in between, until melted and smooth. Dip the bottoms of the cooled cookies in the melted chocolate and place on a waxed paper–lined baking sheet.

1. In a large saucepan over medium heat, bring the coconut milk to a boil. Reduce the heat to medium-low and cook until reduced and slightly thickened, about 10 minutes.

2. Whisk in the sweetener and vanilla. Sprinkle the surface with the xanthan gum and whisk vigorously to combine. Stir in the shredded coconut and set aside.

3. Preheat the oven to 325°F and line a cookie sheet with parchment paper.

4. In a large bowl, beat the egg whites and salt with an electric mixer until the whites hold stiff peaks. Gently fold in the shredded coconut mixture until well combined.

5. Using about 3 tablespoons per cookie, drop in mounds on the prepared cookie sheet. For a perfect rounded look, use a ¼-cup cookie scoop but fill it only three-quarters full.

6. Bake for 20 to 25 minutes, until barely browned around the edges and just firm to the touch. Remove from the oven and let cool completely on the pan.

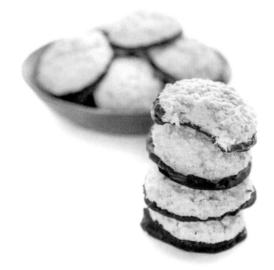

NUTRITIONAL INFORMATION

CALORIES: 120 | FAT: 11.6g | CARBS: 5.1g | FIBER: 2.4g | PROTEIN: 1.6g

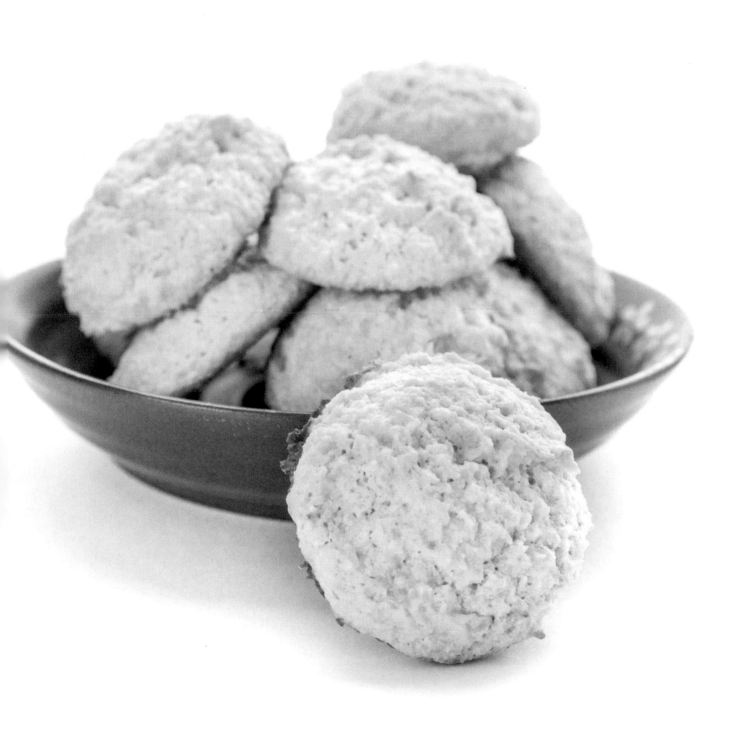

LADYFINGERS

OPTION

Yield: 36 cookies (3 per serving) Prep Time: 25 minutes Cook Time: 17 minutes

These light and airy finger cookies are wonderful on their own and even more wonderful in Classic Tiramisu (page 360).

¾ cup (75g) blanched almond flour

1 tablespoon unflavored whey protein powder

4 large eggs, separated, room temperature

⅛ teaspoon cream of tartar

⅛ teaspoon salt

½ cup granulated erythritol sweetener, divided

½ teaspoon almond or vanilla extract

Powdered erythritol sweetener, for dusting

DAIRY-FREE OPTION:

Replace the whey protein powder with egg white protein powder.

1. Set the oven racks in the middle and second-from-bottom positions. Preheat the oven to 375°F and line two cookie sheets with silicone baking mats or parchment paper. Lightly grease the mat or paper.

2. In a small bowl, whisk together the almond flour and protein powder. Set aside.

3. In a large bowl, use an electric mixer to beat the egg whites with the cream of tartar and salt until foamy. With the mixer running, slowly pour in about ¼ cup of the sweetener. Continue to beat until the egg whites are glossy and hold stiff peaks.

4. In another large bowl, beat the egg yolks with the remaining ¼ cup of sweetener and the extract until thick and pale yellow, 2 to 3 minutes. Beat in the almond flour mixture.

5. Add about one-third of the egg white mixture to the yolk mixture and fold in to lighten it, then fold in the remaining egg whites until no streaks remain.

6. Cut the end off of a piping bag so that the opening is about 1 inch wide. Fill the piping bag with the batter and pipe 3-inch-long lines onto the prepared cookie sheets, about 1 inch apart.

7. Bake for 13 to 17 minutes, until just golden around the edges, switching and rotating the pans halfway through baking. Remove from the oven and let cool completely on the pans before dusting lightly with powdered sweetener.

TIP: *These cookies are delicate, but definitely worth the trouble. Grease the parchment paper or silicone baking mat lightly with a liquid oil or spray. They do like to stick once cool, so use a sharp-edged metal spatula to get underneath them.*

NUTRITIONAL INFORMATION

CALORIES: 68 | FAT: 5g | CARBS: 1.7g | FIBER: 0.8g | PROTEIN: 4g

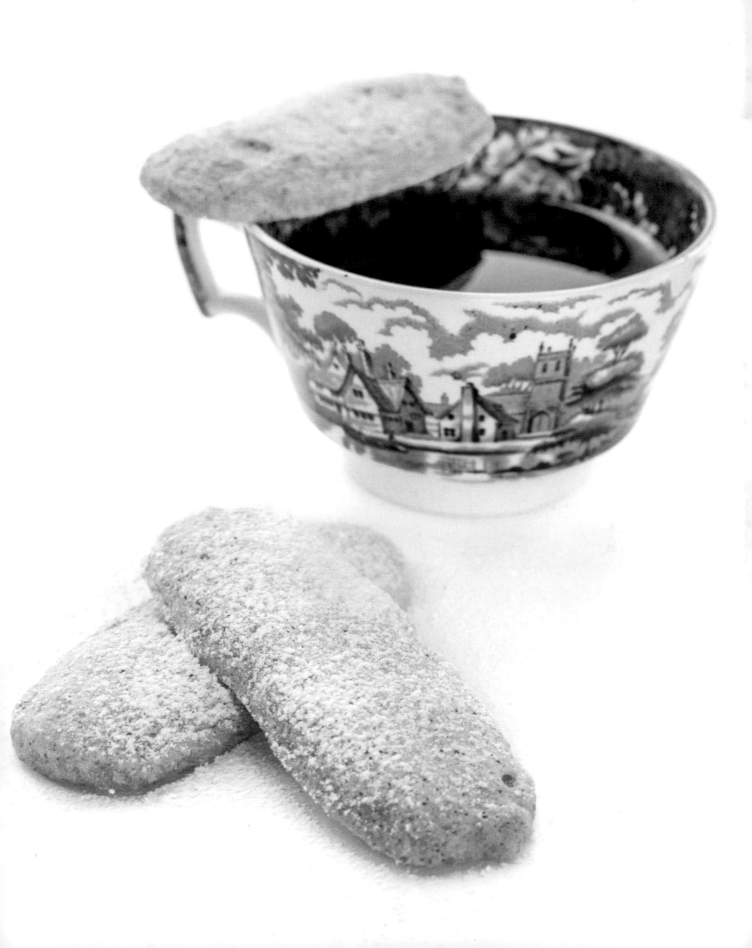

Chapter 8:
BROWNIES & BARS

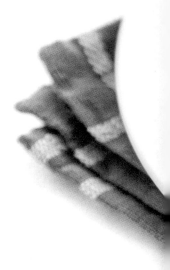

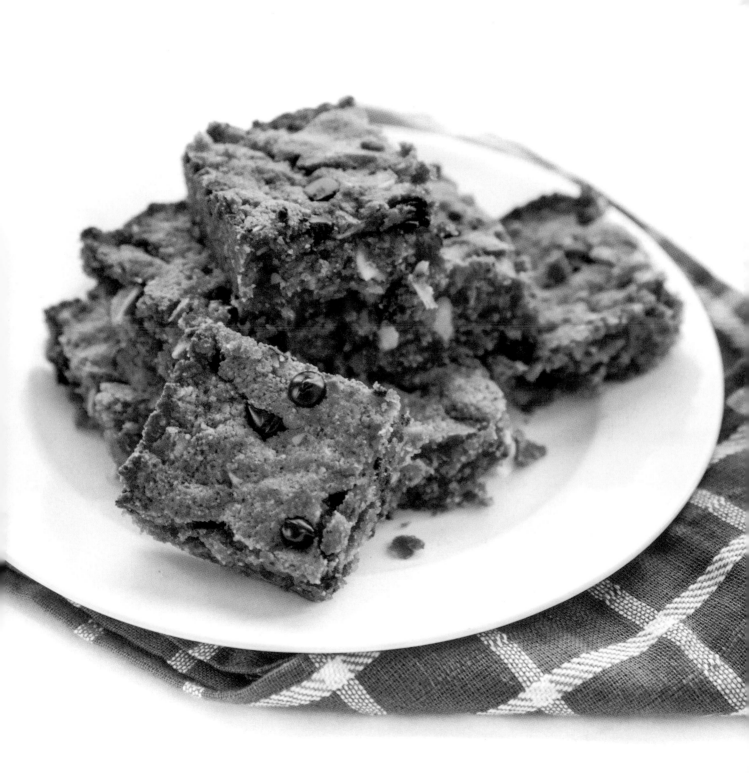

CHEWY KETO BROWNIES

OPTION OPTION

Yield: 16 brownies (1 per serving) **Prep Time:** 10 minutes **Cook Time:** 20 minutes

Once I started adding gelatin to cookies for extra chewiness, I realized it would work in things like brownies as well. It really changes the game for keto baked goods!

⅔ cup granulated sweetener of choice

½ cup (1 stick) unsalted butter, melted

3 large eggs, room temperature

½ teaspoon vanilla extract

½ cup (50g) blanched almond flour

⅓ cup cocoa powder

1 tablespoon grass-fed gelatin (optional)

1 teaspoon baking powder

¼ teaspoon salt

¼ cup water

⅓ cup sugar-free chocolate chips (optional)

1. Preheat the oven to 350°F and grease an 8-inch square baking pan.

2. In a large bowl, whisk together the sweetener, melted butter, eggs, and vanilla.

3. Add the almond flour, cocoa powder, gelatin (if using), baking powder, and salt and whisk until well combined. Stir in the water to thin the batter. Stir in the chocolate chips, if using.

4. Spread the batter in the prepared pan. Bake for 15 to 20 minutes, until the edges are set but the center still seems a tiny bit wet. Remove from the oven and let cool completely in the pan before cutting into bars.

TIPS: *This is a recipe that can handle any sweetener you like. The brownies are meant to be gooey and fudgy.*

The gelatin isn't required, as the brownies will still be tasty and fudgy without it, but I do recommend it. An envelope of unflavored Knox gelatin can sub in if you can't get your hands on the good grass-fed stuff.

DAIRY-FREE OPTION:

Replace the butter with melted ghee or coconut oil.

NUT-FREE OPTION:

Substitute sunflower seed meal or pumpkin seed meal for the almond flour.

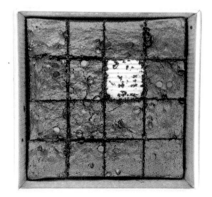

NUTRITIONAL INFORMATION

CALORIES: 110 | FAT: 9.5g | CARBS: 3.6g | FIBER: 2.4g | PROTEIN: 3.1g

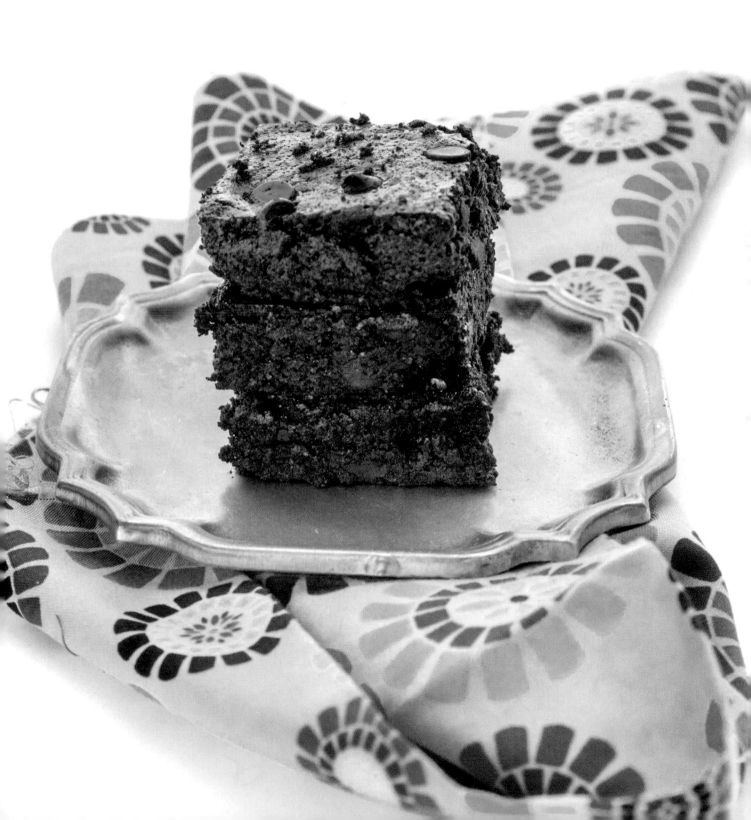

PEANUT BUTTER SWIRL BROWNIES

OPTION OPTION

Yield: 16 brownies (1 per serving) Prep Time: 15 minutes Cook Time: 25 minutes

How do you take the best keto brownies to the next level? By adding peanut butter, of course. Did you even need to ask?

1 recipe Chewy Keto Brownies batter (page 178), without chocolate chips

⅔ cup creamy natural peanut butter

3 tablespoons unsalted butter

3 tablespoons powdered erythritol sweetener

½ teaspoon vanilla extract

DAIRY-FREE OPTION:

Use the dairy-free version of the brownies, and use coconut oil or ghee in place of the butter in the peanut butter swirl.

NUT-FREE OPTION:

Use the nut-free version of the Chewy Keto Brownies.

1. Preheat the oven to 350°F and grease an 8-inch square baking pan.

2. Prepare the brownie batter according to the directions, but without the chocolate chips. Spread the batter in the prepared pan, but don't bake it yet.

3. Place the peanut butter and butter in a microwave-safe bowl. Heat on high in 30-second increments, stirring in between, until melted and smooth. Whisk in the sweetener and vanilla until well combined.

4. Dollop the peanut butter mixture over the brownie batter and swirl with a knife to mix it in. Tap the pan firmly on the counter to even out the batter.

5. Bake for 20 to 25 minutes, until the edges are set but the center still seems a tiny bit wet. Remove from the oven and let cool completely in the pan before cutting into bars.

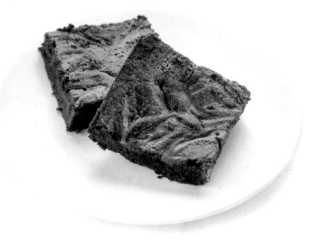

NUTRITIONAL INFORMATION

CALORIES: 176 | FAT: 15.3g | CARBS: 4.4g | FIBER: 1.6g | PROTEIN: 5.1g

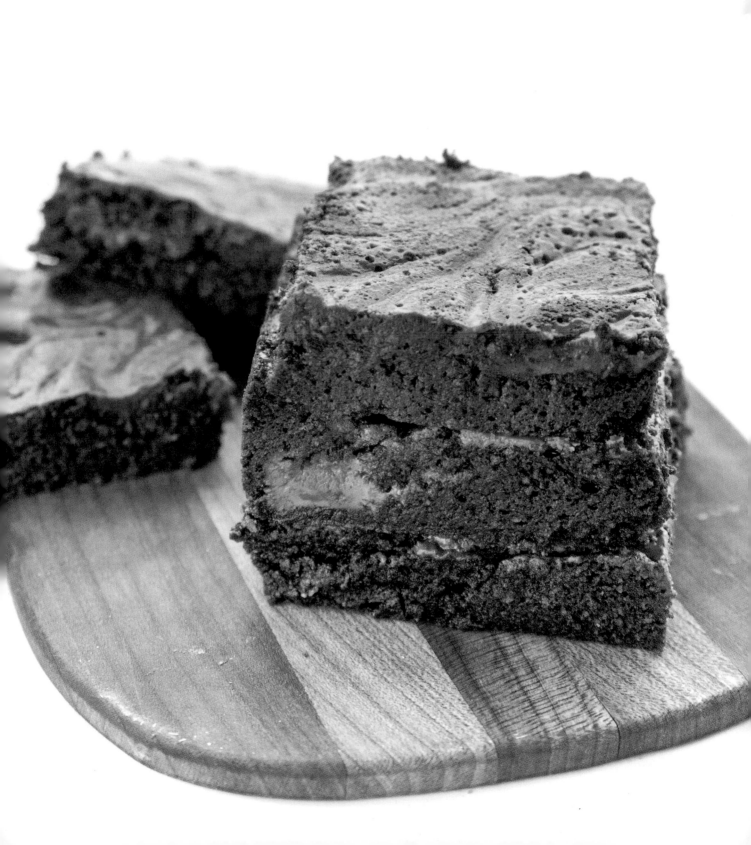

DAIRY-FREE PEPPERMINT PATTY BROWNIES

OPTION

Yield: 16 brownies (1 per serving) Prep Time: 15 minutes, plus 50 minutes to chill Cook Time: 25 minutes

It's like biting into a York Peppermint Patty. No one would ever guess that these brownies are sugar-free and dairy-free.

1 recipe Chewy Keto Brownies (page 178), dairy-free version, without chocolate chips

Filling:

⅔ cup coconut oil, slightly softened

3 tablespoons coconut cream (see tips)

½ cup powdered erythritol sweetener

1½ teaspoons peppermint extract

Topping:

⅓ cup full-fat coconut milk

2 ounces sugar-free dark chocolate, chopped

1. Bake the brownies, without the chocolate chips, as directed, using the dairy-free substitution. Let cool completely in the pan.

2. In a medium bowl, beat the coconut oil and coconut cream with an electric mixer until smooth, then beat in the sweetener and peppermint extract. Spread the filling mixture evenly over the cooled brownies. Refrigerate for 30 minutes.

3. In a small saucepan over medium heat, bring the coconut milk to a boil. Remove from the heat and add the chopped chocolate. Let sit for 4 minutes to melt, then whisk until smooth.

4. Pour the topping over the chilled filling, spreading it to the edges. Refrigerate until set, another 20 minutes or so.

NUT-FREE OPTION:

Use the nut-free version of the Chewy Keto Brownies.

TIPS: *For the coconut cream, simply scoop 3 tablespoons from the thick part at the top of a can of full-fat coconut milk.*

The filling really needs a powdered erythritol-based sweetener to set properly.

NUTRITIONAL INFORMATION

CALORIES: 222 | FAT: 21.7g | CARBS: 5.3g | FIBER: 3.1g | PROTEIN: 3.8g

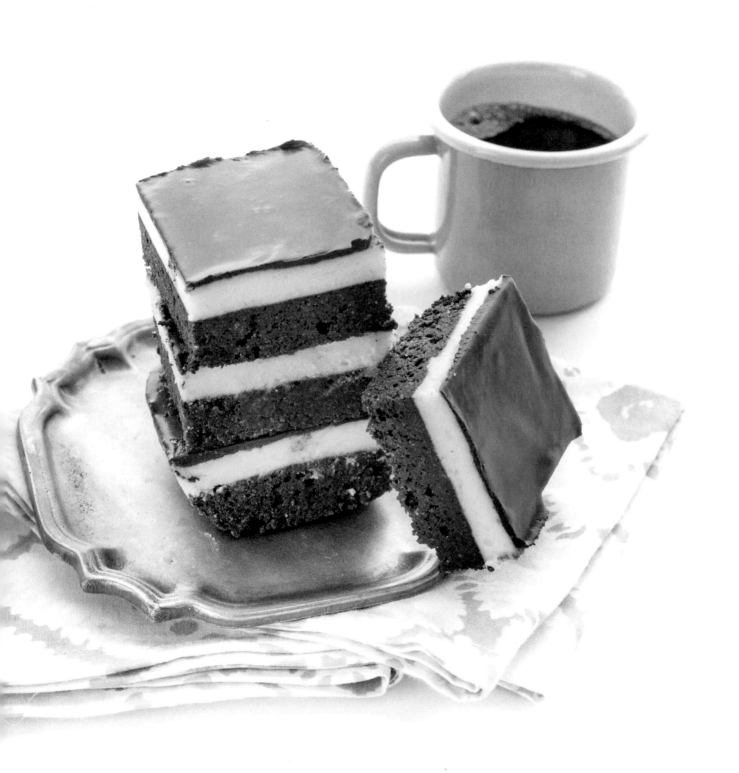

WHITE CHOCOLATE MACADAMIA NUT BLONDIES

OPTION

Yield: 16 blondies (1 per serving) **Prep Time:** 25 minutes **Cook Time:** 25 minutes

---

If you are a white chocolate fan, you're going to love these chewy keto blondies. Since white chocolate is mostly made up of cocoa butter, sugar, and vanilla, I used cocoa butter to mimic that same flavor. But be sure to check out the tips (opposite) for new developments in the keto baking world.

Blondies:

¼ cup (½ stick) unsalted butter

2 ounces cocoa butter, chopped

2 cups (200g) blanched almond flour

½ cup brown sugar substitute

1 tablespoon grass-fed gelatin (optional; adds chewiness)

1 teaspoon baking powder

½ teaspoon salt

½ cup chopped macadamia nuts

1 large egg

½ teaspoon vanilla extract

Drizzle:

1 ounce cocoa butter, chopped

2 tablespoons powdered erythritol sweetener

½ teaspoon vanilla extract

DAIRY-FREE OPTION:

Substitute coconut oil or ghee for the butter. Coconut oil will have a stronger flavor.

TO MAKE THE BLONDIES:

1. Preheat the oven to 325°F and grease an 8-inch square baking pan.

2. In a small microwave-safe bowl, heat the butter and cocoa butter on high in 30-second increments, stirring in between, until melted. Set aside to cool. Alternatively, you can melt them in a heatproof bowl set over a pan of barely simmering water.

3. In a large bowl, whisk together the almond flour, brown sugar substitute, gelatin (if using), baking powder, and salt. Stir in the nuts. Stir in the melted butters, egg, and vanilla until the batter comes together.

4. Spread the batter evenly in the prepared pan and smooth the top. Bake for 20 to 25 minutes, until the edges are just golden and the center is just firm to the touch. Remove from the oven and let cool completely in the pan before cutting into bars.

TO MAKE THE DRIZZLE:

5. Gently melt the cocoa butter in a microwave-safe bowl on high in 30-second increments or in a heatproof bowl set over a pan of barely simmering water. Let cool to lukewarm.

6. Whisk in the sweetener and vanilla until smooth. Immediately drizzle over the cooled bars.

NUTRITIONAL INFORMATION

CALORIES: 191 | FAT: 18.1g | CARBS: 3.7g | FIBER: 1.9g | PROTEIN: 4.1g

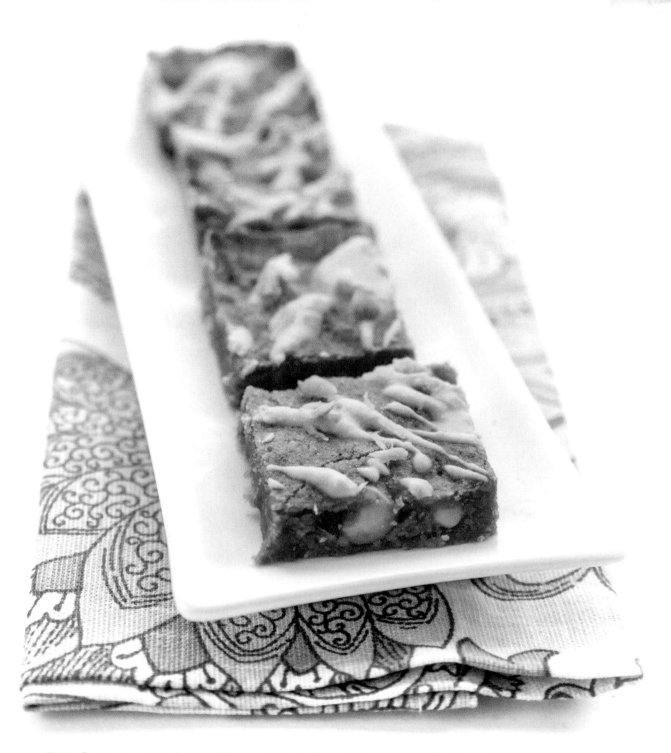

TIPS: *Cocoa butter can be a bit finicky to work with. It doesn't like to combine with other oils or sweeteners and can separate out. For the drizzle, let it cool quite a bit before adding the sweetener.*

When I first developed this recipe, there were no good keto-friendly white chocolate chips on the market. But lo and behold, a few months later, not one but two brands came out with them (see page 402). I've only tried the Bake Believe brand as yet, but they melt nicely and would be perfect for the drizzle in this recipe. I recommend melting them double boiler–style with a little cocoa butter for smoothness.

BUTTERSCOTCH BARS

Yield: 16 bars (1 per serving) **Prep Time:** 20 minutes **Cook Time:** 25 minutes

Most conventional recipes for butterscotch bars call for butterscotch chips, but that's not an option on a keto diet. So I went full steam ahead for *real* butterscotch flavor, with tons of butter and "brown sugar."

½ cup (1 stick) unsalted butter

½ cup brown sugar substitute

¼ cup Bocha Sweet or allulose (see tips)

½ cup heavy whipping cream

1 teaspoon butterscotch or caramel flavoring (see tips)

½ teaspoon salt

1 large egg

1 large egg yolk

1¾ cups (175g) blanched almond flour

1 teaspoon baking powder

⅓ cup sugar-free chocolate chips

1. In a large deep saucepan over medium heat, melt the butter with the sweeteners, stirring until combined. Bring to a boil and cook for 3 minutes, until the mixture is a dark amber color.

2. Remove from the heat and add the cream. The mixture will bubble vigorously. Whisk in the butterscotch flavoring and salt and let cool to lukewarm, about 10 minutes.

3. Preheat the oven to 325°F and grease an 8-inch square baking pan.

4. Whisk the whole egg and egg yolk into the cooled butterscotch, then whisk in the almond flour and baking powder. Stir in the chocolate chips.

5. Spread the batter in the prepared pan and bake for 20 minutes. Remove from the oven and let cool completely in the pan before cutting into bars.

TIPS: *For the real gooeyness of butterscotch bars, a mix of sweeteners is the best approach here. You want a brown sugar substitute for most of it, plus a sweetener that keeps things softer, such as Bocha Sweet or allulose. If you can do only erythritol-based sweeteners, the bars will still be delicious.*

Butterscotch flavoring isn't always easy to find, so you can use caramel flavoring or even vanilla extract here instead. See page 402 for where to find natural and keto-friendly flavorings.

SERVING SUGGESTION: *Drizzle with a little caramel sauce (page 388) for an extra-special treat.*

NUTRITIONAL INFORMATION

CALORIES: 177 | FAT: 16g | CARBS: 4.7g | FIBER: 2.7g | PROTEIN: 3.7g

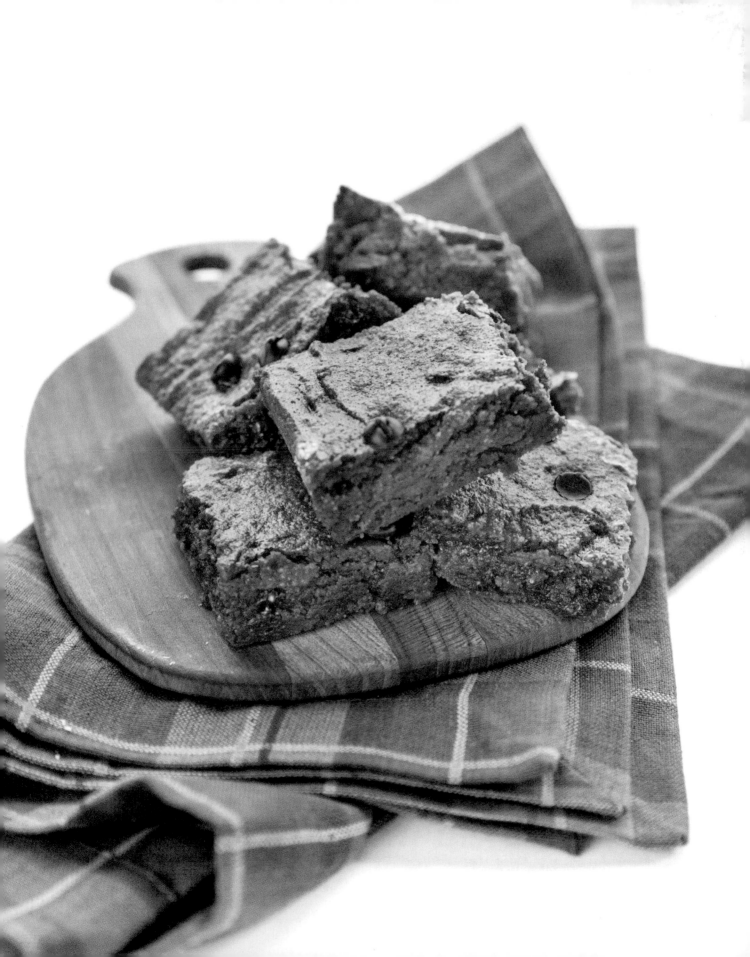

ZUCCHINI SPICE BARS WITH BROWN BUTTER GLAZE

Yield: 16 bars (1 per serving) Prep Time: 10 minutes, plus 1 hour to drain zucchini Cook Time: 40 minutes

Zucchini is a wonderfully versatile vegetable, playing as well with sweet flavors as it does with savory.

Bars:

1 cup lightly packed shredded zucchini

½ teaspoon salt, divided

⅔ cup (73g) coconut flour

½ cup granulated sweetener of choice

2 teaspoons baking powder

1 teaspoon ground cinnamon

½ teaspoon ginger powder

⅛ teaspoon ground cloves

3 large eggs

¼ cup (½ stick) unsalted butter, melted but not hot

¼ cup water

½ teaspoon vanilla extract

Glaze:

¼ cup (½ stick) unsalted butter

¾ cup powdered erythritol sweetener

3 tablespoons heavy whipping cream, room temperature

TO MAKE THE BARS:

1. Place the zucchini in a sieve in the sink or over a bowl. Sprinkle with ¼ teaspoon of the salt and toss to combine. Let drain for 1 hour, then squeeze out as much moisture as possible.

2. Preheat the oven to 325°F and grease a 9-inch square baking pan.

3. In a large bowl, whisk together the coconut flour, granulated sweetener, baking powder, cinnamon, ginger, cloves, and remaining ¼ teaspoon of salt. Add the drained zucchini, eggs, melted butter, water, and vanilla and stir until well combined.

4. Spread the batter evenly in the prepared baking pan. Bake for 30 to 35 minutes, until golden brown around the edges and just firm to the touch on top. Remove from the oven and let cool completely in the pan.

TO MAKE THE GLAZE:

5. Melt the butter in a medium saucepan over medium heat until it browns and becomes fragrant, about 4 minutes. Remove from the heat and let cool for at least 10 minutes, until lukewarm.

6. Place the powdered sweetener in a medium bowl and slowly pour in the browned butter, whisking to combine. Add the cream and beat until a spreadable consistency is achieved.

7. Spread the glaze over the cooled bars.

TIPS: *Do not add the browned butter to the sweetener while it's still hot, or it will clump like crazy. The browned butter should be cooled to lukewarm before being added, but don't let it resolidify.*

You can also use an 8-inch square baking pan, but the bars will take longer to cook through.

NUTRITIONAL INFORMATION

CALORIES: 100 | FAT: 7.8g | CARBS: 3.4g | FIBER: 1.9g | PROTEIN: 2.1g

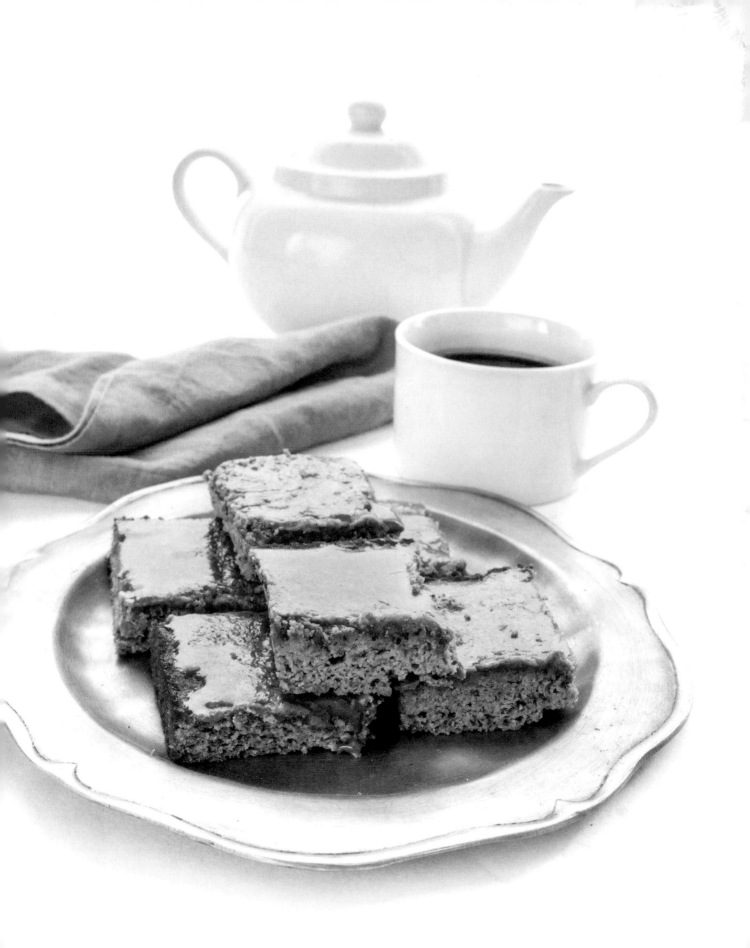

MAPLE WALNUT BARS

Yield: 16 bars (1 per serving) Prep Time: 15 minutes Cook Time: 45 minutes

Maple walnut is one of my favorite flavor combinations. These bars have a delicious shortbread crust and a rich maple-scented filling.

1 recipe Shortbread Crust (page 372)

½ cup (1 stick) unsalted butter

⅓ cup brown sugar substitute (see tips)

⅓ cup Bocha Sweet or allulose

½ cup heavy whipping cream

1½ teaspoons maple extract

2 large eggs

¼ teaspoon salt

1½ cups coarsely chopped walnuts

1. Preheat the oven to 325°F.

2. Prepare the shortbread crust according to the directions and press firmly and evenly into the bottom of an 8-inch square baking pan. Par-bake for 12 to 15 minutes, until just golden brown around the edges. Remove from the oven and let cool in the pan while you prepare the filling.

3. In a medium saucepan over low heat, melt the butter. Stir in the sweeteners and continue to whisk until they have dissolved. Remove the pan from the heat and whisk in the cream and maple extract.

4. Add the eggs and salt and whisk until fully combined.

5. Scatter the walnuts over the crust, then pour the maple filling on top. Shake the pan from side to side a bit to spread the filling over the crust.

6. Bake for 25 to 30 minutes, until the filling is mostly set but still jiggles a little in the middle. Remove from the oven and let cool in the pan for at least 30 minutes before cutting into bars.

TIPS: *Once again, a combination of sweeteners gives the best results here, especially for the filling. Bocha Sweet or allulose will help keep it gooier, and a brown sugar substitute will give it more color and richness. I highly recommend Swerve Brown here, as it has a bit of a maple flavor on its own.*

One of my recipe testers had only an 8-inch square glass baking dish. She found that she needed to bake the crust for 25 minutes and the filling for 30-plus minutes, and even then, the bars were a bit too soft. This supports my idea that keto baked goods need to bake longer in glass and ceramic than they do in metal. Find more on why metal pans are preferred on page 16.

NUTRITIONAL INFORMATION

CALORIES: 236 | FAT: 22g | CARBS: 3.3g | FIBER: 1.7g | PROTEIN: 5.7g

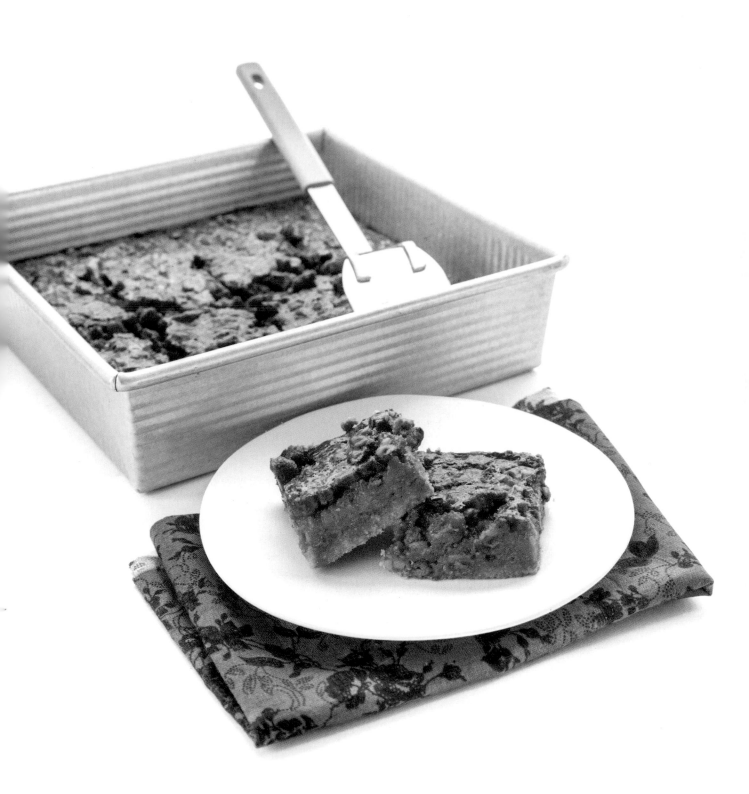

CLASSIC LEMON BARS

OPTION

Yield: 16 bars (1 per serving) Prep Time: 20 minutes Cook Time: 50 minutes

Lemon bars are a classic treat, and these stay true to the original, with a shortbread crust and a tangy sweet filling.

1 recipe Shortbread Crust (page 372)

3 large eggs

2 large egg yolks

¼ cup granulated erythritol sweetener

¼ cup Bocha Sweet or allulose (see tip)

½ teaspoon salt

1 teaspoon grated lemon zest

⅓ cup fresh lemon juice

2 tablespoons coconut flour

Powdered erythritol sweetener, for garnish

Thinly sliced lemon wedges, for garnish (optional)

DAIRY-FREE OPTION:

Use the dairy-free version of the crust.

1. Preheat the oven to 325°F and line an 8-inch square baking pan with parchment paper or foil, leaving some overhanging the sides for easier removal.

2. Prepare the shortbread crust according to the directions and press firmly and evenly into the bottom of the prepared pan. Par-bake for 12 to 15 minutes, until just golden brown around the edges. Remove from the oven and let cool while you prepare the filling.

3. In a large bowl, whisk together the whole eggs, egg yolks, sweeteners, and salt until the mixture turns a pale yellow, about 2 minutes. Whisk in the lemon zest and juice until well combined.

4. Slowly sift the coconut flour over the filling mixture, whisking frequently to combine. Pour the filling over the cooled crust.

5. Bake for 30 to 35 minutes, until the filling is set but isn't browned at all. Remove from the oven and let cool completely in the pan before lifting out with the overhanging parchment or foil.

6. Dust lightly with powdered sweetener and cut into bars. Garnish each bar with a thin lemon wedge, if desired.

TIP: *This filling is quite custardlike, so a combination of sweeteners can help keep recrystallization to a minimum. However, you can use all Swerve or another erythritol-based sweetener if you like. Several of my recipe testers did so and loved the result.*

NUTRITIONAL INFORMATION
CALORIES: 219 | FAT: 20.8g | CARBS: 2.9g | FIBER: 1.3g | PROTEIN: 3.7g

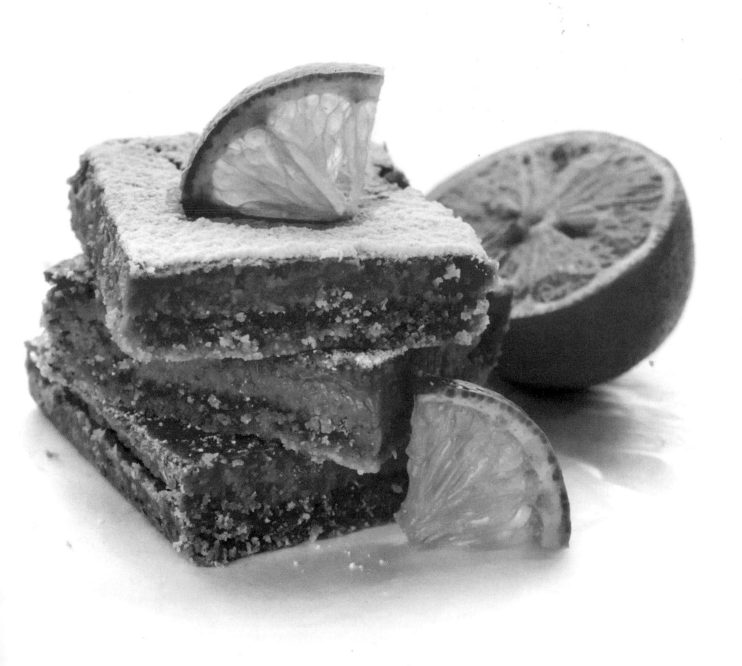

MAGIC COOKIE BARS

Yield: 16 bars (1 per serving) **Prep Time:** 15 minutes (not including time to make condensed milk) **Cook Time:** 50 minutes

Magic Cookie Bars, Seven-Layer Bars, or Hello Dollies—whatever you called them back in the day, you now have a healthy keto version. Gooey and delicious!

1 recipe Shortbread Crust (page 372)

⅓ cup sugar-free chocolate chips

½ cup unsweetened flaked coconut

½ cup chopped pecans or walnuts

1 recipe Keto Sweetened Condensed Milk (page 386)

1. Preheat the oven to 325°F.

2. Prepare the shortbread crust according to the directions and press firmly and evenly into the bottom of an 8-inch square baking pan. Par-bake for 12 to 15 minutes, until just golden brown around the edges. Remove from the oven and let cool completely.

3. Increase the oven temperature to 350°F.

4. Sprinkle the cooled crust with the chocolate chips, coconut, and nuts. Pour the sweetened condensed milk over the top and bake for 25 to 35 minutes, until the mixture is bubbly and beginning to brown.

5. Remove from the oven and let cool completely in the pan before cutting into bars.

TIP: *If you made the condensed milk ahead and refrigerated it, let it come to room temperature before pouring it over the cooled crust.*

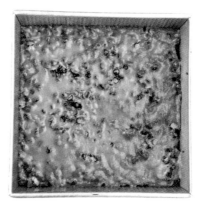

NUTRITIONAL INFORMATION

CALORIES: 232 | FAT: 21.8g | CARBS: 5.4g | FIBER: 3g | PROTEIN: 4.2g

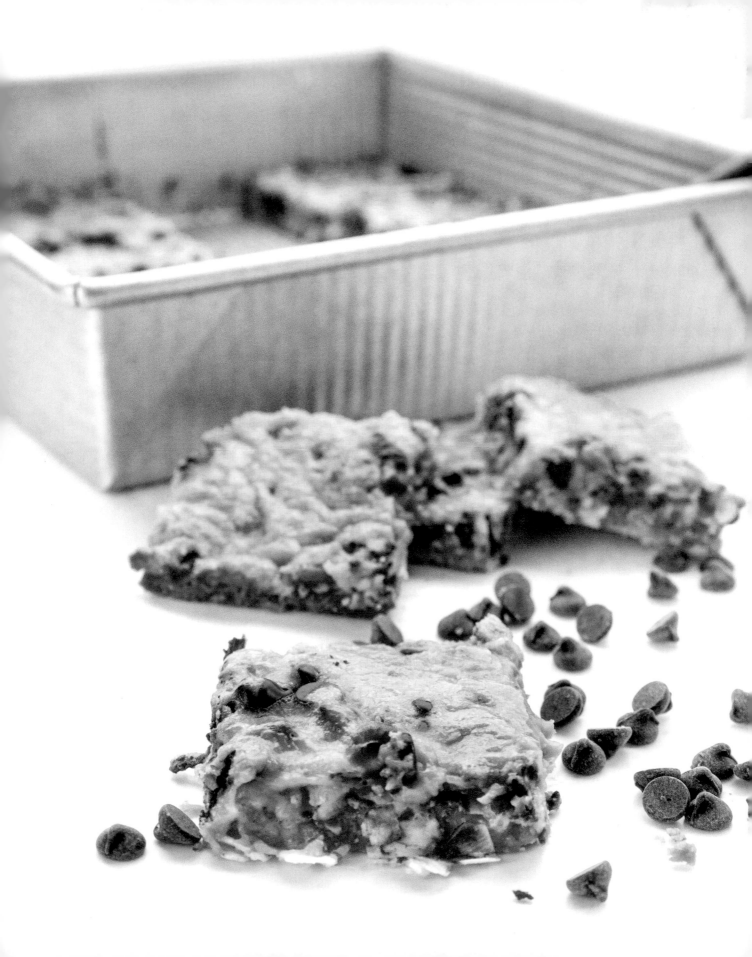

KEY LIME PIE BARS

Yield: 16 bars (1 per serving) Prep Time: 20 minutes, plus 1 hour to chill (not including time to make condensed milk)
Cook Time: 35 minutes

Creamy and tangy, these Key lime pie bars really satisfy that urge for the classic Floridian treat.

1 recipe Shortbread Crust (page 372)

3 ounces cream cheese, softened

2 teaspoons grated Key lime zest

4 large egg yolks, room temperature

1 cup Keto Sweetened Condensed Milk (page 386)

6 tablespoons Key lime juice (see tip)

1. Preheat the oven to 325°F.

2. Prepare the shortbread crust according to the directions and press firmly and evenly into the bottom of an 8-inch square baking pan. Par-bake for 12 to 15 minutes, until just golden brown around the edges. Remove from the oven and let cool while you prepare the filling.

3. In a large bowl, beat the cream cheese and lime zest with an electric mixer until smooth. Beat in the egg yolks until well combined. Slowly beat in the condensed milk and lime juice until the filling mixture is smooth.

4. Spread the filling over the cooled crust and bake for 18 to 20 minutes, watching carefully to make sure it doesn't brown at all. Remove from the oven and let cool completely in the pan, then refrigerate for 1 hour to firm up before cutting into bars.

TIP: *Key limes are so little that it can take quite a few to get enough juice. Feel free to cheat with regular limes!*

SERVING SUGGESTION: *Top the bars with lightly sweetened whipped cream, grated lime zest, and/or lime slices, if desired.*

NUTRITIONAL INFORMATION
CALORIES: 188 | FAT: 17.5g | CARBS: 3.4g | FIBER: 1g | PROTEIN: 3.4g

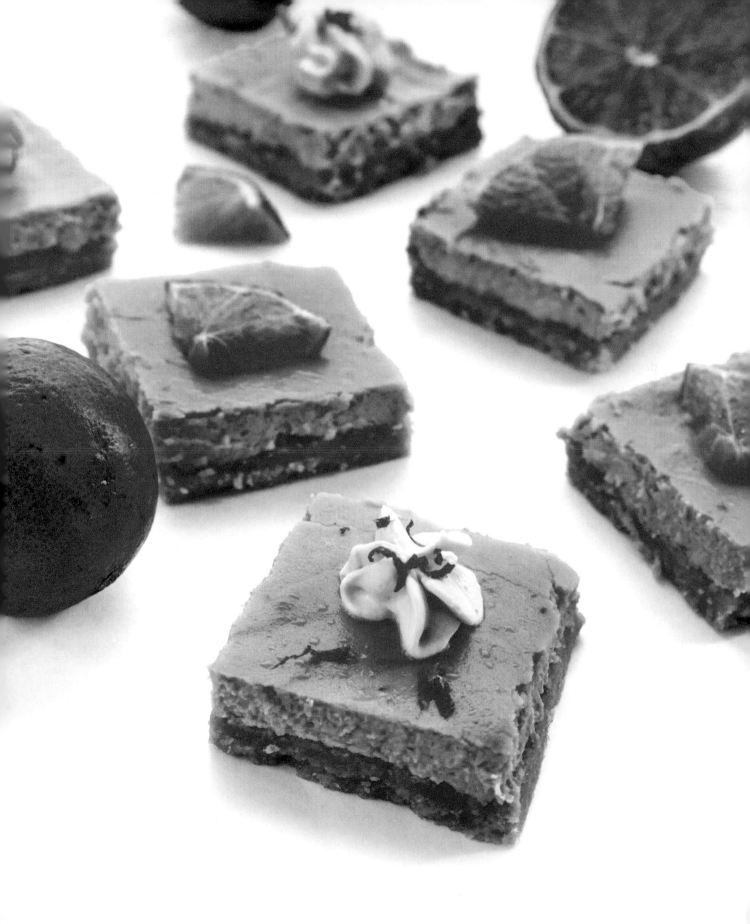

DAIRY-FREE COCONUT CARAMEL BARS

Yield: 16 bars (1 per serving) Prep Time: 20 minutes, plus 1 hour to cool Cook Time: 30 minutes

Delicious dairy-free caramel with toasted coconut and chocolate on a shortbread crust. These delicious bars are reminiscent of the famous Girl Scout Samoa Cookies.

1 recipe Shortbread Crust (page 372), dairy-free version

4 ounces sugar-free dark chocolate, chopped

5 tablespoons coconut oil, divided

1½ cups unsweetened shredded coconut

¼ cup brown sugar substitute

¼ cup Bocha Sweet or allulose (see tips)

¾ cup full-fat coconut milk

½ teaspoon vanilla extract

¼ teaspoon salt

TIPS: *Unlike using butter to make dairy-based caramel, coconut oil won't necessarily come to a boil and darken in the first stage. So just cook it for the length of time stated rather than waiting for it to do something it may not do.*

For the sweeteners, a combination of a brown sugar substitute and a sweetener that stays softer is going to give you the best results and make these bars gooier. But, if you need to use all erythritol-based sweetener, they will still be delicious.

1. Preheat the oven to 325°F.

2. Prepare the shortbread crust according to the directions and press firmly and evenly into the bottom of an 8-inch square baking pan. Par-bake for 12 to 15 minutes, until just golden brown around the edges. Remove from the oven and let cool while you prepare the chocolate filling.

3. In a small microwave-safe bowl, heat the chocolate and 2 tablespoons of the coconut oil on high in 30-second increments, stirring in between, until melted and smooth. Alternatively, you can melt them double boiler–style in a heatproof bowl set over a pan of barely simmering water.

4. Spread about two-thirds of the melted chocolate mixture over the cooled crust. Set the remainder aside for the top.

5. Spread the shredded coconut in a medium skillet and set over medium heat. Toast, stirring frequently, until light golden brown. Set aside.

6. Place the remaining 3 tablespoons of coconut oil and the sweeteners in a large saucepan over medium heat. Stir until the oil is melted and the sweeteners have dissolved, then continue to cook for another 3 minutes.

7. Remove the pan from the heat and add the coconut milk, vanilla, and salt. The mixture may bubble up quite a bit.

8. Stir in the toasted coconut. Spread the mixture over the chocolate-covered crust. Let cool completely (about 1 hour) before cutting into bars.

9. Gently reheat the remaining chocolate mixture and drizzle over the bars.

NUTRITIONAL INFORMATION
CALORIES: 219 | FAT: 22g | CARBS: 7g | FIBER: 3.4g | PROTEIN: 2.9g

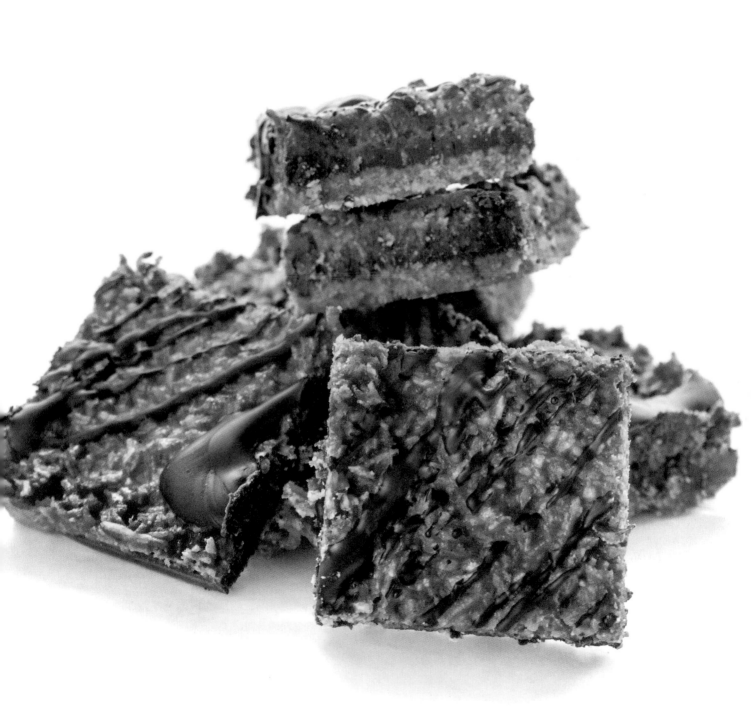

DAIRY-FREE FUDGE CRUMB BARS

Yield: 16 bars (1 per serving) Prep Time: 20 minutes, plus 1 hour to chill Cook Time: 26 minutes

With a crumbly oatmeal-like crust and a fudgy dairy-free filling, these bars are seriously decadent!

Crust:

1¼ cups (125g) blanched almond flour

⅓ cup unsweetened shredded coconut

⅓ cup brown sugar substitute

¼ teaspoon salt

¼ cup melted coconut oil

1 to 2 tablespoons water

Filling:

1 cup full-fat canned coconut milk

3 ounces unsweetened chocolate, chopped

½ cup powdered erythritol sweetener

½ teaspoon vanilla extract

¼ teaspoon glucomannan or xanthan gum

1. Preheat the oven to 325°F.

2. In a large bowl, whisk together the almond flour, shredded coconut, brown sugar substitute, and salt. Stir in the melted coconut oil until well combined.

3. Add 1 tablespoon of water and mix until combined. The mixture should be crumbly but hold together a bit when you squeeze it. If it does not, add another tablespoon of water.

4. Press about two-thirds of the crust mixture into the bottom of an 8-inch square baking pan and par-bake for 8 minutes. Remove from the oven and let cool while you prepare the filling.

5. Heat the coconut milk in a large saucepan over medium-low heat until just simmering. Remove from the heat and add the chocolate. Let sit for 5 minutes to melt.

6. Add the powdered sweetener and vanilla and whisk until smooth. Sprinkle the surface with the glucomannan and whisk to combine. Pour the filling over the crust.

7. Sprinkle the remaining crust mixture over the top of the filling and press lightly into the filling. Bake for another 15 to 18 minutes, until the top crust is light golden brown.

8. Remove from the oven and let cool completely, then chill for 1 hour to set before cutting into bars.

TIP: *You really do need to add a thickener here, such as glucomannan or xanthan gum. It will help stabilize the filling so it doesn't goo all over the place.*

NUTRITIONAL INFORMATION

CALORIES: 156 | FAT: 14.5g | CARBS: 4.2g | FIBER: 2g | PROTEIN: 3g

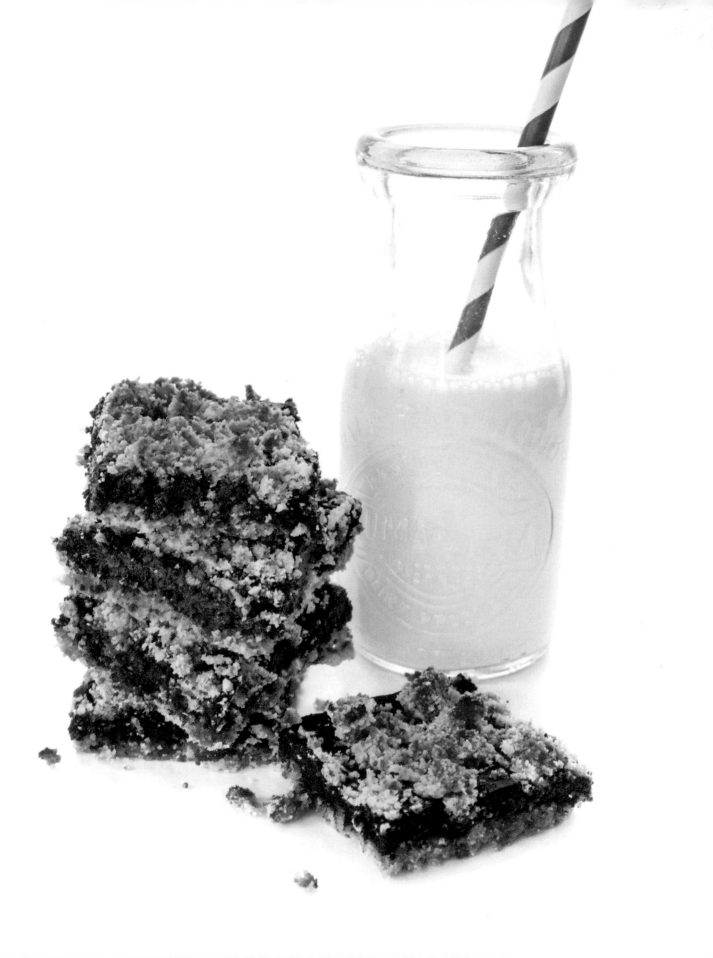

FLAG SUGAR COOKIE BARS

Yield: 16 bars (1 per serving) **Prep Time:** 25 minutes (not including time to make frosting) **Cook Time:** 15 minutes

Get all patriotic *and* healthy with these cute little bars. They're fun and easy to make. And a shout-out to my fellow Canucks: you could just use red berries and decorate it as a Canadian flag, too.

Crust:

2 cups (200g) blanched almond flour

½ cup granulated erythritol sweetener

¼ cup (28g) coconut flour

1 teaspoon baking powder

½ teaspoon salt

1 large egg

½ cup (1 stick) unsalted butter, melted

½ teaspoon vanilla extract

Toppings:

½ recipe Cream Cheese Frosting (page 380)

⅓ cup fresh blueberries

½ cup fresh raspberries

6 medium-sized fresh strawberries, sliced

TO MAKE THE CRUST:

1. Preheat the oven to 325°F and place a silicone baking mat or a large piece of parchment paper on a work surface.

2. In a large bowl, whisk together the almond flour, sweetener, coconut flour, baking powder, and salt. Stir in the egg, melted butter, and vanilla until the dough comes together.

3. Transfer the dough to the prepared work surface and pat into a rough rectangle. Cover with a piece of parchment paper and roll out to 9 by 11 inches (about ¼ inch thick). Remove the top piece of parchment.

4. Transfer the baking mat or parchment paper to a cookie sheet and bake for 12 to 15 minutes, until the edges are just golden brown. Remove from the oven and let cool completely.

TO ADD THE TOPPINGS:

5. Spread the frosting evenly over the cooled crust, leaving a ½-inch border.

6. In the upper-left corner, arrange the blueberries in a square. Then arrange the raspberries and strawberries in alternating horizontal rows.

NUTRITIONAL INFORMATION

CALORIES: 203 | FAT: 18g | CARBS: 5.7g | FIBER: 2.5g | PROTEIN: 4.3g

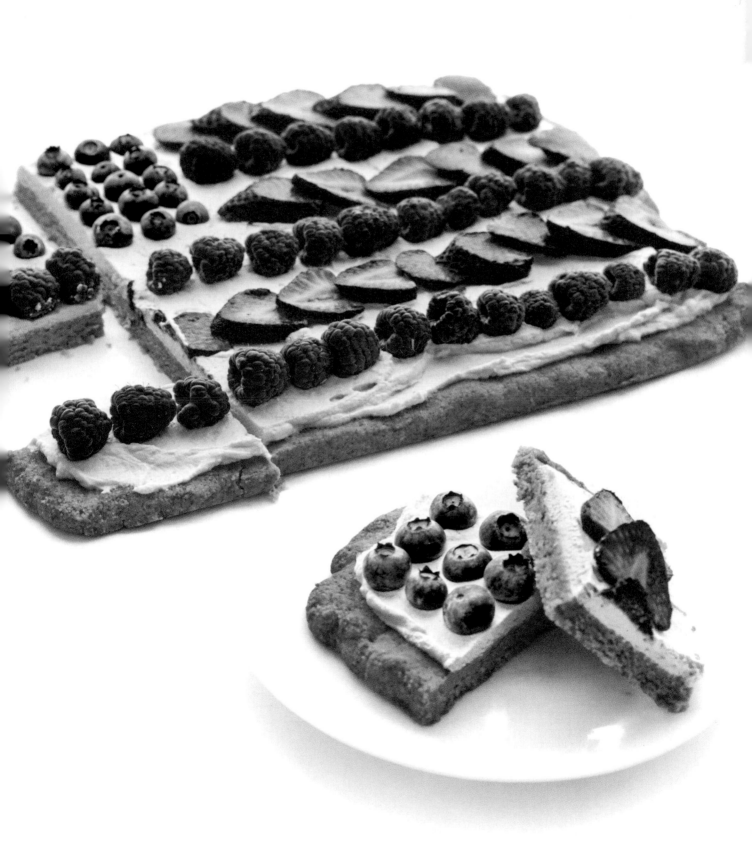

TRIPLE CHOCOLATE CHEESECAKE BARS

OPTION

Yield: 16 bars (1 per serving)   Prep Time: 30 minutes, plus 3 hours to chill bars and 30 minutes to set glaze   Cook Time: 52 minutes

Heavenly chocolate cheesecake squares. Enough said!

1 recipe Keto Chocolate Pie Crust (page 370)

1 tablespoon unsalted butter

2 ounces unsweetened chocolate, chopped

2 (8-ounce) packages cream cheese, softened

¾ cup powdered erythritol sweetener (see tip)

1 teaspoon vanilla extract

2 large eggs, room temperature

¼ cup cocoa powder

¼ cup heavy whipping cream, room temperature

1 recipe Easy Chocolate Glaze (page 390)

NUT-FREE OPTION:

Use the nut-free version of the crust.

1. Preheat the oven to 325°F.

2. Prepare the chocolate crust according to the directions and press firmly into the bottom of an 8-inch square baking pan. Par-bake for 12 minutes, then remove from the oven and reduce the oven temperature to 300°F. Let the crust cool while you prepare the filling.

3. In a small saucepan over low heat, melt the butter and chocolate, stirring until smooth.

4. In a large bowl, beat the cream cheese and sweetener with an electric mixer until well combined. Beat in the vanilla, then beat in the eggs one at a time, scraping down the sides of the bowl and the beaters as needed.

5. Add the cocoa powder and melted chocolate mixture and beat until smooth. The mixture may be very thick at this point. Add the cream and mix slowly to avoid splashing, then increase the speed and beat until just combined.

6. Lightly grease the sides of the baking pan, taking care not to disturb the crust. Pour the cheesecake filling over the crust and bake for 30 to 40 minutes, until the sides are set but the center still jiggles slightly. Remove from the oven and let cool completely, then refrigerate for at least 3 hours.

7. Prepare the glaze and pour it over the completely chilled cheesecake, spreading it to the edges with an offset spatula. Let set for about 30 minutes before cutting into squares.

TIP: *You can use powdered Swerve here, or you can use a 50/50 combination of Swerve and Bocha Sweet or allulose. Using a combination of sweeteners helps keep the filling softer and less likely to recrystallize.*

NUTRITIONAL INFORMATION

CALORIES: 276 | FAT: 23.7g | CARBS: 7g | FIBER: 3.1g | PROTEIN: 6.1g

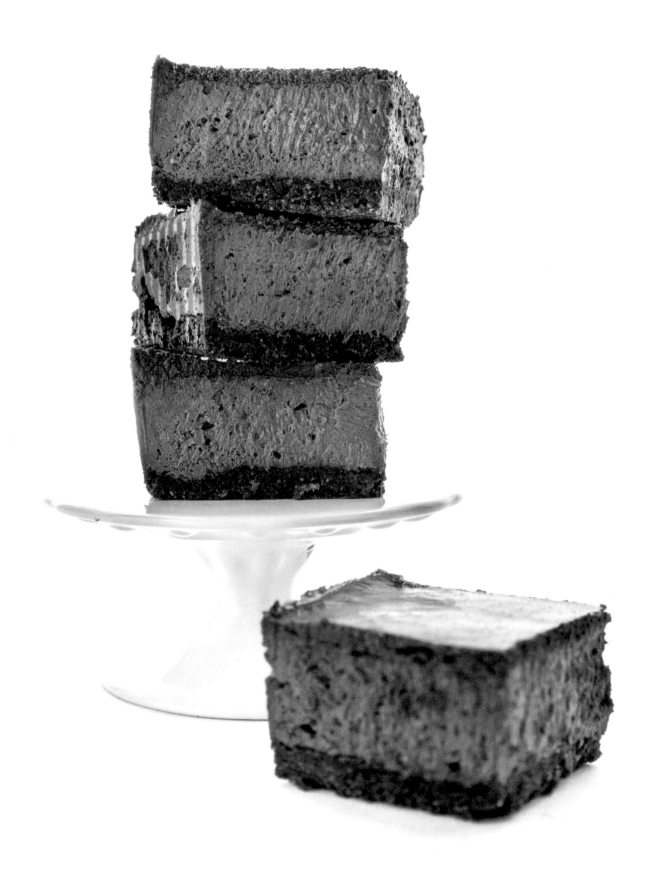

GRANOLA BARS

Yield: 12 bars (1 per serving) Prep Time: 15 minutes Cook Time: 35 minutes

My family has always loved granola bars, and now we can enjoy them again, keto style. That makes this snacking mama very happy.

1 cup unsweetened flaked coconut

1 cup almonds

½ cup pecan halves

½ cup shelled pumpkin seeds

2 tablespoons grass-fed collagen peptides (optional)

½ teaspoon salt

½ cup (1 stick) unsalted butter

2 tablespoons brown sugar substitute

⅓ cup powdered erythritol sweetener (see tips)

½ teaspoon vanilla extract

1. Preheat the oven to 300°F and line an 8-inch square baking pan with parchment paper, leaving some overhanging the sides for easier removal.

2. Place the coconut, almonds, pecans, and pumpkin seeds in a food processor and grind until the mixture resembles coarse crumbs with some larger chunks. Add the collagen (if using) and salt and pulse a few times to combine.

3. In a large saucepan, melt the butter and brown sugar substitute, whisking until smooth and the sweetener has mostly dissolved. Remove the pan from the heat and stir in the powdered sweetener and vanilla until well combined.

4. Add the nut mixture to the saucepan and stir until well coated. Press the mixture firmly and evenly into the bottom of the prepared pan, pressing down with a flat-bottomed glass.

5. Bake for 25 to 30 minutes, until golden brown. Remove from the oven and let cool completely in the pan, then use the parchment paper to lift the granola mixture out of the pan and cut into bars.

TIPS: *Do not—I repeat, do NOT—use Bocha Sweet or allulose in this recipe. I tried that and ended up with delicious granola goo that I could hardly pick up. This recipe needs erythritol to firm up properly.*

The collagen helps hold the bars together as they bake and cool. I highly recommend it.

NUTRITIONAL INFORMATION

CALORIES: 239 | FAT: 21.4g | CARBS: 5.1g | FIBER: 2.9g | PROTEIN: 7g

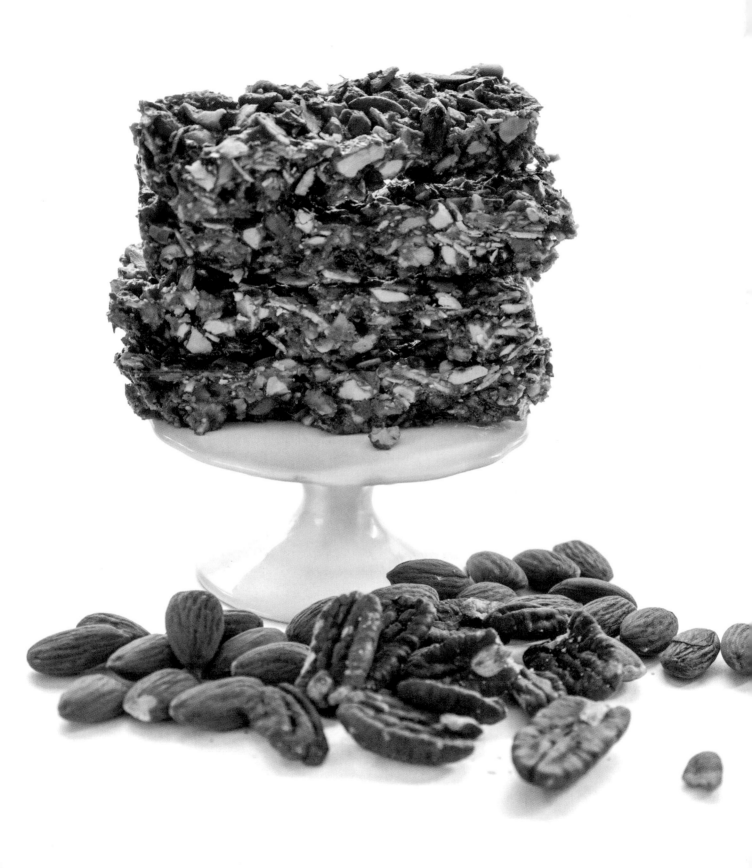

PEANUT BUTTER "OATMEAL" BARS

OPTION BEG

Yield: 16 bars (1 per serving) Prep Time: 20 minutes Cook Time: 25 minutes

No oats were hurt in the making of these "oatmeal" bars. I've found that grinding up coconut and sliced almonds creates a very oatmeal-like consistency. These bars can be breakfast or dessert.

¾ cup unsweetened flaked coconut

½ cup sliced almonds

½ cup creamy natural peanut butter

¼ cup (½ stick) unsalted butter

½ cup brown sugar substitute

2 large eggs, room temperature

½ teaspoon vanilla extract

1 cup (100g) blanched almond flour

1 teaspoon baking powder

¼ teaspoon salt

⅓ cup sugar-free chocolate chips

1. Preheat the oven to 325°F and grease an 8-inch square baking pan.

2. In a food processor, grind the coconut and sliced almonds until the mixture resembles oats.

3. In a large microwave-safe bowl, heat the peanut butter and butter on high in 30-second increments, stirring in between, until melted and smooth. Whisk in the sweetener, eggs, and vanilla.

4. Add the coconut and almond mixture, then stir in the almond flour, baking powder, and salt. Stir in the chocolate chips.

5. Press the mixture into the prepared pan and bake for 20 to 25 minutes, until the edges are golden brown and the top is just firm to the touch. Remove from the oven and let cool completely in the pan before cutting into bars.

DAIRY-FREE OPTION:

Use coconut oil or ghee in place of the butter.

TIP: *These bars aren't overly sweet, so we like to eat them for breakfast. If you want to make them more of a treat, try adding an additional ¼ cup of sweetener. Any type will do.*

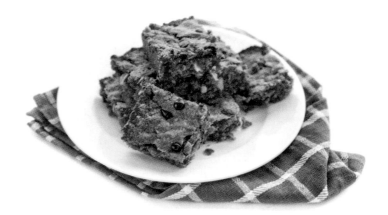

NUTRITIONAL INFORMATION

CALORIES: 187 | FAT: 16g | CARBS: 6.8g | FIBER: 3.3g | PROTEIN: 5.5g

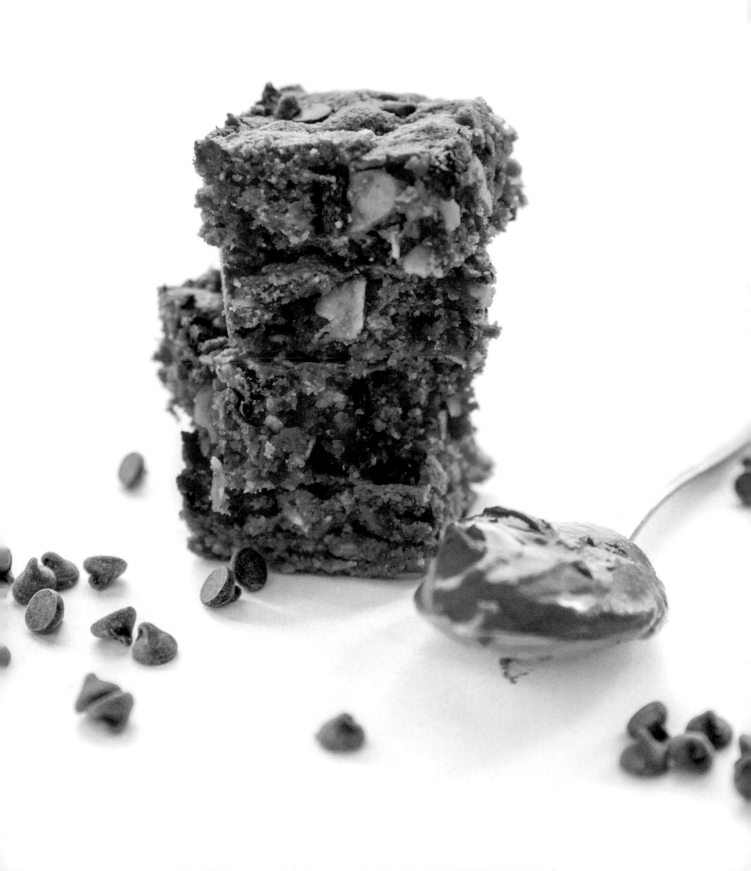

Chapter 9: MUFFINS & DONUTS

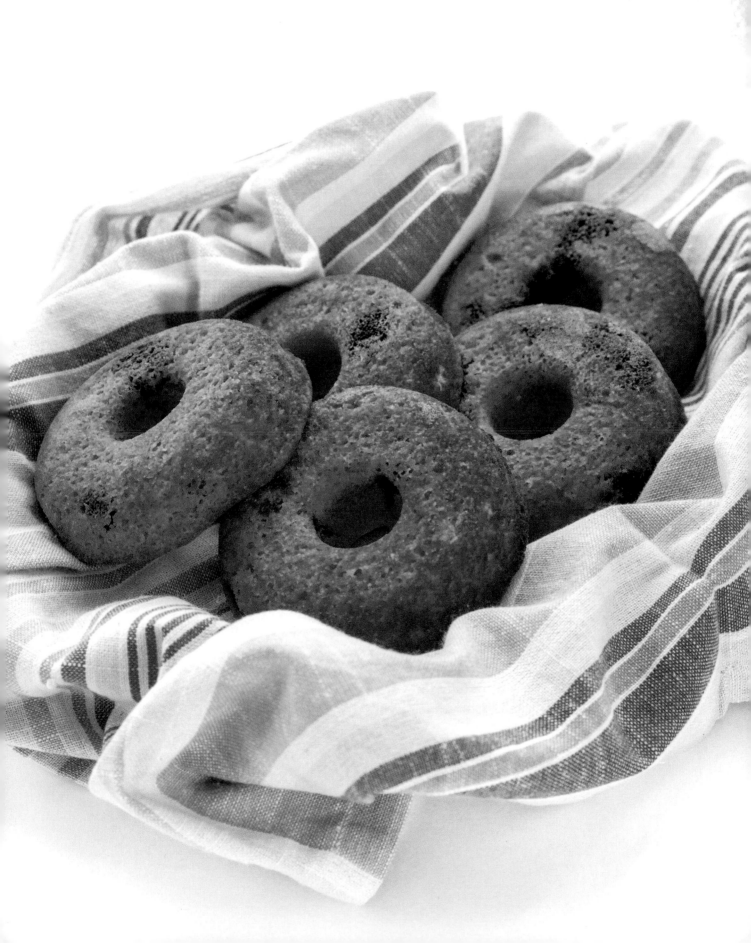

BASIC ALMOND FLOUR MUFFINS

OPTION

Yield: 12 muffins (1 per serving) Prep Time: 12 minutes Cook Time: 25 minutes

Muffins are one of my favorite keto snacks, and I don't discriminate. I love all kinds of muffins, from sweet to savory. For this book, I wanted to create a really great basic muffin that you could adapt to your favorite flavors. This one was the winner!

2½ cups (250g) blanched almond flour

⅓ cup granulated sweetener of choice

¼ cup unflavored whey protein powder

2 teaspoons baking powder

¼ teaspoon salt

3 large eggs

½ cup (1 stick) unsalted butter, melted but not hot

½ cup unsweetened almond milk

½ teaspoon vanilla extract

1. Preheat the oven to 325°F and line a standard muffin pan with 12 silicone or parchment paper liners.

2. In a large bowl, whisk together the almond flour, sweetener, protein powder, baking powder, and salt.

3. Stir in the eggs, melted butter, almond milk, and vanilla until well combined.

4. Divide the batter among the prepared muffin cups, filling each about two-thirds full. Bake for 20 to 25 minutes, until the tops are golden and firm to the touch. Remove from the oven and let cool in the pan.

DAIRY-FREE OPTION:

Use egg white protein powder for the whey protein and melted ghee or coconut oil or avocado oil in place of the butter.

TIP: *Feel free to mix in whatever add-ins you want. Blueberries, chocolate chips, nuts, different extracts—it's all good! You could even make some lovely lemon poppyseed muffins by adding 2 teaspoons grated lemon zest and 2 tablespoons poppyseeds and replacing the vanilla extract with lemon extract.*

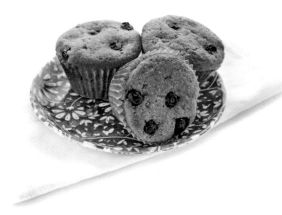

NUTRITIONAL INFORMATION

CALORIES: 229 | FAT: 20.1g | CARBS: 5.5g | FIBER: 2.5g | PROTEIN: 8.1g

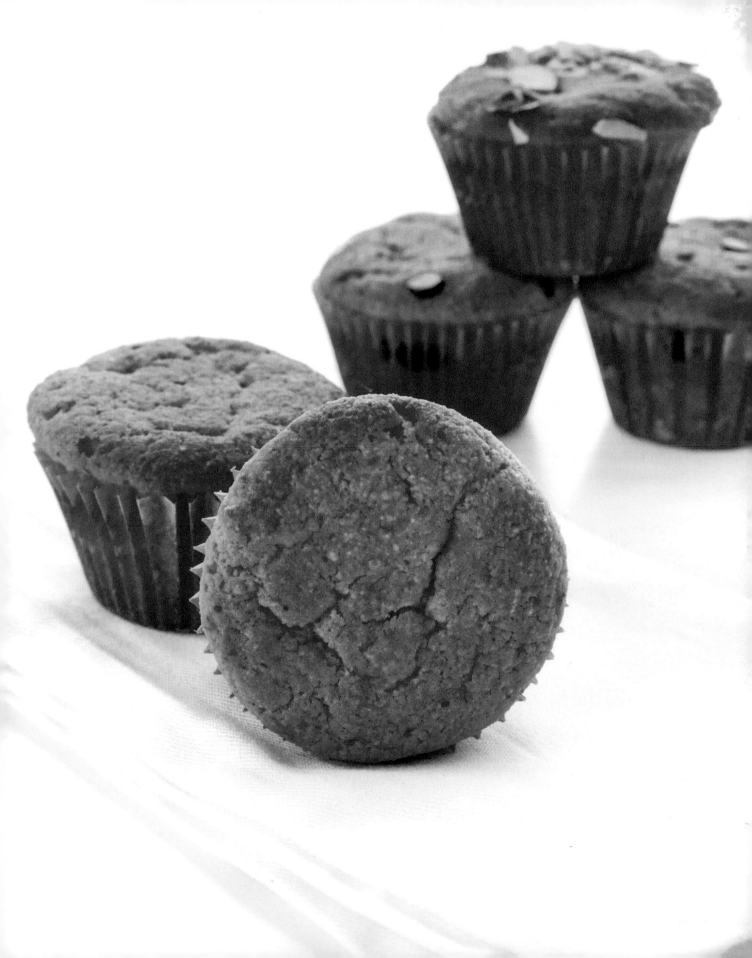

HAZELNUT CHOCOLATE CHIP MUFFINS

Yield: 12 muffins (1 per serving) Prep Time: 15 minutes Cook Time: 30 minutes

Hazelnut meal is fun to play with and produces lovely baked goods. It is a little more coarse than blanched almond meal, but in things like muffins, that hardly matters.

2¼ cups hazelnut meal

½ cup granulated sweetener of choice

¼ cup unflavored egg white protein powder

2 teaspoons baking powder

¼ teaspoon salt

3 large eggs

⅓ cup toasted hazelnut oil

⅓ cup water

½ teaspoon hazelnut or vanilla extract

⅓ cup sugar-free chocolate chips

1. Preheat the oven to 325°F and line a standard muffin pan with 12 silicone or parchment paper liners.

2. In a large bowl, whisk together the hazelnut meal, sweetener, protein powder, baking powder, and salt. Stir in the eggs, hazelnut oil, water, and extract until well combined. Stir in the chocolate chips.

3. Divide the batter among the prepared muffin cups, filling each about two-thirds full. Bake for 25 to 30 minutes, until the tops are golden and firm to the touch. Remove from the oven and let cool in the pan.

TIP: *If you don't have a dairy intolerance, feel free to use whey protein powder instead of egg white. Using hazelnut oil does give these muffins a more intense hazelnut flavor, but melted butter would work fine as well.*

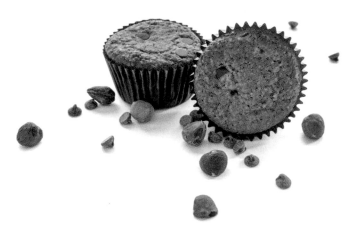

 214 *Chapter 9:* MUFFINS & DONUTS

NUTRITIONAL INFORMATION

CALORIES: 241 | FAT: 21.5g | CARBS: 6.5g | FIBER: 4g | PROTEIN: 6.4g

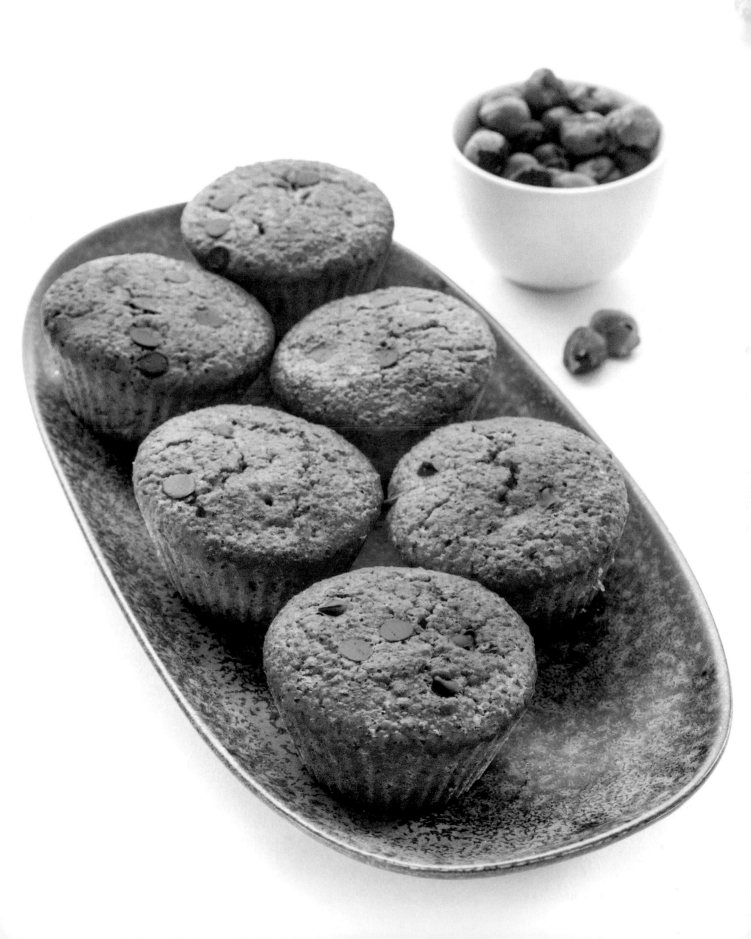

DOUBLE CHOCOLATE ALMOND BUTTER MUFFINS

Yield: 12 muffins (1 per serving) **Prep Time:** 15 minutes **Cook Time:** 25 minutes

These muffins are rich and delicious, but they can become dry if overbaked. Make sure to watch them and take them out of the oven just when they seem to have firmed up. They can be made with any nut butter you like.

1 cup creamy unsalted almond butter (see tips)

¼ cup melted coconut oil

½ cup granulated sweetener of choice

¼ teaspoon salt

2 large eggs

½ teaspoon vanilla extract

¼ cup cocoa powder

2 teaspoons baking powder

¼ cup unsweetened almond milk

2 ounces sugar-free dark chocolate, coarsely chopped

1. Preheat the oven to 325°F and line a standard muffin pan with 12 silicone or parchment paper liners.

2. In a large bowl, whisk together the almond butter, coconut oil, sweetener, and salt. Add the eggs and vanilla and stir until well combined.

3. Stir in the cocoa powder and baking powder, then whisk in the almond milk. Add the chopped chocolate and mix well.

4. Divide the batter among the prepared muffin cups, filling each about two-thirds full. Bake for 18 to 25 minutes, until the muffins are puffed and just barely firm to the touch. Remove from the oven and let cool in the pan.

NUT-FREE OPTION:

Use sunflower seed butter in place of the almond butter and hemp milk or another nut-free nondairy milk in place of the almond milk. Even water or cold coffee should work!

TIPS: *Nut butters vary so much from brand to brand. Some are very oily, some much less so. That's why the baking time range is wide here. Use your best judgment, and take them out when they have risen but aren't super firm.*

If your nut butter is salted, you may want to leave out the ¼ teaspoon salt.

Have a little fun with the chopped chocolate. I used Lily's salted almond extra-dark since it goes so well with the almond butter theme.

NUTRITIONAL INFORMATION
CALORIES: 206 | FAT: 17.9g | CARBS: 7.2g | FIBER: 3.8g | PROTEIN: 6g

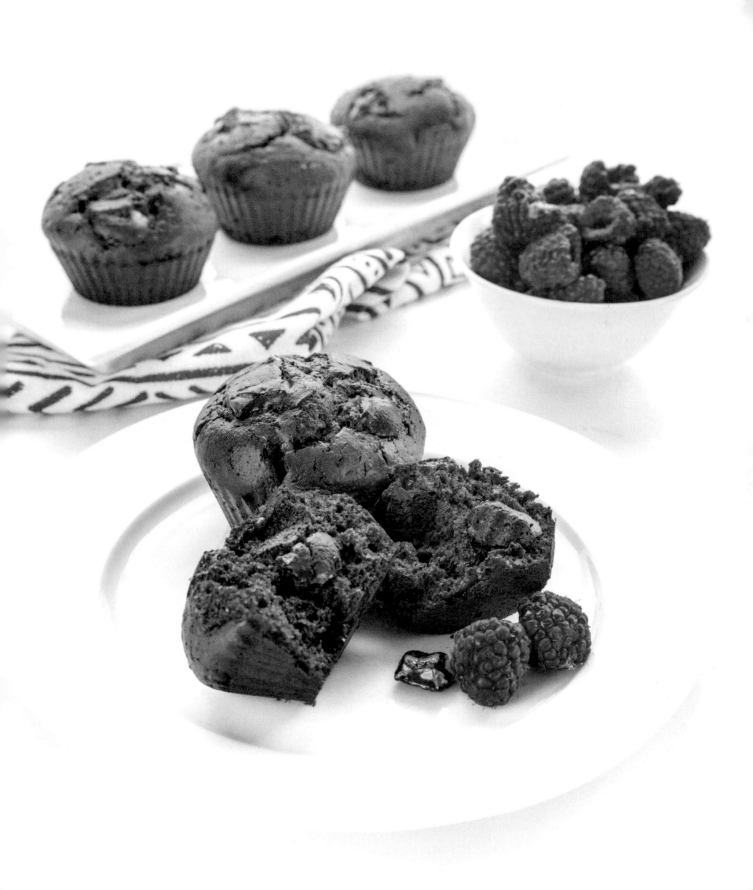

LEMON RICOTTA MUFFINS

Yield: 12 muffins (1 per serving) **Prep Time:** 20 minutes **Cook Time:** 30 minutes

Can muffins be called creamy? If so, these are deliciously creamy and tangy lemon muffins.

Muffins:

⅔ cup whole-milk ricotta cheese, room temperature

½ cup granulated sweetener of choice

3 large eggs

1 teaspoon grated lemon zest

¾ teaspoon lemon extract

½ teaspoon vanilla extract

2 cups (200g) blanched almond flour

¼ cup (28g) coconut flour

1 tablespoon baking powder

¼ teaspoon salt

2 to 4 tablespoons water

Glaze (Optional):

¼ cup powdered erythritol sweetener

1½ tablespoons fresh lemon juice

1. Preheat the oven to 325°F and line a standard muffin pan with 12 silicone or parchment paper liners.

2. Place the ricotta, granulated sweetener, eggs, lemon zest, and extracts in a blender or food processor. Blend until smooth.

3. Add the almond flour, coconut flour, baking powder, and salt and blend until smooth. Add 2 tablespoons of water and blend again. If the batter is very thick, add 1 or 2 tablespoons more water and blend.

4. Divide the batter among the prepared muffin cups, filling each about three-quarters full. Bake for 25 to 30 minutes, until the tops are firm to the touch. Remove from the oven and let cool in the pan.

5. To make the glaze, if using, whisk the powdered sweetener with the lemon juice until smooth. Drizzle over the cooled muffins.

TIP: *If you decide to skip the glaze but you really love lemon, replace the water with lemon juice for extra zing.*

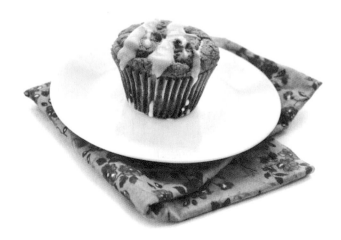

NUTRITIONAL INFORMATION

CALORIES: 163 | FAT: 12.5g | CARBS: 6.4g | FIBER: 2.9g | PROTEIN: 7.5g

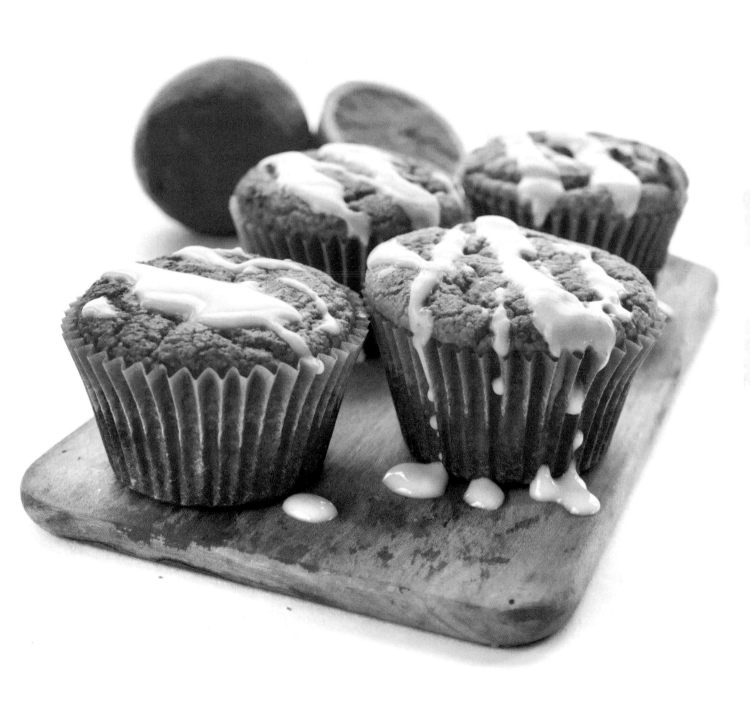

RASPBERRY COCONUT MUFFINS

Yield: 12 muffins (1 per serving)   Prep Time: 15 minutes   Cook Time: 25 minutes

If you've never worked with coconut flour, muffins are a good place to start because the method is straightforward. But yes, it really does take that little flour and that many eggs!

¾ cup (83g) coconut flour

¾ cup granulated sweetener of choice

½ cup unsweetened shredded coconut

1 tablespoon baking powder

¼ teaspoon salt

6 large eggs

⅓ cup coconut oil, melted but not hot

½ cup full-fat coconut milk

1 teaspoon vanilla or coconut extract

1 cup fresh raspberries

1. Preheat the oven to 350°F and line a standard muffin pan with 12 silicone or parchment paper liners.

2. In a large bowl, whisk together the coconut flour, sweetener, shredded coconut, baking powder, and salt.

3. Stir in the eggs, coconut oil, coconut milk, and extract, then carefully fold in the raspberries, taking care not to crush them.

4. Divide the batter among the prepared muffin cups, filling each about two-thirds full. Bake for 20 to 25 minutes, until lightly browned and firm to the touch. Remove from the oven and let cool in the pan for 15 minutes before serving.

TIPS: *You can use frozen raspberries here. Fresh berries tend to crush more easily when folded into a batter. But oddly, frozen raspberries tend to have more carbs than fresh ones. I suspect it has to do with some shrinkage during the freezing process, which means that more frozen berries fit into a measuring cup.*

I used vanilla extract in these muffins, but if you want a stronger coconut flavor, try coconut extract.

NUTRITIONAL INFORMATION

CALORIES: 170 | FAT: 13.6g | CARBS: 6.9g | FIBER: 3.6g | PROTEIN: 4.7g

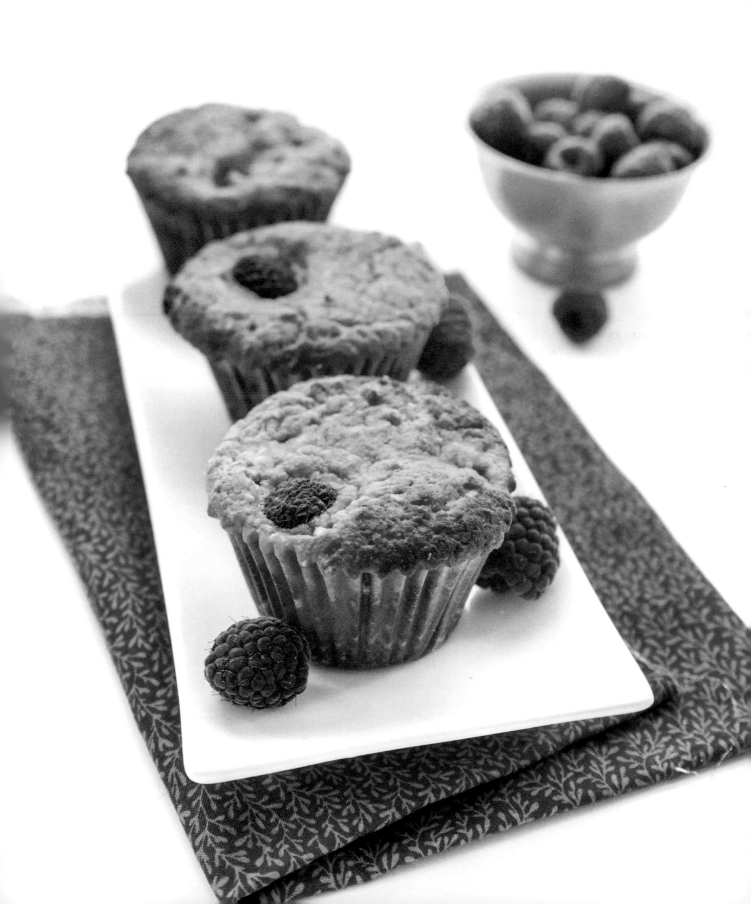

PIÑA COLADA MUFFINS

Yield: 12 muffins (1 per serving) Prep Time: 20 minutes Cook Time: 25 minutes

Your favorite cocktail, now in muffin form!

Muffins:

1¾ cups (175g) blanched almond flour

½ cup granulated erythritol sweetener

⅓ cup unsweetened shredded coconut

¼ cup (28g) coconut flour

¼ cup unflavored egg white protein powder

1 tablespoon baking powder

¼ teaspoon salt

4 large eggs

½ cup melted (but not hot) coconut oil

½ cup water

1½ teaspoons pineapple extract

Glaze:

½ cup powdered erythritol sweetener

3 tablespoons water

½ teaspoon coconut extract

½ teaspoon pineapple extract

¼ cup unsweetened flaked coconut, for garnish

1. Preheat the oven to 325°F and line a standard muffin pan with 12 silicone or parchment paper liners.

2. In a large bowl, whisk together the almond flour, sweetener, shredded coconut, coconut flour, protein powder, baking powder, and salt. Stir in the eggs, coconut oil, water, and pineapple extract until well combined.

3. Divide the batter among the prepared muffin cups, filling each almost to the top. Bake for 20 to 25 minutes, until the tops are golden and firm to the touch. Remove from the oven and let cool in the pan.

4. For the glaze, whisk together the sweetener, water, and extracts in a medium bowl. Drizzle over the cooled muffins, then sprinkle immediately with the flaked coconut. Press lightly to adhere.

TIP: *Flavorings like pineapple come as extracts or emulsions. Extracts are alcohol based, whereas emulsions are water based. It is technically a 1:1 substitution, but many people find that emulsions taste stronger, so use your own judgment when adding an emulsion to a recipe.*

NUTRITIONAL INFORMATION
CALORIES: 223 | FAT: 21.1g | CARBS: 5.1g | FIBER: 1.8g | PROTEIN: 7.4g

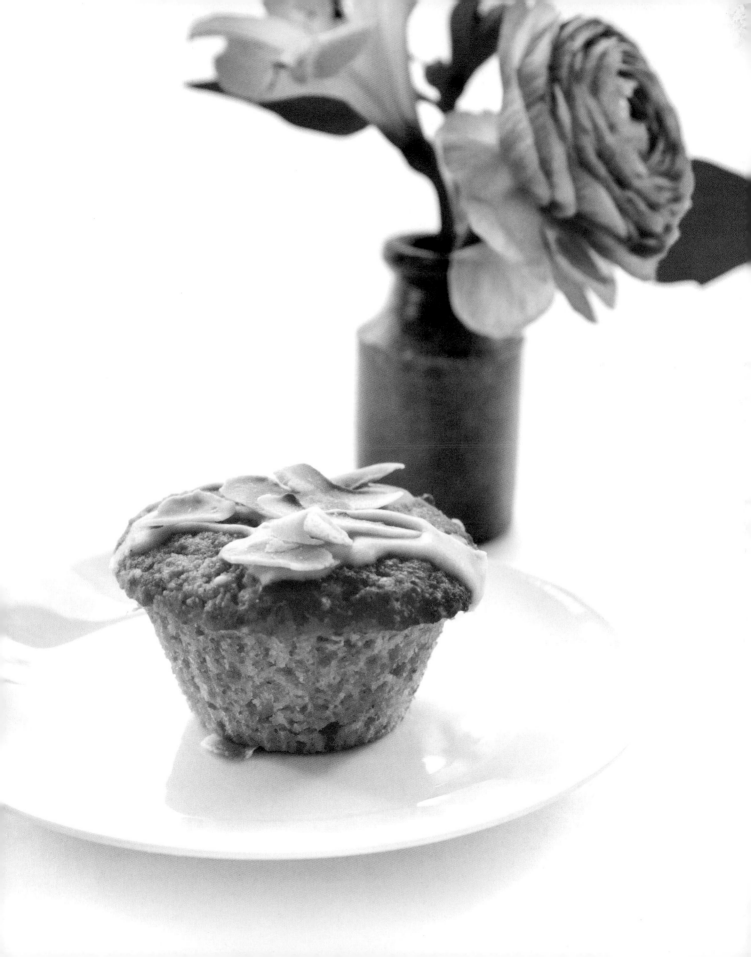

PIZZA MUFFINS

Yield: 12 muffins (1 per serving) Prep Time: 20 minutes Cook Time: 25 minutes

Who says you can't have pizza on a keto diet? These pizza muffins are as fun to eat as they are to make. And very kid-friendly!

¾ cup (83g) coconut flour

¼ cup unflavored whey or egg white protein powder

1½ cups shredded mozzarella cheese (about 6 ounces), divided

½ cup diced pepperoni

1 tablespoon pizza or Italian seasoning

1 tablespoon baking powder

¾ teaspoon garlic powder

½ teaspoon salt

¼ teaspoon red pepper flakes

6 large eggs

½ cup olive oil or melted (but not hot) unsalted butter

½ cup water

12 slices pepperoni, for the top

1. Preheat the oven to 350°F and line a standard muffin pan with 12 silicone or parchment paper liners.

2. In a large bowl, whisk together the coconut flour, protein powder, 1 cup of the mozzarella, the pepperoni, pizza seasoning, baking powder, garlic powder, salt, and red pepper flakes.

3. Stir in the eggs, olive oil, and water. If the batter is very thick, add more water 1 tablespoon at a time until it thins out a bit. It should be scoopable but not pourable.

4. Divide the batter among the prepared muffin cups, filling each about two-thirds full. Sprinkle the remaining ½ cup of mozzarella over the muffins and top each with a slice of pepperoni.

5. Bake for 20 to 25 minutes, until the tops are turning golden and are firm to the touch. Remove from the oven and let cool in the pan.

SERVING SUGGESTION: *Grab some low-carb marinara sauce for dipping!*

NUTRITIONAL INFORMATION
CALORIES: 230 | FAT: 17.4g | CARBS: 5.1g | FIBER: 2.5g | PROTEIN: 10.3g

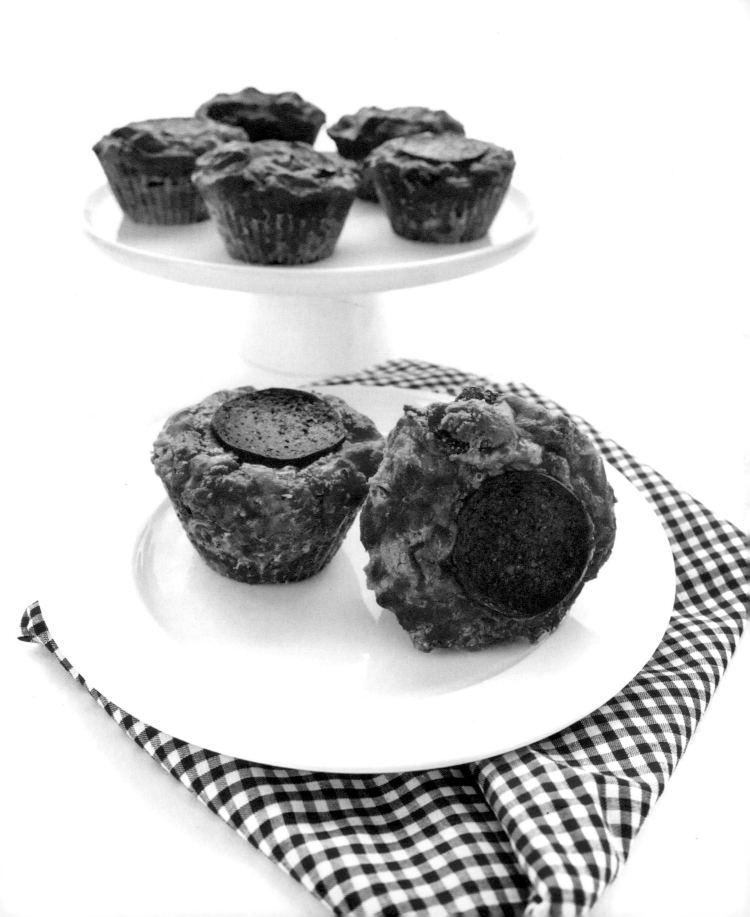

CHEESY GARLIC BREAD MUFFINS

Yield: 12 muffins (1 per serving) Prep Time: 25 minutes Cook Time: 30 minutes

Buttery and garlicky, these delicious savory muffins are the perfect companion to any keto soup, stew, or salad.

6 tablespoons unsalted butter, melted

5 cloves garlic, minced, divided

½ cup sour cream

4 large eggs

1 teaspoon salt

3 cups (300g) blanched almond flour

2 teaspoons baking powder

1 cup shredded cheddar cheese (about 4 ounces)

¼ cup chopped fresh parsley

1 cup shredded mozzarella cheese (about 4 ounces)

Coarse sea salt, for sprinkling

1. Preheat the oven to 325°F and grease a standard nonstick muffin pan very well. Set the muffin pan on a large rimmed baking sheet.

2. In a small bowl, combine the melted butter and 3 cloves of the minced garlic. Set aside.

3. Place the sour cream, eggs, salt, and remaining minced garlic in a blender or food processor. Process until well combined. Add the almond flour, baking powder, cheddar cheese, and parsley and process again until smooth.

4. Divide half of the batter among the prepared muffin cups, filling each about one-third full. Use a spoon to make a small well in the center of each.

5. Divide the shredded mozzarella among the wells in the muffin batter, pressing it into the wells. Drizzle about 1 teaspoon of the garlic butter into each.

6. Divide the remaining batter among the muffin cups, covering the cheese as best you can. Brush the tops with the remaining garlic butter and sprinkle with coarse salt.

7. Bake for 25 to 30 minutes, until the tops are golden brown and just firm to the touch. (These will drip a lot of oil as they bake, and it may spill over the sides a bit; the baking sheet is there to catch the spills.) Remove from the oven and let cool in the pan for 10 minutes before serving.

TIPS: *You can use liners for these if you like, but they brown and crisp up deliciously when the batter is directly against the metal pan.*

Be sure to set the muffin pan on a rimmed baking sheet before putting it in the oven. The amount of butter used in these delectable muffins means that it sometimes leaks out a bit during baking. Better to clean a pan than your whole oven!

SERVING SUGGESTION: *These muffins are fantastic still warm from the oven with the gooey cheese center. They are also fine at room temperature and warm up nicely in the microwave.*

NUTRITIONAL INFORMATION
CALORIES: 322 | FAT: 27.2g | CARBS: 7.4g | FIBER: 3.1g | PROTEIN: 12.8g

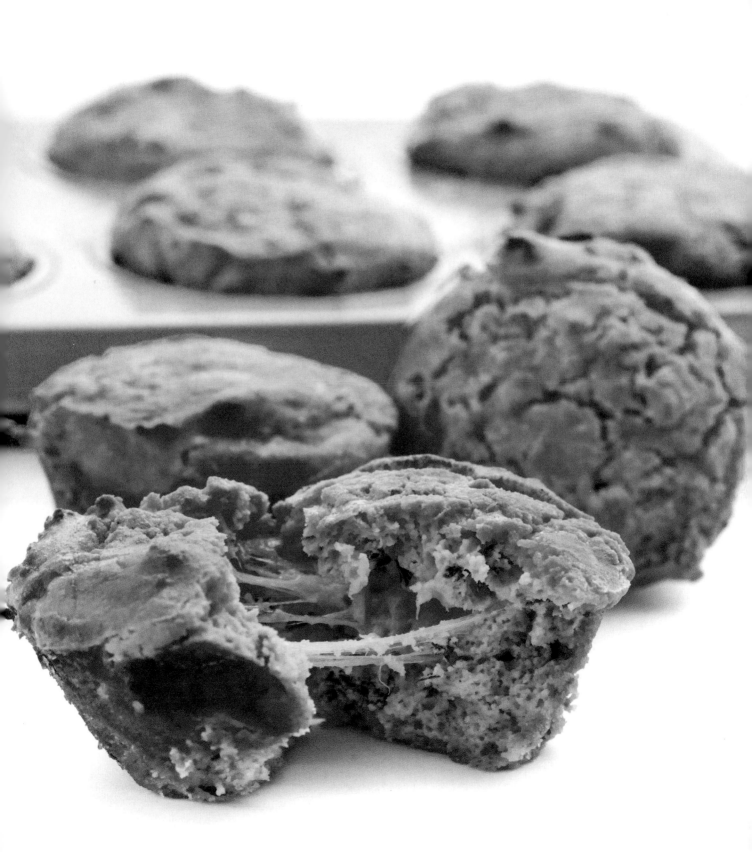

MINI CORNDOG MUFFINS

Yield: 24 mini muffins (3 per serving) Prep Time: 15 minutes Cook Time: 20 minutes

Keto corndogs! Well, sort of. These are such fun finger foods for kids.

½ cup (55g) coconut flour

2 tablespoons granulated sweetener of choice (optional; see tips)

1½ teaspoons baking powder

½ teaspoon salt

4 large eggs

¼ cup (½ stick) unsalted butter, melted but not hot

½ cup water

½ teaspoon cornbread flavoring (optional; see tips)

1 cup shredded cheddar cheese (about 4 ounces), divided

4 hot dogs, each cut into 6 even pieces

1. Preheat the oven to 325°F and grease a nonstick mini muffin pan very well.

2. In a large bowl, combine the coconut flour, sweetener (if using), baking powder, and salt, breaking up any clumps with the back of a fork.

3. Stir in the eggs, melted butter, water, and cornbread flavoring, if using, until well combined. Stir in ¾ cup of the shredded cheese.

4. Divide the batter among the prepared muffin cups, filling each about two-thirds full. Press a piece of hot dog into the center of each. Sprinkle the tops with the remaining cheese.

5. Bake for 15 to 20 minutes, until the cheese is melted and the muffins are firm to the touch. Remove from the oven and let cool in the pan for 15 minutes, then gently run a knife around the edge of each muffin and remove from the pan.

TIPS: *Cornmeal has a bit of a sweet flavor, which is why there is sweetener in this recipe. But many people prefer to leave it out and just let these be savory mini muffins.*

The cornbread flavoring is not required, but it does help give the illusion of real corndogs.

SERVING SUGGESTION: *Dip these mini muffins into some keto-friendly ketchup. I like the unsweetened one from Primal Kitchen.*

NUTRITIONAL INFORMATION

CALORIES: 193 | FAT: 12.8g | CARBS: 5.7g | FIBER: 2.5g | PROTEIN: 10.8g

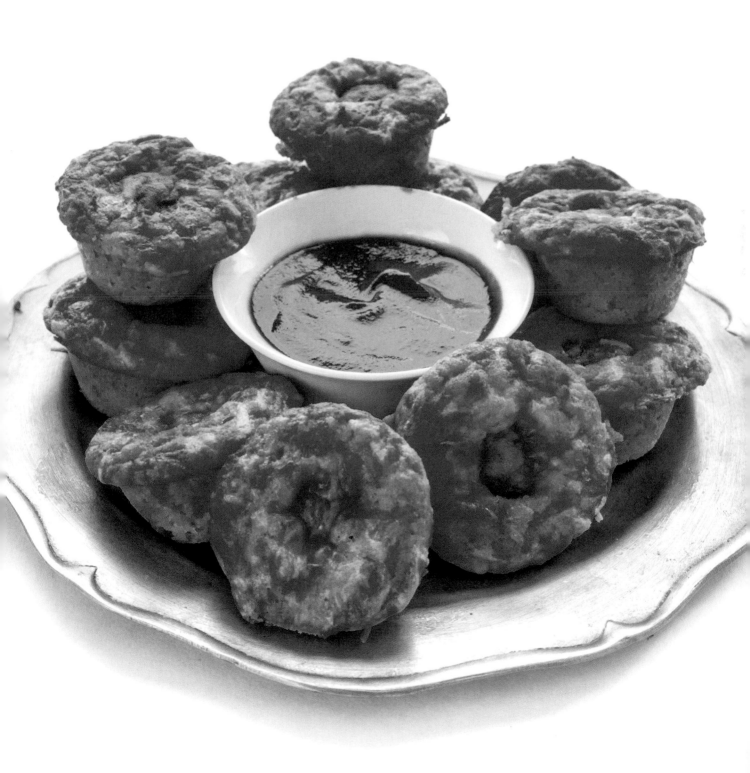

BLUEBERRY VANILLA DONUTS

Yield: 10 donuts (1 per serving) Prep Time: 15 minutes Cook Time: 20 minutes

Time to make dairy-free keto donuts! This is a very basic coconut flour donut recipe, and you can really switch things up flavorwise. (See the variations below for some ideas.) This recipe makes 10 donuts, so if you have only one pan that holds six, you will need to work in two batches. You could also make a half batch.

4 large eggs

2 large egg whites

½ cup unsweetened coconut or hemp milk

¼ cup avocado oil

1 teaspoon vanilla extract

¾ cup (83g) coconut flour

½ cup granulated erythritol sweetener

¼ cup unflavored egg white protein powder

2 teaspoons baking powder

¼ teaspoon salt

½ cup fresh blueberries

Special equipment: one 12-cavity or two 6-cavity donut pan(s)

1. Preheat the oven to 325°F and grease 10 wells of one 12-cavity donut pan or two 6-cavity donut pans.

2. Crack the whole eggs into a blender, then add the egg whites, coconut milk, avocado oil, and vanilla. Blend until well combined.

3. Add the coconut flour, sweetener, protein powder, baking powder, and salt and blend again until smooth. Spoon the batter into the prepared pan(s), filling the cavities about three-quarters full. Divide the blueberries among the cavities, pressing them into the batter.

4. Bake for 15 to 20 minutes, until golden brown and firm to the touch. Remove from the oven and let cool completely in the pan(s) before flipping out onto a wire rack.

VARIATIONS:

LEMON BLUEBERRY DONUTS.

Add 1 teaspoon lemon extract and reduce the vanilla extract to ½ teaspoon.

CLASSIC VANILLA DONUTS.

Simply omit the blueberries and dust with powdered sweetener.

NUTRITIONAL INFORMATION
CALORIES: 112 | FAT: 8.8g | CARBS: 6.5g | FIBER: 3.3g | PROTEIN: 6.2g

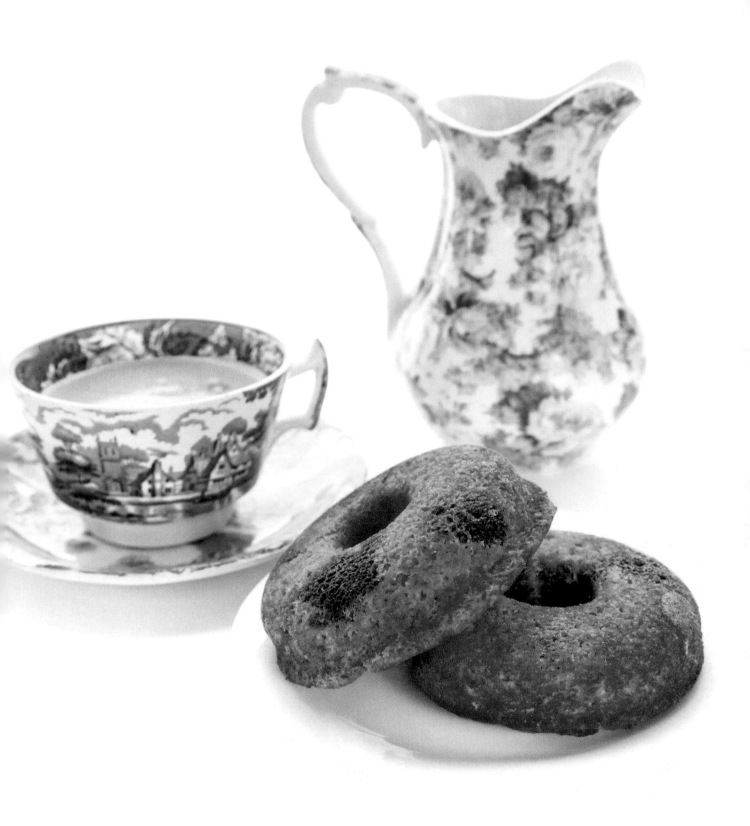

CHOCOLATE DONUTS WITH PEANUT BUTTER GLAZE

Yield: 10 donuts (1 per serving) Prep Time: 25 minutes Cook Time: 23 minutes

How can you go wrong with chocolate peanut butter donuts? This recipe makes 10 donuts, so if you have only one pan that holds six, you will need to work in two batches. You could also make a half batch.

Donuts:

2 cups (200g) blanched almond flour

¼ cup plus 2 tablespoons granulated sweetener of choice

¼ cup cocoa powder

2 teaspoons baking powder

¼ teaspoon salt

3 large eggs, room temperature

½ cup unsweetened almond milk

6 tablespoons unsalted butter, melted

½ teaspoon vanilla extract

Glaze:

3 tablespoons creamy natural peanut butter

2 tablespoons unsalted butter

3 tablespoons powdered erythritol sweetener

2 tablespoons heavy whipping cream, room temperature

¼ teaspoon vanilla extract

Pinch of salt (omit if using salted peanut butter)

Warm water to thin, as needed

2 tablespoons finely chopped roasted peanuts, for garnish

Special equipment: one 12-cavity or two 6-cavity donut pan(s)

TO MAKE THE DONUTS:

1. Preheat the oven to 325°F and grease 10 wells of one 12-cavity donut pan or two 6-cavity donut pans.

2. In a large bowl, whisk together the almond flour, sweetener, cocoa powder, baking powder, and salt. Add the eggs, almond milk, melted butter, and vanilla and stir until well combined.

3. Spoon the batter into the prepared pan(s), filling the cavities about three-quarters full. Bake for 18 to 23 minutes, until set and firm to the touch. Remove from the oven and let cool completely in the pan(s) before flipping out onto a wire rack.

TO MAKE THE GLAZE:

4. In a microwave-safe bowl, heat the peanut butter and butter on high in 30-second increments, stirring in between, until melted and smooth.

5. Whisk in the sweetener, cream, vanilla, and salt, if using. If the glaze is very thick, whisk in warm water a few teaspoons at a time until a dippable consistency is achieved.

6. Working quickly, dip the tops of the cooled donuts into the glaze and place on the wire rack to set. If the glaze thickens up too quickly, you can simply spread it onto the donuts.

7. Sprinkle with the chopped peanuts and let set, about 20 minutes.

NUTRITIONAL INFORMATION

CALORIES: 285 | FAT: 25.4g | CARBS: 7.7g | FIBER: 3.5g | PROTEIN: 8.4g

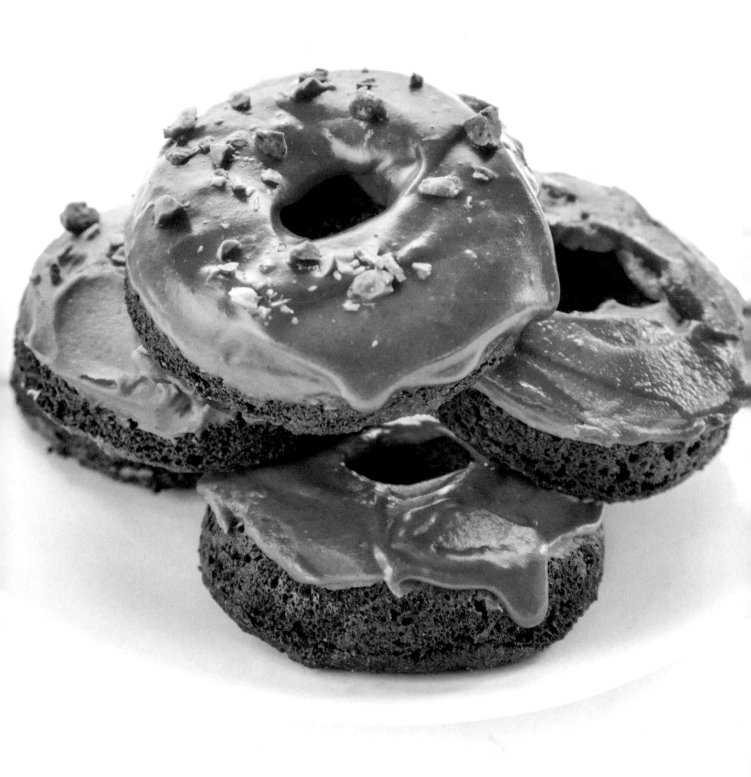

MAPLE-GLAZED DONUTS

Yield: 12 donuts (1 per serving) Prep Time: 20 minutes Cook Time: 23 minutes

One thing you need to know about me is that I am a maple fanatic. I love maple-flavored cakes, cookies, and donuts. I do miss real maple syrup, but I am ever so grateful that an extract exists so that I can still get my maple fix!

This recipe makes 12 donuts, so if you have only one pan that holds six, you will need to work in two batches. You could also make a half batch.

Donuts:

4 large eggs

¼ cup plus 2 tablespoons water

¼ cup heavy whipping cream

½ teaspoon vanilla extract

1¼ cups (125g) blanched almond flour

½ cup granulated sweetener of choice

¼ cup plus 1 tablespoon (34g) coconut flour

2 teaspoons baking powder

¼ teaspoon salt

Glaze:

½ cup powdered erythritol sweetener

¼ cup heavy whipping cream

1 teaspoon yacón syrup or molasses (optional; improves color)

1 teaspoon maple extract

Special equipment: one 12-cavity or two 6-cavity donut pan(s)

TO MAKE THE DONUTS:

1. Preheat the oven to 325°F and grease one 12-cavity donut pan or two 6-cavity donut pans.

2. Crack the eggs into a blender and add the water, cream, and vanilla. Blend to combine.

3. Add the almond flour, granulated sweetener, coconut flour, baking powder, and salt and blend again until smooth.

4. Spoon the batter into the prepared pan, filling the wells about two-thirds full. Bake for 18 to 23 minutes, until set and firm to the touch. Remove from the oven and let cool completely in the pan before flipping out onto a wire rack.

TO MAKE THE GLAZE:

5. Whisk together the powdered sweetener, cream, yacón syrup (if using), and maple extract until well combined. Dip the tops of the cooled donuts in the glaze and place on the wire rack until set, about 20 minutes.

TIPS: *Yacón syrup comes from the yacón, or* Smallanthus sonchifolius *plant, native to South America. Although it is a sugar, it is said to have a very low glycemic index. I can't really speak to the supposed health benefits, but it is useful as an alternative to molasses when trying to achieve a caramel color. Using only 1 teaspoon in a recipe such as this adds about 0.5 gram of carbs per serving. Molasses also adds only 0.5 gram to each serving. However, if you aren't comfortable with either of these additions, leave them out. The glaze will be paler in color but will still taste great.*

NUTRITIONAL INFORMATION

CALORIES: 143 | FAT: 11.2g | CARBS: 5.2g | FIBER: 2.3g | PROTEIN: 5.2g

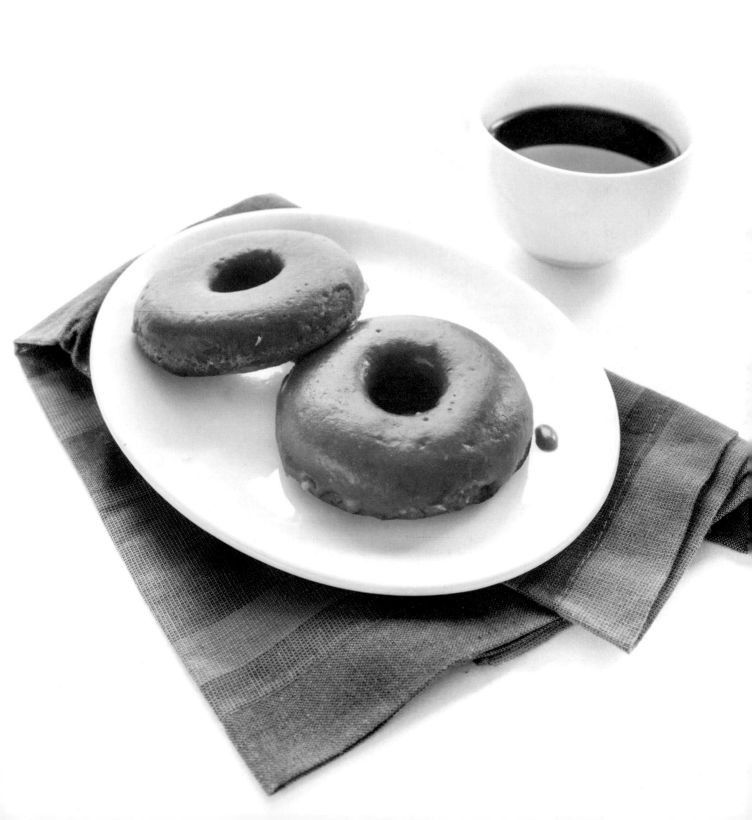

PUMPKIN SPICE DONUT HOLES

Yield: 24 donut holes (3 per serving) Prep Time: 25 minutes Cook Time: 20 minutes

Okay, you caught me. These donut "holes" are really just mini muffins in disguise. But your taste buds won't care, and it's just more fun to call them donut holes.

Donut Holes:

¼ cup plus 2 tablespoons (41g) coconut flour

¼ cup granulated sweetener of choice, divided

2 tablespoons unflavored whey or egg white protein powder

1 teaspoon baking powder

1 teaspoon pumpkin pie spice

¼ teaspoon salt

½ cup pumpkin puree

3 large eggs, room temperature

3 tablespoons unsalted butter, melted but not hot

Water to thin, as needed

Cinnamon "Sugar" Coating:

2 tablespoons granulated sweetener of choice

1 teaspoon ground cinnamon

¼ cup (½ stick) unsalted butter, melted

TO MAKE THE DONUT HOLES:

1. Preheat the oven to 350°F and grease a nonstick mini muffin pan very well.

2. In a large bowl, whisk together the coconut flour, sweetener, protein powder, baking powder, pumpkin pie spice, and salt.

3. Stir in the pumpkin puree, eggs, and melted butter until well combined. If the batter is very thick, add water 1 tablespoon at a time. The batter should be scoopable but not pourable.

4. Divide the batter among the prepared muffin cups, filling them almost to the top. Bake for 15 to 20 minutes, until the tops are golden and firm to the touch. Remove from the oven and let cool in the pan for 10 minutes, then transfer to a wire rack to cool completely.

TO COAT IN CINNAMON "SUGAR":

5. In a shallow bowl, whisk together the sweetener and cinnamon. Roll the donut holes in the melted butter, then roll in the cinnamon mixture to coat.

TIPS: *Pumpkin pie spice is really just a blend of cinnamon, ginger, cloves, and/or nutmeg. If you want to make your own, try using about ½ teaspoon each of cinnamon and ginger and ⅛ teaspoon each of cloves and/or nutmeg.*

If your mini muffin pan is not a very good nonstick one, try using silicone or parchment paper liners. The resulting donut holes will have little ridges, but it's better than having them stick to the pan.

NUTRITIONAL INFORMATION
CALORIES: 153 | FAT: 11.9g | CARBS: 5.1g | FIBER: 2.5g | PROTEIN: 4.5g

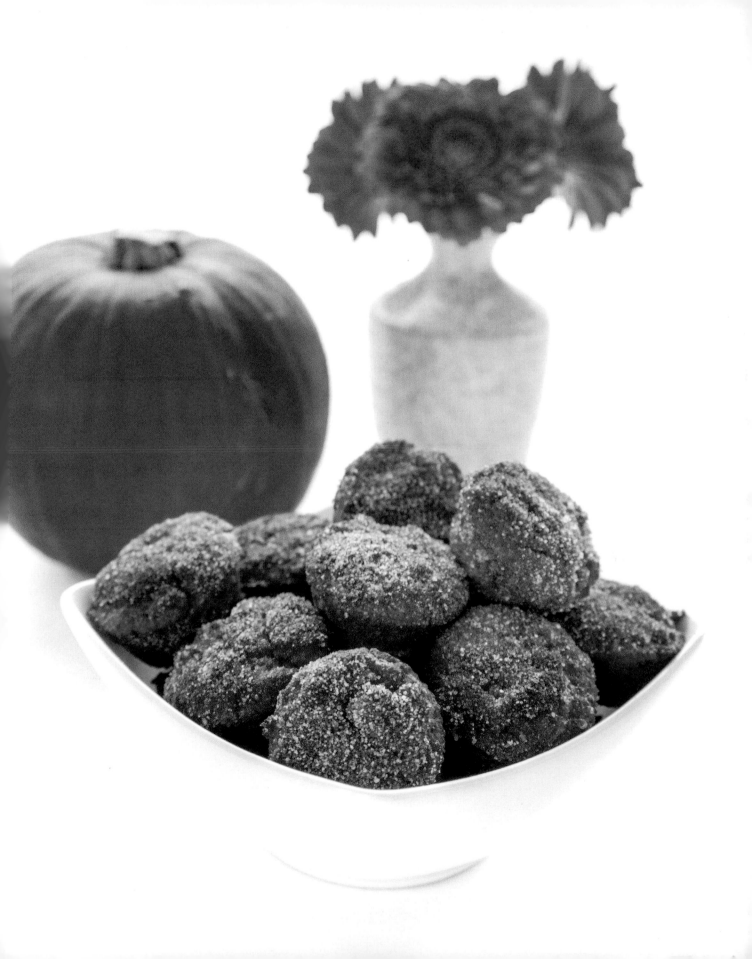

Chapter 10:
BISCUITS &
SCONES

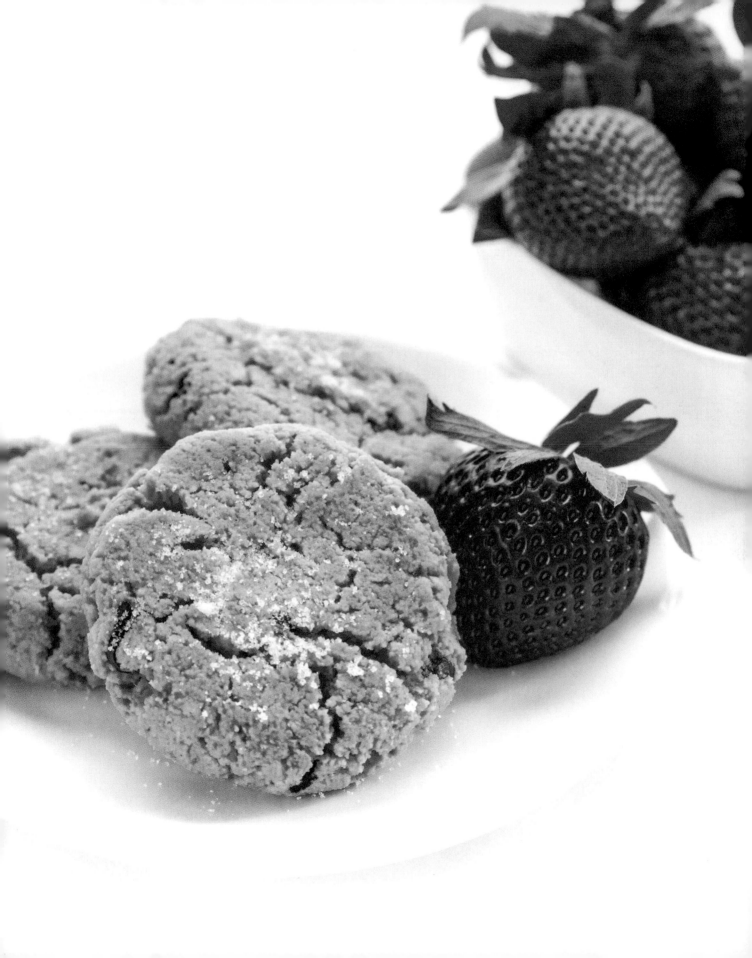

CREAM CHEESE BISCUITS

OPTION

Yield: 10 biscuits (1 per serving) Prep Time: 15 minutes Cook Time: 15 minutes

Cream cheese makes these biscuits unbelievably tender, yet they still hold together well. I added garlic powder to make them savory, but you can omit it and have a more basic biscuit that's perfect with a little butter or sugar-free jam.

1¾ cups (175g) blanched almond flour, plus more for dusting

¼ cup unflavored egg white protein powder

1 tablespoon baking powder

½ teaspoon salt

½ teaspoon garlic powder (optional)

6 ounces cold cream cheese, cut into chunks

1 large egg

DAIRY-FREE OPTION:

You can use Kite Hill almond milk cream cheese in place of the regular cream cheese. My dairy-free recipe tester said it worked perfectly.

1. Preheat the oven to 350°F and line a baking sheet with a silicone baking mat or parchment paper.

2. Place the almond flour, protein powder, baking powder, salt, and garlic powder, if using, in a food processor and pulse to combine. Scatter the cream cheese chunks over the dry ingredients and process until the mixture resembles coarse crumbs.

3. Transfer the mixture to a large bowl and stir in the egg until just combined.

4. Dust a work surface lightly with almond flour and transfer the dough to the work surface. Knead a few times, adding a bit more flour until the dough is no longer sticky. The dough will be soft.

5. Roll the dough into a thick log about 10 inches long. Use a sharp knife to cut the log into 1-inch-thick slices and place on the prepared baking sheet, about 2 inches apart.

6. Bake for 15 minutes, or until the biscuits are firm to the touch and the tops and sides are golden. Let cool on the pan for at least 15 minutes before serving.

TIPS: *I tried this recipe a few different ways and found that rolling the dough into a log and slicing it worked best. If, after completing Step 4, you find the dough too difficult to work with, transfer it to a large sheet of parchment paper and use the paper to help you roll it into a log.*

You can make these biscuits with whey protein, but I found that they tended to spread more.

SERVING SUGGESTION: *Brush the biscuits with a little melted butter and sprinkle with sea salt after baking.*

NUTRITIONAL INFORMATION

CALORIES: 187 | FAT: 15.3g | CARBS: 5.6g | FIBER: 2.1g | PROTEIN: 7.6g

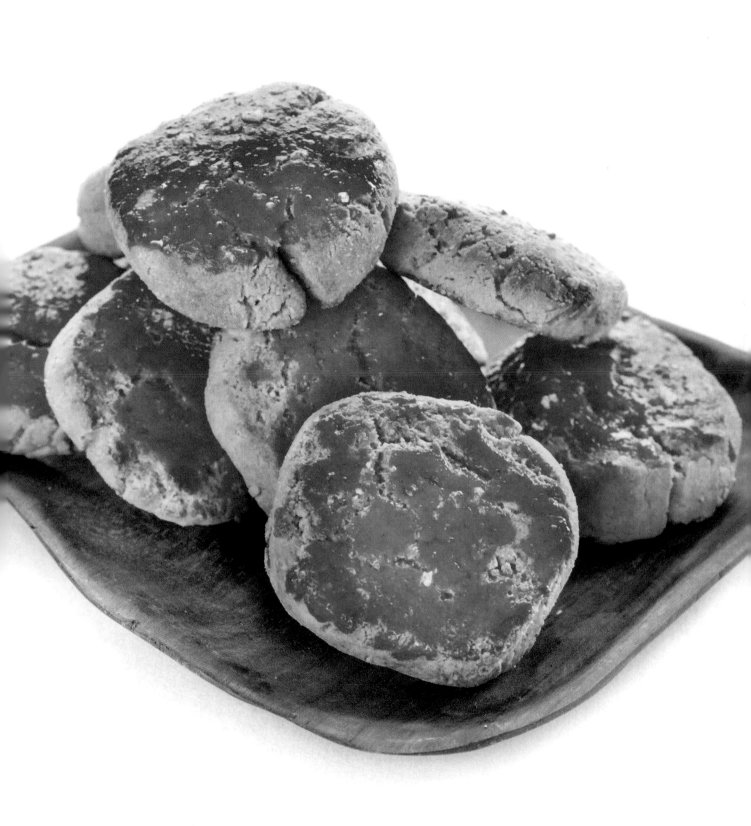

CHEDDAR GARLIC DROP BISCUITS

Yield: 12 biscuits (1 per serving) **Prep Time:** 15 minutes **Cook Time:** 22 minutes

---

The famous Cheddar Bay Biscuits from Red Lobster are now keto-friendly. How can you go wrong with an easy drop biscuit drenched in garlic butter?

1½ cups (150g) blanched almond flour

½ cup ground pork rinds (see tip)

1 tablespoon baking powder

1½ tablespoons dried parsley, divided

1½ teaspoons garlic powder, divided

¼ teaspoon salt

1½ cups shredded cheddar cheese (about 6 ounces)

2 large eggs

⅓ cup heavy whipping cream

½ cup (1 stick) unsalted butter, melted, divided

1 tablespoon apple cider vinegar

1. Preheat the oven to 375°F and line a baking sheet with a silicone baking mat or parchment paper.

2. In a large bowl, combine the almond flour, pork rinds, baking powder, 1 tablespoon of the parsley, 1 teaspoon of the garlic powder, and the salt. Stir in the cheese, eggs, cream, ¼ cup of the melted butter, and the apple cider vinegar until well combined.

3. Let sit for 5 minutes to thicken, then drop the dough by large rounded spoonfuls onto the prepared baking sheet, about 2 inches apart.

4. Bake for 17 to 22 minutes, until golden brown and firm to the touch. Remove from the oven and let cool on the pan for 10 minutes.

5. Combine the remaining ¼ cup of melted butter, remaining ½ tablespoon of parsley, and remaining ½ teaspoon of garlic powder and brush over the warm biscuits just before serving.

TIP: *You can grind your own pork rinds in a food processor or purchase them already ground (see page 401). If you grind your own, it will take about 2 ounces to make ½ cup. Be sure to measure them out after grinding them.*

NUTRITIONAL INFORMATION

CALORIES: 268 | FAT: 22.7g | CARBS: 4.2g | FIBER: 1.6g | PROTEIN: 10.7g

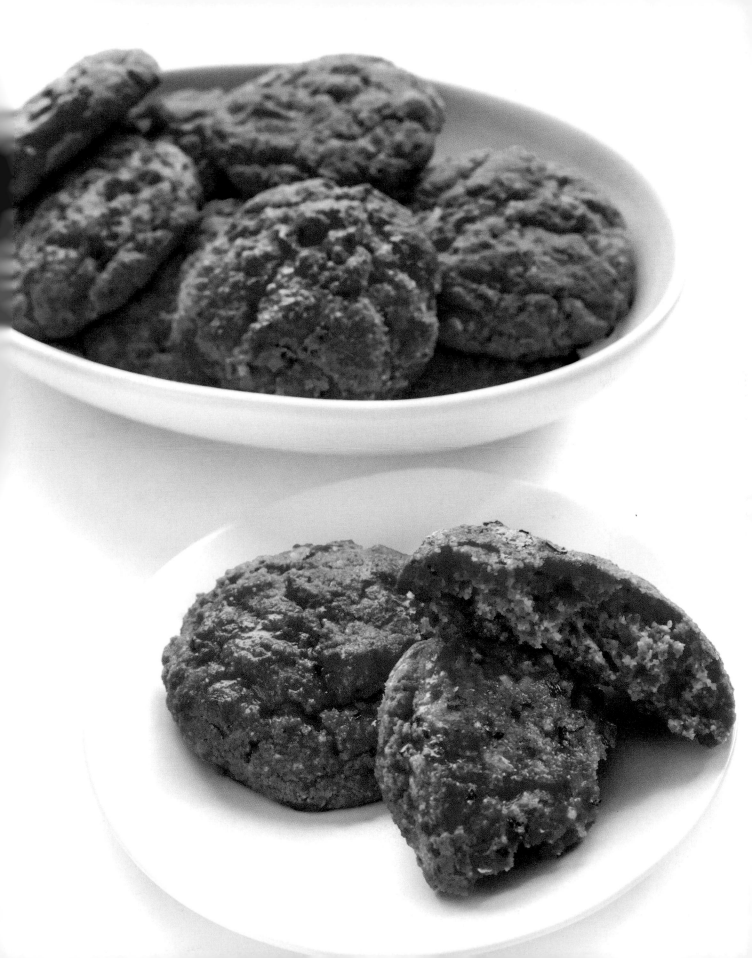

CLASSIC CREAM SCONES

OPTION

Yield: 10 scones (1 per serving) Prep Time: 20 minutes Cook Time: 23 minutes

I'm a bit of a scone fanatic and decided that I needed to make over classic cream scones. You could get all fancy and serve these with clotted cream and some sugar-free jam. Then you can sip tea and imagine yourself dining with the Queen.

2 cups (200g) blanched almond flour

⅓ cup granulated erythritol sweetener

¼ cup (28g) coconut flour

1 tablespoon baking powder

¼ teaspoon salt

1 large egg

1 large egg white

¼ cup plus 2 tablespoons heavy whipping cream

½ teaspoon vanilla extract

1. Preheat the oven to 325°F and line a baking sheet with a silicone baking mat or parchment paper.

2. In a large bowl, whisk together the almond flour, sweetener, coconut flour, baking powder, and salt. Stir in the whole egg, egg white, cream, and vanilla until the dough comes together. To cut the dough with cookie cutters, complete Step 3; to form the dough into scones by hand, skip to Step 4.

3. Turn the dough out onto the prepared baking sheet and pat into a rough rectangle about 1 inch thick. Use a 2½-inch round cookie cutter to cut into scones. Gather up the scraps, pat out again, and cut more scones. Place the scones around the baking sheet, about 2 inches apart.

4. Alternatively, you can divide the dough into 10 pieces and roll into balls, then press down to a 1-inch thickness with the palm of your hand.

5. Bake for 18 to 23 minutes, until the scones are golden brown on the bottom and just firm to the touch. Remove from the oven and let cool on the pan for 10 minutes before serving.

DAIRY-FREE OPTION:

While it may not be "classic" at all, you can substitute full-fat coconut milk for the heavy cream.

VARIATION: CHOCOLATE CHIP SCONES.

Stir ⅓ cup sugar-free chocolate chips into the dry ingredients. Sprinkle the tops with some granulated sweetener as soon as they come out of the oven.

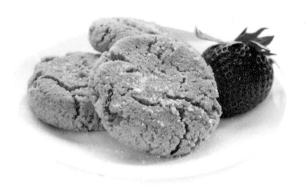

NUTRITIONAL INFORMATION
CALORIES: 182 | FAT: 15.2g | CARBS: 7.1g | FIBER: 3.4g | PROTEIN: 6.4g

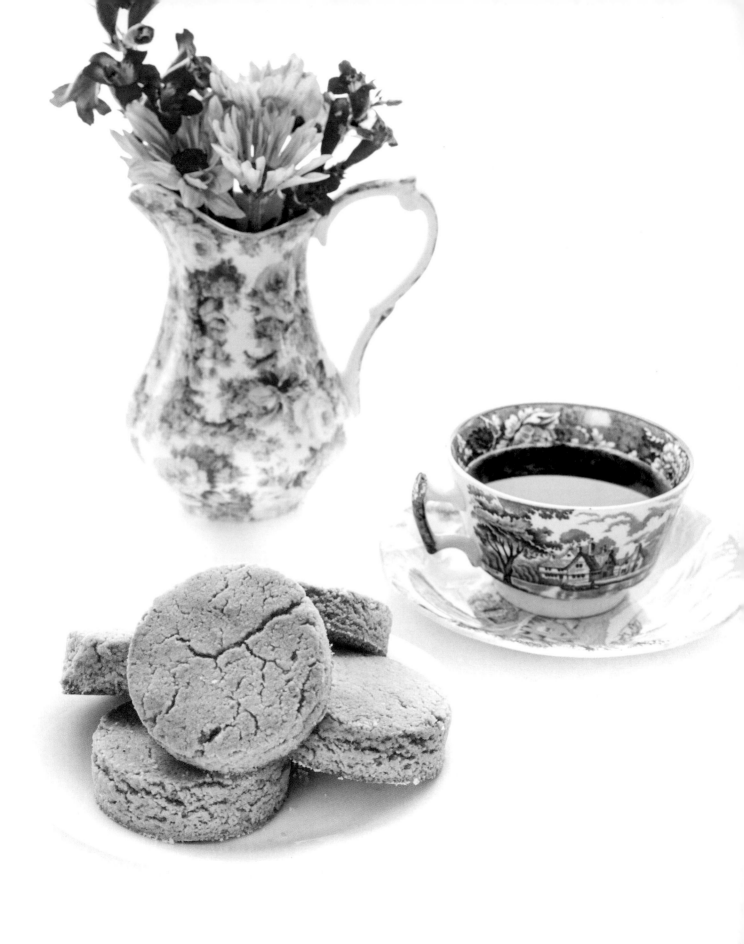

CINNAMON ROLL SCONES

Yield: 8 scones (1 per serving) Prep Time: 20 minutes Cook Time: 25 minutes

Two of my favorite breakfast treats in one delicious package.

Scones:

2 cups (200g) blanched almond flour

¼ cup plus 2 tablespoons granulated sweetener of choice, divided

2 teaspoons baking powder

½ teaspoon salt

1 large egg, room temperature

¼ cup (½ stick) unsalted butter, melted but not hot

2 tablespoons heavy whipping cream

½ teaspoon vanilla extract

2 teaspoons ground cinnamon

Drizzle:

1 ounce cream cheese, softened

1 tablespoon powdered erythritol sweetener

1 tablespoon heavy whipping cream, room temperature

¼ teaspoon vanilla extract

TO MAKE THE SCONES:

1. Preheat the oven to 325°F and line a baking sheet with a silicone baking mat or parchment paper.

2. In a large bowl, whisk together the almond flour, ¼ cup of the sweetener, the baking powder, and salt. Stir in the egg, melted butter, cream, and vanilla until the dough comes together.

3. In a small bowl, whisk the remaining 2 tablespoons of sweetener with the cinnamon. Sprinkle half of this mixture into the dough and mix in a little but do not fully incorporate so that it remains a bit streaky.

4. Turn the dough out onto the prepared baking sheet and pat into an 8-inch circle. Sprinkle with the remaining cinnamon mixture. Using a large sharp knife, cut into 8 even wedges. Wiggle a small knife or an offset spatula under the wedges to carefully separate them, then space the wedges evenly around the baking sheet.

5. Bake for 20 to 25 minutes, until lightly browned and firm to the touch. Remove from the oven and let cool on the pan for 5 minutes, then transfer to a wire rack to cool completely.

TO MAKE THE DRIZZLE:

6. In a medium bowl, beat the cream cheese and sweetener with an electric mixer until well combined. Beat in the cream and vanilla until smooth.

7. Place the drizzle in a small resealable plastic bag and snip off the very tip of one corner. Pipe the drizzle decoratively over the cooled scones.

TIP: *When using a large knife to cut the dough into wedges, be sure to cut straight up and down rather than dragging the knife through the dough. This will help the scones keep their wedge shape.*

NUTRITIONAL INFORMATION

CALORIES: 252 | FAT: 23.4g | CARBS: 7.1g | FIBER: 3.4g | PROTEIN: 6.7g

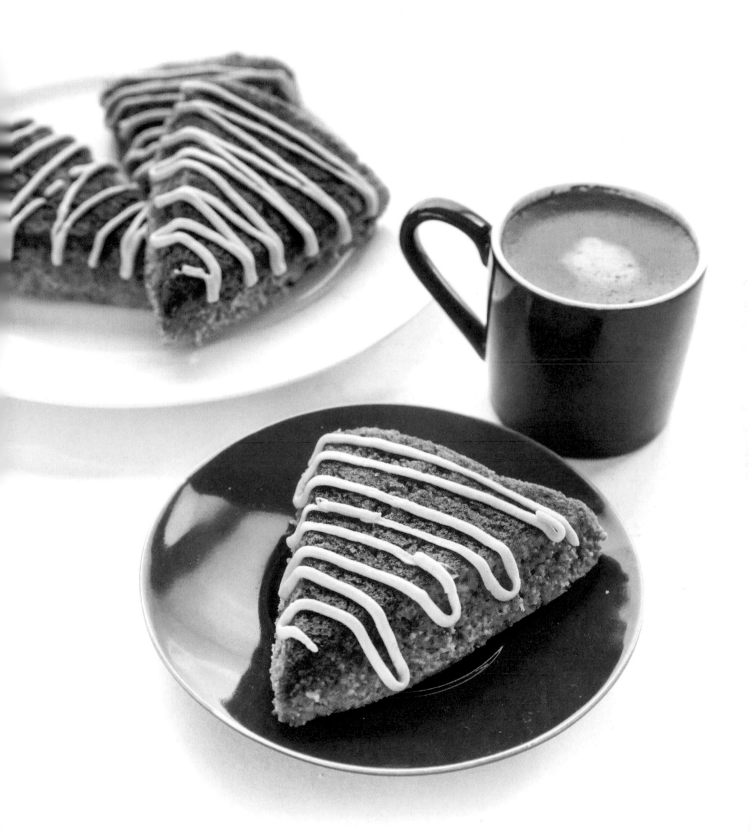

FRESH HERB AND RICOTTA SCONES

Yield: 6 scones (1 per serving) Prep Time: 25 minutes Cook Time: 27 minutes

Ricotta makes these scones moist and delicious. They are a wonderful accompaniment to soups, stews, or salad.

1¼ cups (125g) blanched almond flour

2 green onions, white and light green parts only, chopped

1 tablespoon chopped fresh parsley

2 teaspoons chopped fresh rosemary

2 teaspoons fresh thyme leaves

1½ teaspoons baking powder

¾ teaspoon salt

½ teaspoon black pepper

¼ cup whole-milk ricotta cheese, room temperature

1 large egg

¼ teaspoon paprika

¼ teaspoon coarse sea salt

1. Preheat the oven to 325°F and line a baking sheet with a silicone baking mat or parchment paper. Lightly grease the mat or paper.

2. In a large bowl, whisk together the almond flour, green onions, herbs, baking powder, salt, and pepper. Stir in the ricotta and egg until the dough comes together.

3. Turn the dough out onto the prepared baking sheet and pat into a 6-inch circle. Using a sharp knife, cut into 6 even wedges. Do not separate. Sprinkle with the paprika and coarse salt.

4. Bake for about 20 minutes, until the tops are firm to the touch. Remove from the oven and carefully separate the scones, then bake for another 5 to 7 minutes, until the sides are dry to the touch.

5. Remove from the oven and let cool completely on the pan.

TIP: *Salt is very much a matter of taste. One recipe tester found these scones a bit too salty, while the others loved them as is. Use your judgment and decrease the salt to ½ teaspoon if you prefer less salty savory breads.*

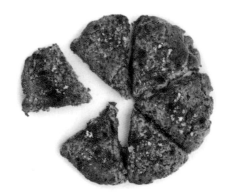

NUTRITIONAL INFORMATION

CALORIES: 168 | FAT: 13.8g | CARBS: 6.8g | FIBER: 3.1g | PROTEIN: 7.4g

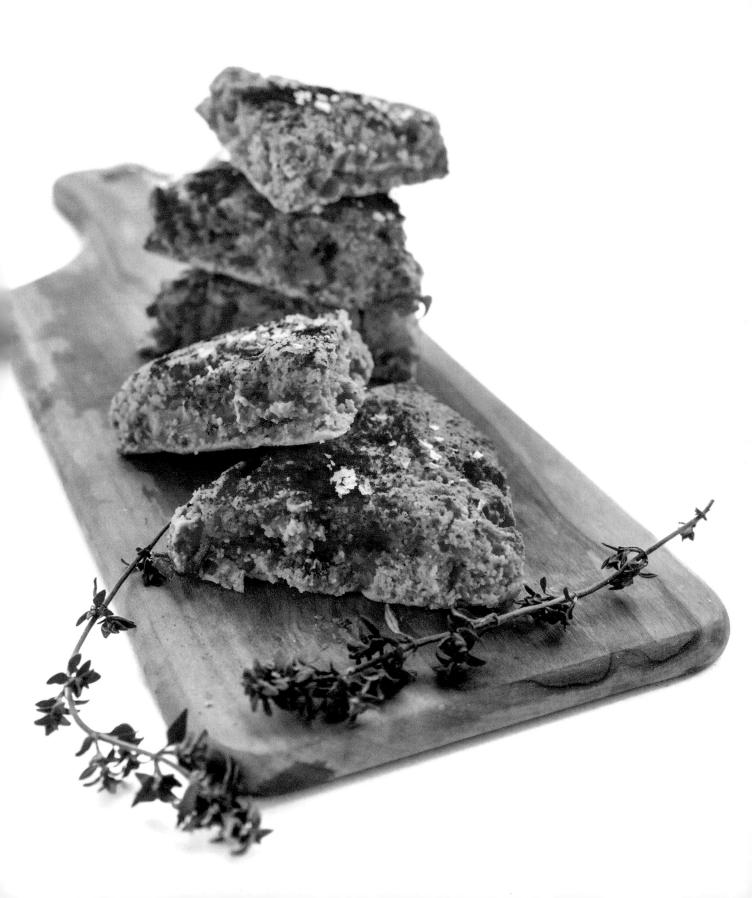

TOASTED COCONUT CHOCOLATE CHUNK DROP SCONES

Yield: 12 scones (1 per serving) Prep Time: 15 minutes Cook Time: 35 minutes

And now for something completely different! I decided to get a little creative with a basic drop scone recipe. These could almost be called breakfast cookies. Whatever you want to call them, they are delicious.

½ cup unsweetened flaked coconut

½ cup (55g) coconut flour

½ cup (50g) blanched almond flour

⅓ cup granulated sweetener of choice

2 teaspoons baking powder

½ teaspoon salt

4 large eggs, room temperature

½ cup coconut cream, softened (see tip)

2 tablespoons coconut water (see tip)

½ teaspoon coconut extract

½ teaspoon vanilla extract

2 ounces sugar-free dark chocolate, coarsely chopped

1. Spread the coconut in a medium skillet and set over medium heat. Toast, stirring frequently, until light golden brown and fragrant, 3 to 5 minutes. Remove the coconut from the pan and let cool.

2. Preheat the oven to 350°F and line a baking sheet with a silicone baking mat or parchment paper.

3. In a large bowl, whisk together the coconut flour, almond flour, sweetener, baking powder, and salt. Stir in the eggs, coconut cream, coconut water, and extracts. Fold in the chopped chocolate and ⅓ cup of the toasted coconut.

4. Using about 3 tablespoons at a time, drop the dough onto the prepared baking sheet, leaving about 2 inches between mounds. Press a few pieces of toasted coconut into the top of each scone.

5. Bake for 26 to 30 minutes, until golden brown and firm to the touch. Remove from the oven and let cool completely on the pan.

TIP: *For the coconut cream, scoop the thick white part from the top of a can of full-fat coconut milk. For the coconut water, simply measure out some of the thinner liquid from the can.*

NUTRITIONAL INFORMATION

CALORIES: 127 | FAT: 9.8g | CARBS: 6.9g | FIBER: 3.5g | PROTEIN: 4.4g

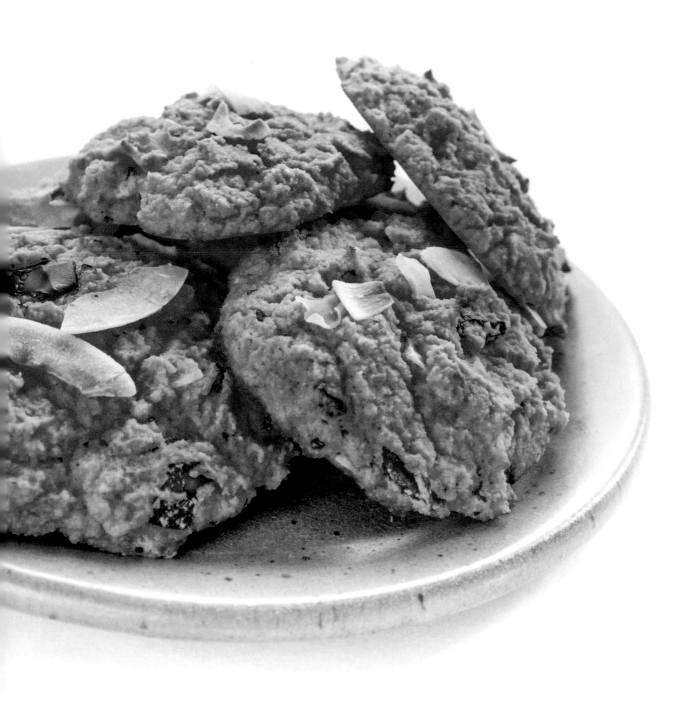

POPOVERS

Yield: 7 popovers (1 per serving) Prep Time: 10 minutes Cook Time: 30 minutes

I'm not going to lie: I may have danced for joy around my kitchen after making these popovers. They worked far better than I could have hoped, and they taste so good with a smear of butter.

6 tablespoons unflavored whey protein powder

6 tablespoons lupin flour (see tips)

½ teaspoon salt

¼ teaspoon garlic powder

⅛ teaspoon xanthan gum

2 large eggs

½ cup water

¼ cup heavy whipping cream

2 tablespoons unsalted butter, melted

Butter, for the pan

1. Preheat the oven to 425°F.

2. In a medium bowl, whisk together the protein powder, lupin flour, salt, garlic powder, and xanthan gum.

3. Place the eggs, water, cream, and melted butter in a blender and blend briefly to combine. Add the dry ingredients and blend until smooth.

4. Place a small piece of butter (about ½ teaspoon) in each of 7 wells of a standard muffin pan. Place the pan in the oven for the last few minutes of preheating, until the butter is melted. Remove the pan from the oven and brush the melted butter onto the sides of each well.

5. Quickly pour the batter into the wells, filling each about two-thirds full. Place the pan back in the oven and bake for 15 minutes. Do not open the oven door.

6. Reduce the oven temperature to 350°F and bake for another 15 minutes, or until the popovers are golden brown all over.

7. Remove from the oven and let cool in the pan for 10 minutes before serving.

TIPS: *I tried making these popovers with both lupin flour and almond flour. They worked out all right with almond flour but were far lighter and fluffier with the lupin flour.*

You really need to add the batter to a hot pan, so be sure to work quickly once you take the pan out of the oven.

These popovers are remarkably crisp when they first come out of the oven but lose their crispness as they sit. It's best to eat them fresh, which is why I created a recipe that makes only a few. They are still good warmed up with some butter, but they won't really get crisp again.

NUTRITIONAL INFORMATION

CALORIES: 106 | FAT: 7.7g | CARBS: 2.1g | FIBER: 1.2g | PROTEIN: 7g

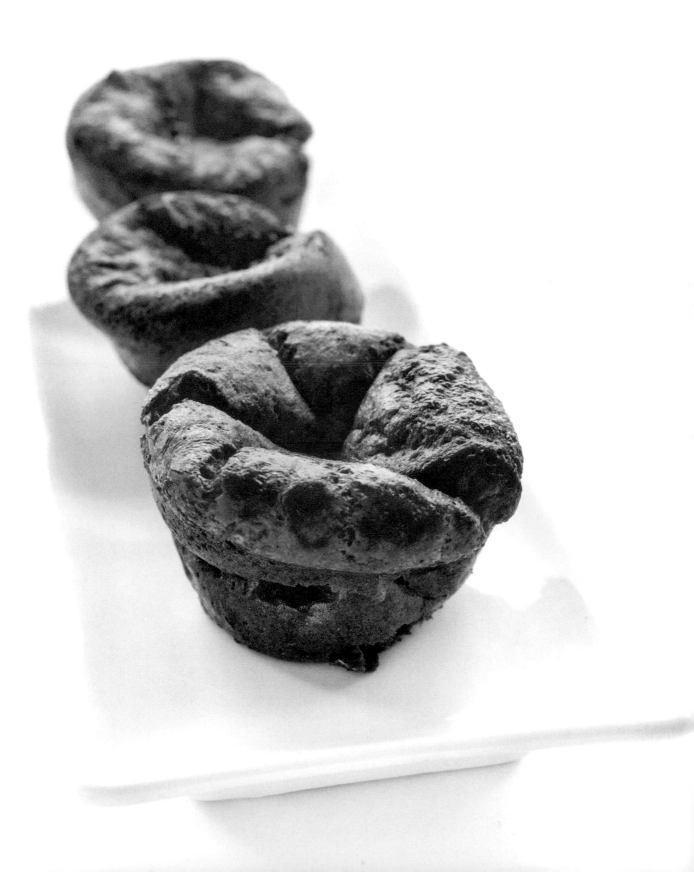

Chapter 11:
BREADS & ROLLS

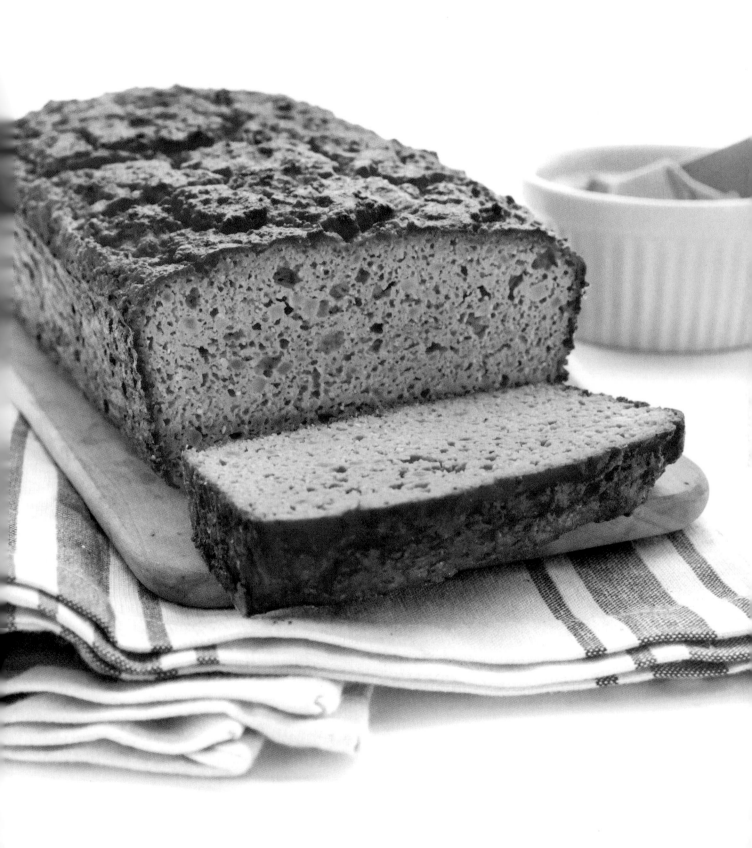

CRANBERRY ORANGE LOAF

OPTION

Yield: 12 servings   Prep Time: 20 minutes   Cook Time: 70 minutes

A holiday classic! This delicious loaf makes a great breakfast or accompaniment to brunch.

3 cups (300g) blanched almond flour

¾ cup granulated sweetener of choice

¼ cup unflavored whey or egg white protein powder

2 teaspoons baking powder

¼ teaspoon salt

1 cup fresh cranberries, coarsely chopped

2 teaspoons grated orange zest

3 large eggs

½ cup (1 stick) unsalted butter, melted but not hot

½ cup water

¾ teaspoon orange extract

½ teaspoon vanilla extract

1. Preheat the oven to 325°F and grease a 9 by 5-inch loaf pan. (An 8 by 4-inch pan also works, but the loaf will take longer to bake through.)

2. In a large bowl, whisk together the almond flour, sweetener, protein powder, baking powder, and salt. Stir in the cranberries and orange zest.

3. Add the eggs, melted butter, water, and extracts and stir until well combined. Spread the batter in the prepared loaf pan and cover the top with foil, shiny side up.

4. Bake for 45 minutes, then remove the foil and bake for another 15 to 25 minutes, until the top is golden brown and firm to the touch. A tester inserted in the center of the loaf should come out clean.

5. Let cool in the pan for at least 20 minutes, then use a knife to loosen the sides and flip out onto a wire rack to cool completely before slicing.

DAIRY-FREE OPTION:

Use egg white protein powder and replace the butter with melted coconut oil or ghee.

TIPS: *Chopping the cranberries a bit before adding them to the batter makes it easier to slice the loaf without tearing the bread.*

You can also make muffins with this recipe. They will take about 25 minutes to bake in a standard muffin pan lined with silicone or parchment paper liners.

NUTRITIONAL INFORMATION
CALORIES: 261 | FAT: 22.3g | CARBS: 7.6g | FIBER: 3.4g | PROTEIN: 9.1g

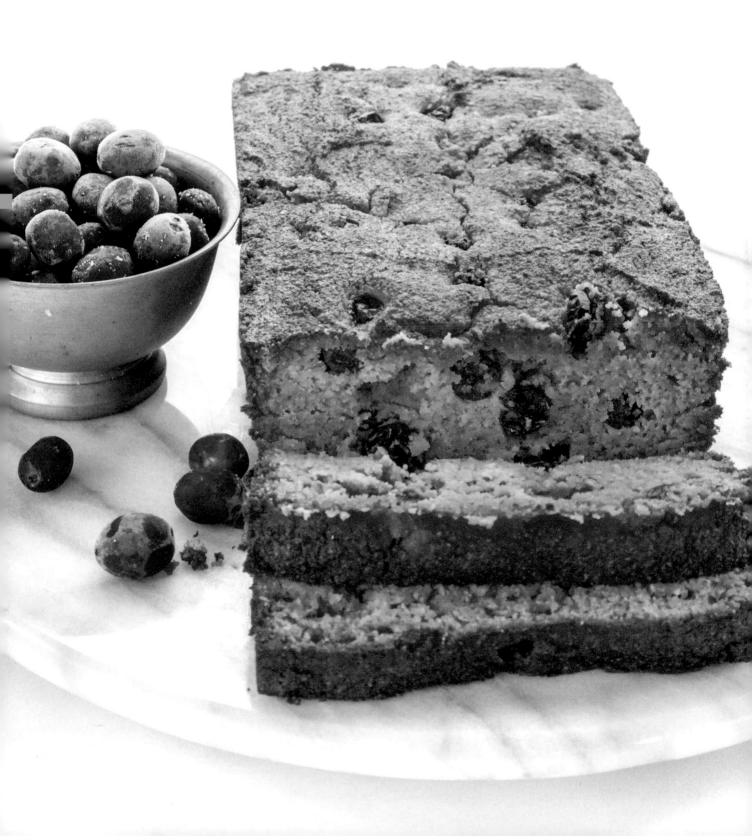

CLASSIC PUMPKIN BREAD

OPTION

Yield: 12 servings Prep Time: 15 minutes Cook Time: 70 minutes

I love pumpkin bread in the fall. This sweet bread reminds me of the pumpkin loaf from Starbucks, an old favorite.

2 cups (200g) blanched almond flour

⅔ cup granulated sweetener of choice

¼ cup (28g) coconut flour

¼ cup unflavored whey or egg white protein powder

2 teaspoons baking powder

1½ teaspoons ground cinnamon

1 teaspoon ginger powder

½ teaspoon salt

¼ teaspoon ground cloves

3 large eggs, room temperature

¾ cup pumpkin puree

¼ cup (½ stick) unsalted butter, melted but not hot

1 teaspoon vanilla extract

2 to 6 tablespoons water

2 tablespoons shelled pumpkin seeds, for garnish (optional)

1. Preheat the oven to 350°F and grease an 8 by 4-inch loaf pan. (A 9 by 5-inch pan also works, but the bread will bake faster, so keep an eye on it.)

2. In a large bowl, whisk together the almond flour, sweetener, coconut flour, protein powder, baking powder, cinnamon, ginger, salt, and cloves.

3. Add the eggs, pumpkin puree, melted butter, and vanilla. Stir in 2 tablespoons of water. Add more water if needed, 1 tablespoon at a time, until a spreadable consistency is achieved.

4. Spread the batter in the prepared loaf pan and sprinkle with the pumpkin seeds, if using. Bake for 55 to 70 minutes, until the top is golden brown and firm to the touch. A tester inserted in the center should come out clean.

5. Let cool in the pan for at least 20 minutes, then use a knife to loosen the sides and flip out onto a wire rack to cool completely before slicing.

DAIRY-FREE OPTION:

Use egg white protein powder and replace the butter with melted coconut oil or ghee.

TIP: *How much water you need to add depends very much on how thick or watery your pumpkin puree is. The batter should not be pourable, but it shouldn't be so thick that you can't spread it easily in the pan.*

NUTRITIONAL INFORMATION
CALORIES: 186 | FAT: 14.4g | CARBS: 7.5g | FIBER: 3.5g | PROTEIN: 7.6g

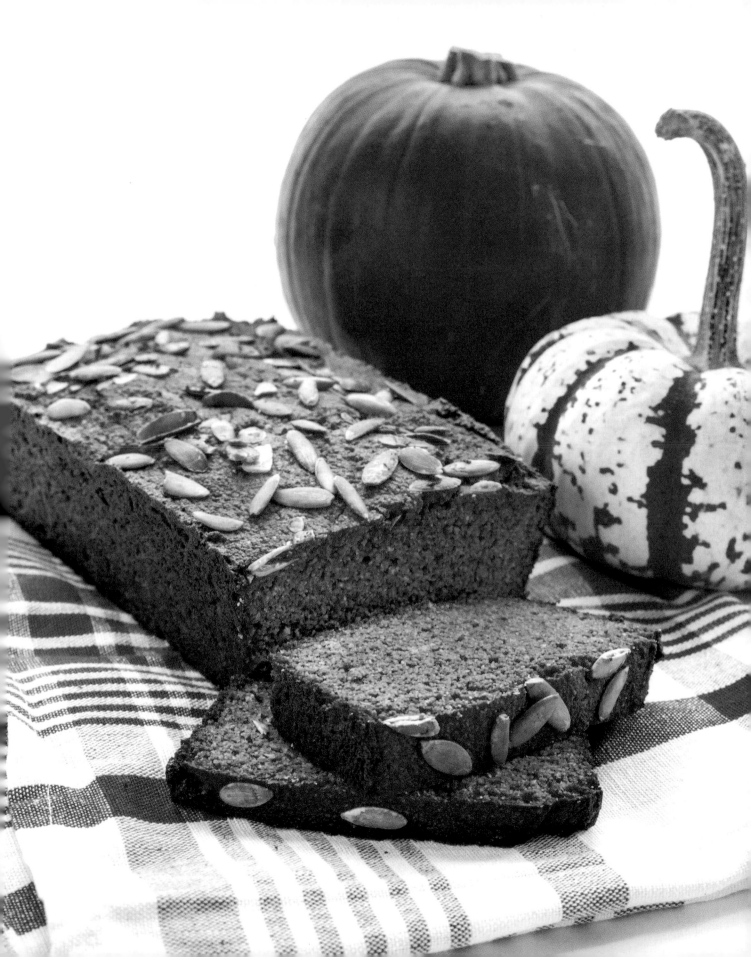

BROWN BUTTER BANANA BREAD

Yield: 12 servings   Prep Time: 15 minutes   Cook Time: 79 minutes

Chia seeds and water create a thick paste that is similar in consistency to mashed bananas. I figured this out a while back, and it's been my trick for keto "banana" bread ever since.

1⅓ cups water, divided

⅓ cup chia seeds, finely ground (see tips)

½ cup (1 stick) unsalted butter

2 cups (200g) blanched almond flour

⅔ cup granulated sweetener of choice

⅓ cup (37g) coconut flour

⅓ cup unflavored whey protein powder

1 tablespoon baking powder

½ teaspoon salt

3 large eggs

1½ teaspoons banana extract

½ teaspoon vanilla extract

1. Preheat the oven to 325°F and grease an 8 by 4-inch loaf pan well. (A 9 by 5-inch pan also works, but the bread will bake faster, so keep an eye on it.)

2. In a small bowl, whisk together ⅔ cup of the water and the ground chia seeds. Let sit until thickened, about 5 minutes.

3. In a medium saucepan over medium heat, melt the butter. Continue cooking until browned and fragrant, about 4 minutes. Let cool for 5 minutes.

4. In a large bowl, whisk together the almond flour, sweetener, coconut flour, protein powder, baking powder, and salt. Stir in the eggs, cooled browned butter, extracts, and remaining ⅔ cup of water until well combined.

5. Spread the batter in the prepared loaf pan and bake for 70 to 75 minutes, until the top is golden brown and firm to the touch. A tester inserted in the center should come out clean.

6. Let cool in the pan for at least 20 minutes, then use a knife to loosen the sides and flip out onto a wire rack to cool completely before slicing.

TIPS: *You can purchase ground chia seeds or grind your own. They are best ground in a coffee grinder because a food processor doesn't seem to catch all the little seeds.*

If you'd prefer to leave the chia seeds out, simply skip Step 2. You may find that you need to add a little more water in Step 4. The batter should be scoopable but not pourable.

NUTRITIONAL INFORMATION
CALORIES: 247 | FAT: 20.1g | CARBS: 8.7g | FIBER: 5.3g | PROTEIN: 9.3g

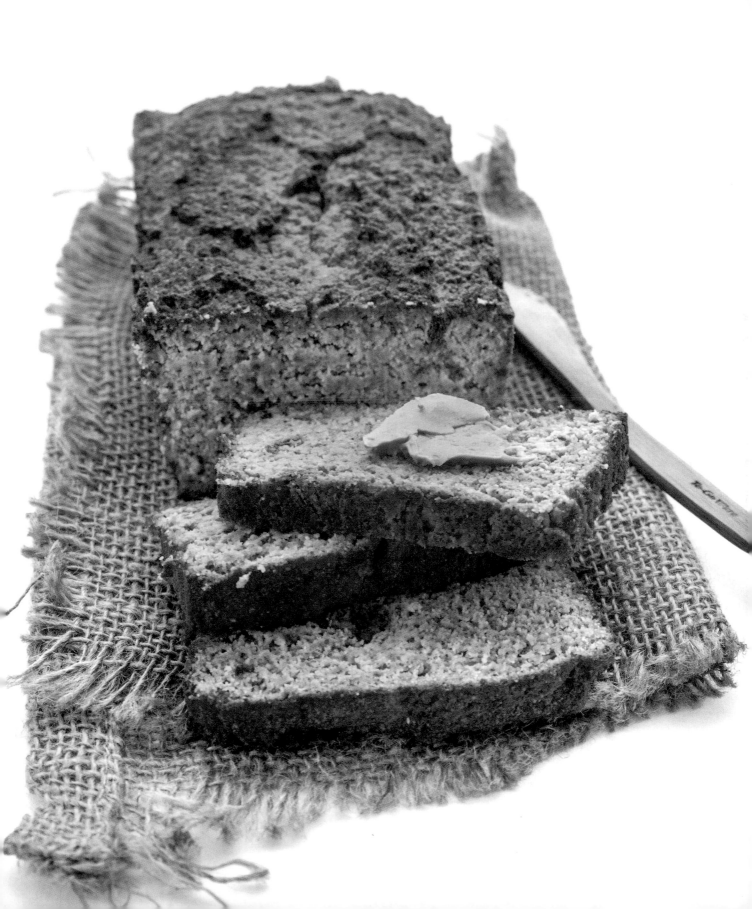

CINNAMON SWIRL BREAD

Yield: 12 servings Prep Time: 20 minutes Cook Time: 1 hour

You can't go wrong with a tender sweet bread that contains a cinnamon swirl. Pro tip: It makes fabulous French toast. We had it that way for Christmas brunch.

Cinnamon "Sugar" Filling/Topping:

2 tablespoons brown sugar substitute

1 tablespoon ground cinnamon

Bread:

¾ cup (83g) coconut flour

⅔ cup granulated erythritol sweetener

¼ cup unflavored whey protein powder

2 teaspoons baking powder

¼ teaspoon salt

½ cup (1 stick) plus 1 tablespoon unsalted butter, melted but not hot, divided

½ cup water

4 large egg whites

2 large eggs

1½ teaspoons vanilla extract

1. Preheat the oven to 350°F and grease a 9 by 5-inch loaf pan. Line the pan with parchment paper, leaving some overhanging the long sides for easier removal.

2. In a small bowl, whisk together the brown sugar substitute and cinnamon.

3. In a large bowl, whisk together the coconut flour, granulated sweetener, protein powder, baking powder, and salt, breaking up any clumps with the back of a wooden spoon.

4. Stir in ½ cup of the melted butter, the water, egg whites, whole eggs, and vanilla until well combined.

5. Spread one-third of the batter in the prepared loaf pan, then sprinkle with one-third of the cinnamon "sugar." Repeat two more times. Drizzle the top of the bread with the remaining 1 tablespoon of melted butter.

6. Bake for 50 to 60 minutes, until the top is firm to the touch and a tester inserted in the center comes out clean. Remove from the oven and let cool in the pan for at least 20 minutes before using the parchment paper to lift the bread out. Transfer to a wire rack to cool completely before slicing.

TIP: *You can use the parchment paper trick for any kind of loaf bread. It makes this tender coconut flour bread much easier to lift out of the pan.*

NUTRITIONAL INFORMATION

CALORIES: 139 | FAT: 10g | CARBS: 5.2g | FIBER: 2.9g | PROTEIN: 4.8g

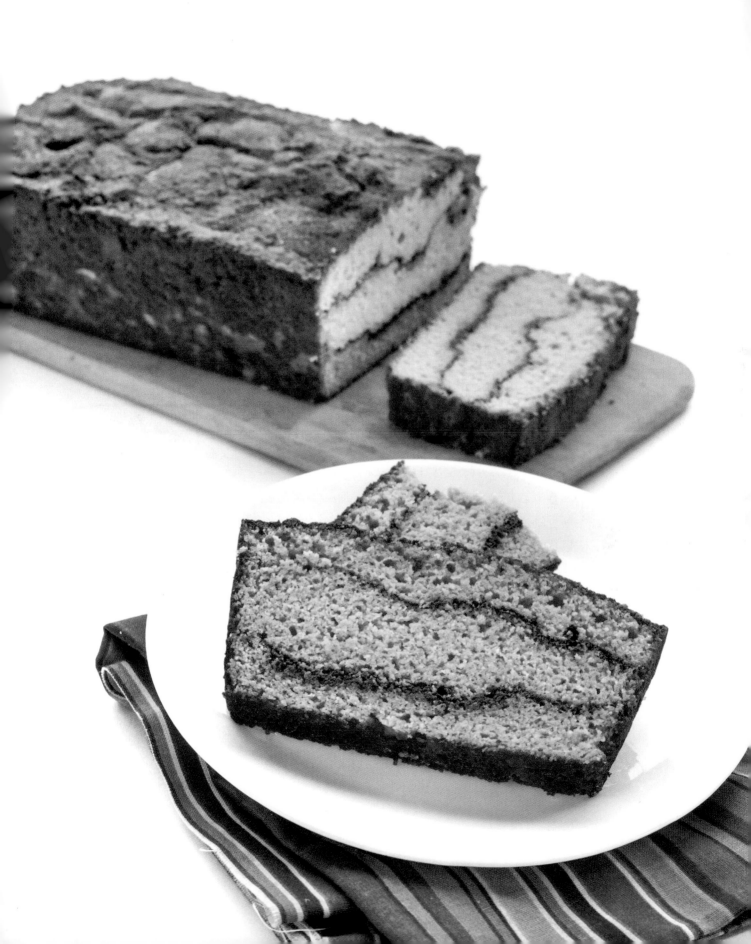

SWEET ALABAMA PECAN BREAD

Yield: 16 servings   Prep Time: 10 minutes   Cook Time: 25 minutes

When I was researching recipes to make for this book, I stumbled upon this pecan bread. I'd never heard of it, but I am a die-hard pecan lover, so I had to try creating a keto version. It's more cake than bread, but it's meant to be served alongside Southern BBQ. I love that idea!

½ cup (1 stick) unsalted butter, melted but not hot

3 large eggs, room temperature

½ cup brown sugar substitute

⅓ cup granulated sweetener of choice

½ teaspoon vanilla extract

1½ cups (150g) blanched almond flour

1½ teaspoons baking powder

½ teaspoon salt

¾ cup chopped pecans

1. Preheat the oven to 325°F and grease a 9-inch square baking pan well.

2. In a large bowl, whisk together the melted butter, eggs, sweeteners, and vanilla. Whisk in the almond flour, baking powder, and salt, then stir in the pecans.

3. Spread the batter evenly in the prepared pan and bake for 20 to 25 minutes, until the edges are golden and the top is just firm to the touch.

4. Remove from the oven and let cool completely in the pan before cutting into squares.

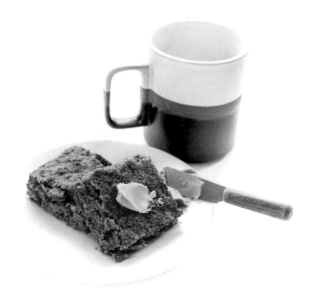

NUTRITIONAL INFORMATION
CALORIES: 159 | FAT: 14.6g | CARBS: 3.1g | FIBER: 1.6g | PROTEIN: 3.9g

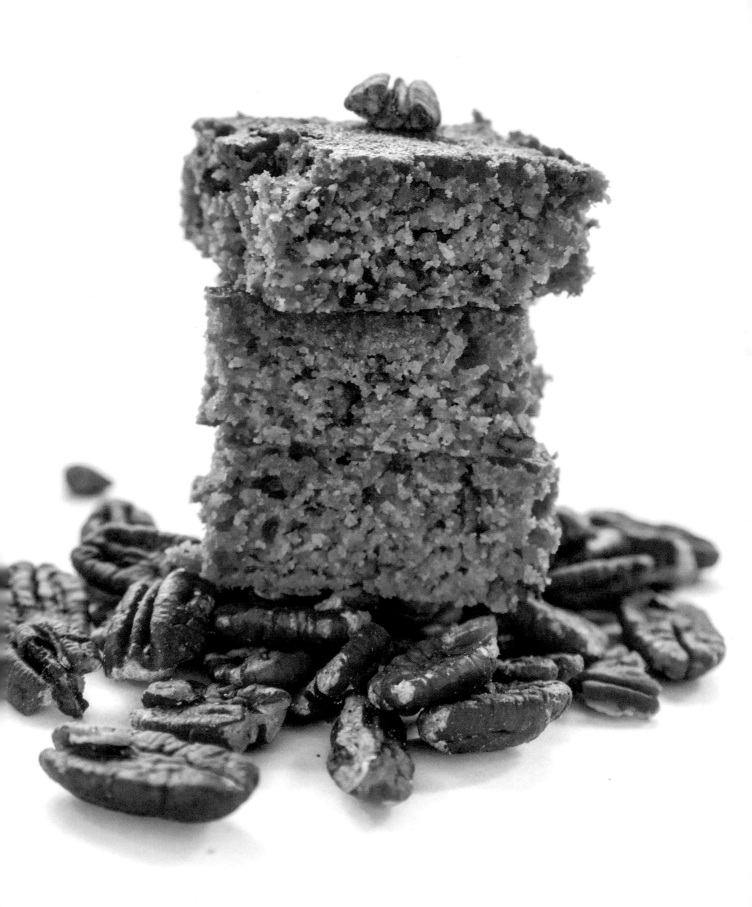

ROSEMARY OLIVE OIL BREAD

Yield: 16 servings Prep Time: 15 minutes Cook Time: 45 minutes

Classic Italian flavors in a savory quick bread. It's good on its own, paired with soup, or turned into sandwiches.

2 cups (200g) blanched almond flour

⅓ cup unflavored egg white protein powder

¼ cup (28g) coconut flour

2 tablespoons psyllium husk powder

2 tablespoons chopped fresh rosemary

1 tablespoon baking powder

1 teaspoon salt

½ teaspoon garlic powder

2 large eggs, room temperature

1 large egg white, room temperature

½ cup plus 1 tablespoon extra-virgin olive oil, divided

⅓ to ½ cup water

Coarse sea salt, for sprinkling

1. Preheat the oven to 350°F and grease an 8 by 4-inch loaf pan very well. (A 9 by 5-inch pan also works, but the bread will bake faster, so keep an eye on it.)

2. In a large bowl, whisk together the almond flour, protein powder, coconut flour, psyllium husk powder, rosemary, baking powder, salt, and garlic powder.

3. Stir in the whole eggs, egg white, ½ cup of the oil, and ⅓ cup water. If the batter is very thick, add more water 1 tablespoon at a time until the batter is spreadable but not pourable.

4. Spread the batter in the prepared loaf pan and bake for 30 minutes. Remove and brush with the remaining 1 tablespoon of oil and sprinkle with the coarse salt. Bake for another 5 to 15 minutes, until the edges are browned and the top is firm to the touch.

5. Remove from the oven and let cool completely in the pan before slicing.

VARIATION: OLIVE AND ROSEMARY BREAD.

Add 4 ounces pitted and sliced black olives to the batter along with the rosemary. Bake as directed.

TIPS: *Psyllium husk powder is a strange ingredient, but it does help create a bready texture. If you want to leave it out, the bread will still be delicious.*

One of my recipe testers turned the leftover bread into croutons by cubing it and baking it in a low-temperature oven until it was dry. A delicious salad topper!

NUTRITIONAL INFORMATION
CALORIES: 170 | FAT: 14.5g | CARBS: 5.8g | FIBER: 3.2g | PROTEIN: 5.7g

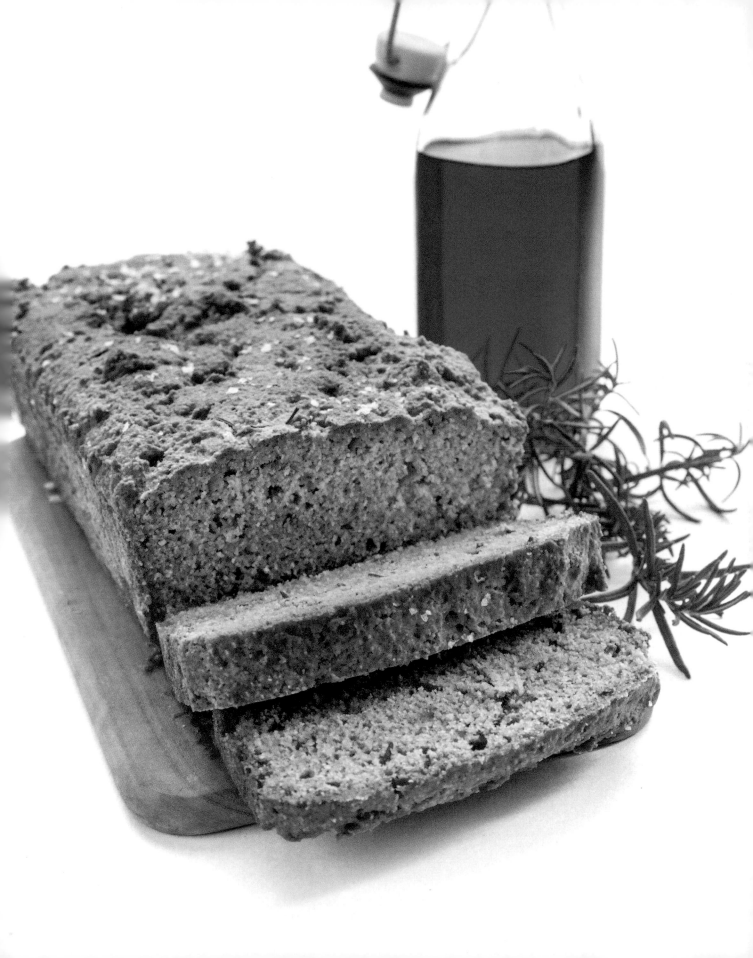

CHEDDAR JALAPEÑO ZUCCHINI BREAD

OPTION

Yield: 12 servings Prep Time: 20 minutes, plus 1 hour to drain zucchini Cook Time: 70 minutes

Zucchini bread doesn't have to be sweet. This cheesy and spicy version is a great way to enjoy that summer zucchini in a tender savory baked good.

2 cups lightly packed shredded zucchini

½ teaspoon salt, divided

2 cups (200g) blanched almond flour

⅓ cup unflavored whey protein powder

¼ cup (28g) coconut flour

1 tablespoon baking powder

1 teaspoon garlic powder

2 cups shredded sharp cheddar cheese (about 8 ounces), divided

2 medium jalapeño peppers, minced (see tips)

3 large eggs

¼ cup (½ stick) unsalted butter, melted but not hot

½ cup to 1 cup unsweetened almond milk

COCONUT-FREE OPTION:

Replace the coconut flour with ⅓ cup (36g) of oat fiber.

1. Place the shredded zucchini in a sieve over a bowl or in the sink. Sprinkle with ¼ teaspoon of the salt and toss to combine. Let drain for 1 hour, then press down firmly to remove as much moisture as possible.

2. Preheat the oven to 325°F and grease a 9 by 5-inch metal loaf pan very well. You can also line the pan with parchment paper, leaving some overhanging the long sides for easier removal.

3. In a large bowl, whisk together the almond flour, protein powder, coconut flour, baking powder, garlic powder, and remaining ¼ teaspoon of salt. Stir in 1½ cups of the shredded cheese and the minced jalapeños.

4. Add the eggs, melted butter, and squeezed zucchini and stir to combine well. Stir in ½ cup almond milk. If the batter is very thick, add more almond milk 1 tablespoon at a time until the batter is spreadable but not pourable.

5. Spread the batter in the prepared loaf pan and sprinkle the remaining ½ cup of cheese over the top. Bake for 60 to 70 minutes, until the bread is risen and golden brown and a tester inserted in the center comes out clean.

6. Remove from the oven and let cool in the pan for 20 minutes, then flip out onto a wire rack to cool completely before slicing.

TIPS: *Heat is a matter of taste. I always leave the seeds in my jalapeños because they contain the most heat and I like things spicy. You can seed yours if you like things milder. You can also skip the peppers altogether if you prefer.*

One of my recipe testers had trouble getting this bread to bake through properly. Turned out she was using a glass loaf pan. I highly recommend using metal here, because zucchini tends to make breads very moist.

NUTRITIONAL INFORMATION

CALORIES: 263 | FAT: 20.2g | CARBS: 7.6g | FIBER: 3.3g | PROTEIN: 12.9g

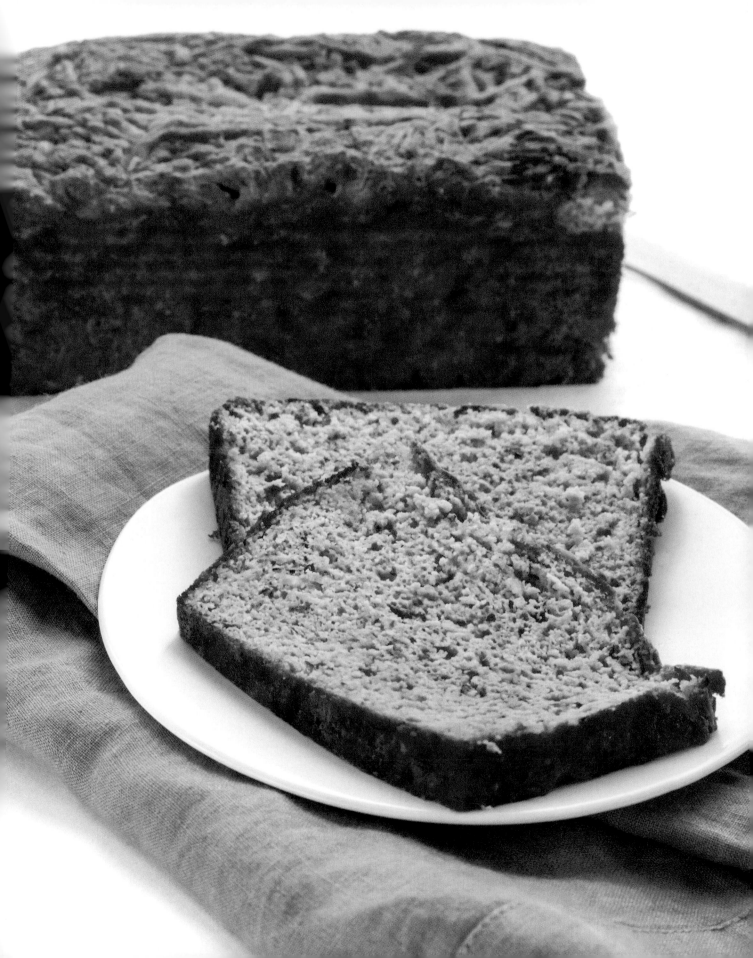

GARLIC PARMESAN CAULIFLOWER BREAD

OPTION

Yield: 12 servings   Prep Time: 20 minutes   Cook Time: 70 minutes

I went out on a limb with this cauliflower bread and was delighted with the results. It's definitely moister than other breads, but it toasts really nicely and makes fabulous garlic bread. My kids ate it happily even after they were informed it was made with cauliflower.

12 ounces riced cauliflower

1 ounce Parmesan cheese, grated (about 1 cup)

4 cloves garlic, minced

1 teaspoon salt

½ teaspoon black pepper

6 large eggs

1 cup (100g) blanched almond flour

¼ cup (28g) coconut flour

1 tablespoon baking powder

COCONUT-FREE OPTION:

Replace the coconut flour with ⅓ cup (36g) of oat fiber.

1. Place the riced cauliflower in a microwave-safe bowl and cover with plastic wrap. Heat on high for 10 minutes, until very tender. Be careful when removing the plastic wrap, as the escaping steam can burn you.

2. Line a sieve with a tea towel and set it in the sink, then transfer the cauliflower to the tea towel. Let sit until it's cool enough to handle, at least 10 minutes. Then gather the ends of the towel and squeeze out as much moisture as possible.

3. Preheat the oven to 350°F and grease a 9 by 5-inch loaf pan. Line the pan with parchment paper, leaving some overhanging the long sides for easier removal.

4. In a large bowl, stir together the squeezed cauliflower, Parmesan, garlic, salt, and pepper, breaking up any clumps of cauliflower. Add the eggs and mix until fully incorporated.

5. Stir in the almond flour, coconut flour, and baking powder until well combined. Spread the batter in the prepared loaf pan and bake for 50 to 60 minutes, until golden brown on top and firm to the touch. A tester inserted in the center should come out clean.

6. Remove from the oven and let cool completely in the pan. Use the parchment to lift the bread out before slicing.

TIPS: *A 9 by 5-inch loaf pan works best because the bread is so moist. The larger pan allows it to bake through a little better.*

Unlike most quick breads, which are fine left on the counter for a few days, this bread should be stored in the fridge.

NUTRITIONAL INFORMATION

CALORIES: 117 | FAT: 7.8g | CARBS: 5.4g | FIBER: 2.5g | PROTEIN: 6.9g

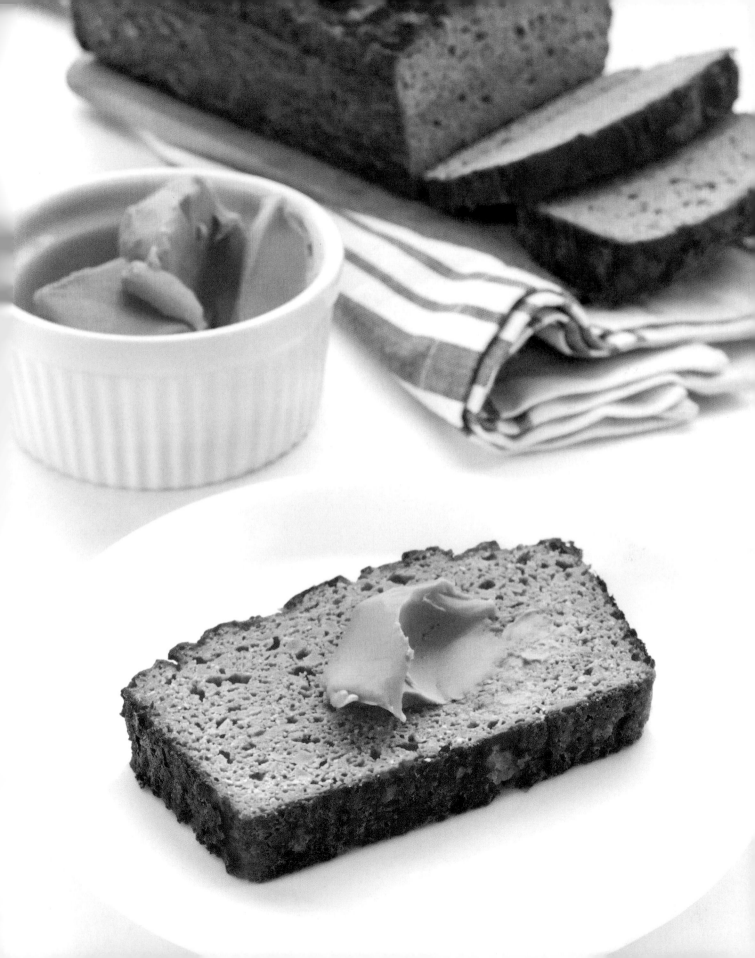

KETO YEAST BREAD

OPTION

Yield: 16 servings Prep Time: 25 minutes, plus 1 hour to rise Cook Time: 50 minutes

I won't lie: this recipe took a lot of tries to get right. And it's a bit of a finicky one. But you end up with a delicious gluten-free keto bread that has all the great yeasty flavor of traditional bread.

¾ cup plus 2 tablespoons warm water (110 to 120°F)

2 teaspoons honey or sugar

2 (¼-ounce) envelopes active dry yeast (about 4½ teaspoons)

1 cup (100g) blanched almond flour

½ cup lupin flour or oat fiber

½ cup unflavored egg white or whey protein powder

¼ cup psyllium husk powder

1 tablespoon baking powder

1 teaspoon salt

2 large eggs

¼ cup (½ stick) unsalted butter, melted but not hot

DAIRY-FREE OPTION:

Use egg white protein powder rather than whey protein powder. Any oil will do in place of the butter. Avocado or olive oil would be delicious!

1. Grease an 8 by 4-inch metal loaf pan well.

2. Place the warm water in a bowl or measuring cup and stir in the honey until dissolved. Sprinkle with the yeast and let sit for 10 minutes.

3. In a large bowl, whisk together the almond flour, lupin flour, protein powder, psyllium husk powder, baking powder, and salt.

4. Add the eggs, melted butter, and yeast mixture all at once and whisk until most of the lumps are gone.

5. Pour the batter into the prepared loaf pan, cover with a tea towel, and set in a warm spot to rise for 40 to 60 minutes. The dough should rise just above the rim of the pan.

6. In the last 10 minutes of rising, start preheating the oven to 350°F. Place the pan in the center of the oven and bake for 40 to 50 minutes, until golden brown and firm to the touch. If the bread begins to brown too quickly, cover with foil, shiny side up.

7. Remove from the oven and let cool completely in the pan before slicing.

TIPS: *Do not panic when you see honey or sugar in this recipe. Yeast feeds on sugar and turns it into the carbon dioxide necessary to make the bread rise properly.*

The bread rises during the first stage but then stops and won't keep rising in the oven. So once you see the dough approaching the rim of the loaf pan, start preheating the oven. Once it reaches just above the rim, that's about as high as it will rise.

Yeast bread really does need a warm place to rise. Your house should be 70°F or warmer to get this bread to rise properly. And don't use a glass loaf pan. The bread simply won't rise or bake as well.

NUTRITIONAL INFORMATION

CALORIES: 107 | FAT: 7.1g | CARBS: 6.5g | FIBER: 4g | PROTEIN: 6.2g

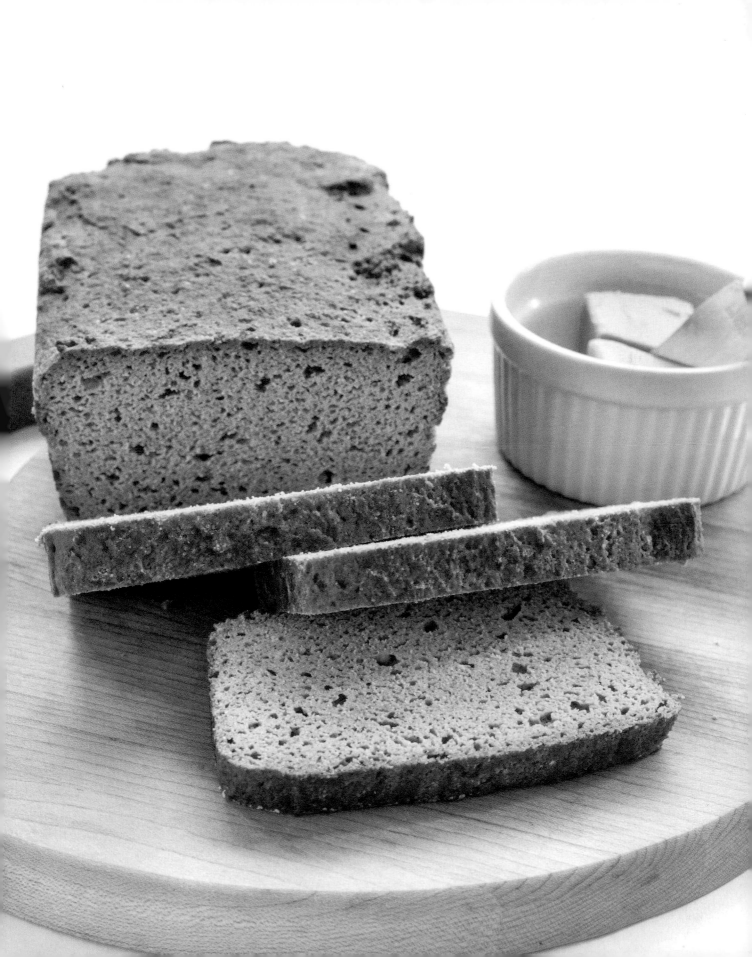

CHEESY PORK RIND BREADSTICKS

Yield: 8 servings Prep Time: 15 minutes Cook Time: 17 minutes

It's shocking to think that something so bready can come from pork rinds. This recipe has no other flours in it, so it's extremely low in carbs.

1½ cups ground pork rinds

2 teaspoons baking powder

½ teaspoon garlic powder

¼ teaspoon black pepper

2 large eggs

¼ cup heavy cream

1 cup shredded mozzarella cheese (about 4 ounces)

1 tablespoon chopped fresh parsley, for garnish

1. Preheat the oven to 425°F and line a baking sheet with a silicone baking mat or parchment paper.

2. In a large bowl, whisk together the ground pork rinds, baking powder, garlic powder, and pepper. Assuming your pork rinds are salted, there should be no need for additional salt.

3. Stir in the eggs and cream until well combined. Turn the dough out onto the prepared baking sheet and pat into a 9 by 7-inch rectangle.

4. Bake for 12 minutes, until puffed and golden. Remove from the oven and sprinkle with the mozzarella, then bake for another 5 minutes to melt the cheese. Turn on the broiler and broil for 1 to 2 minutes to brown the cheese a bit, if desired.

5. Sprinkle with the chopped parsley. Cut lengthwise down the center, then cut slices from each side for breadsticks.

TIP: *It takes quite a lot of pork rinds to get 1½ cups ground. If you're grinding your own, expect to use 5 to 6 ounces.*

SERVING SUGGESTION: *Serve with low-carb marinara sauce for dipping, if desired.*

NUTRITIONAL INFORMATION

CALORIES: 183 | FAT: 11.8g | CARBS: 1.1g | PROTEIN: 15.7g

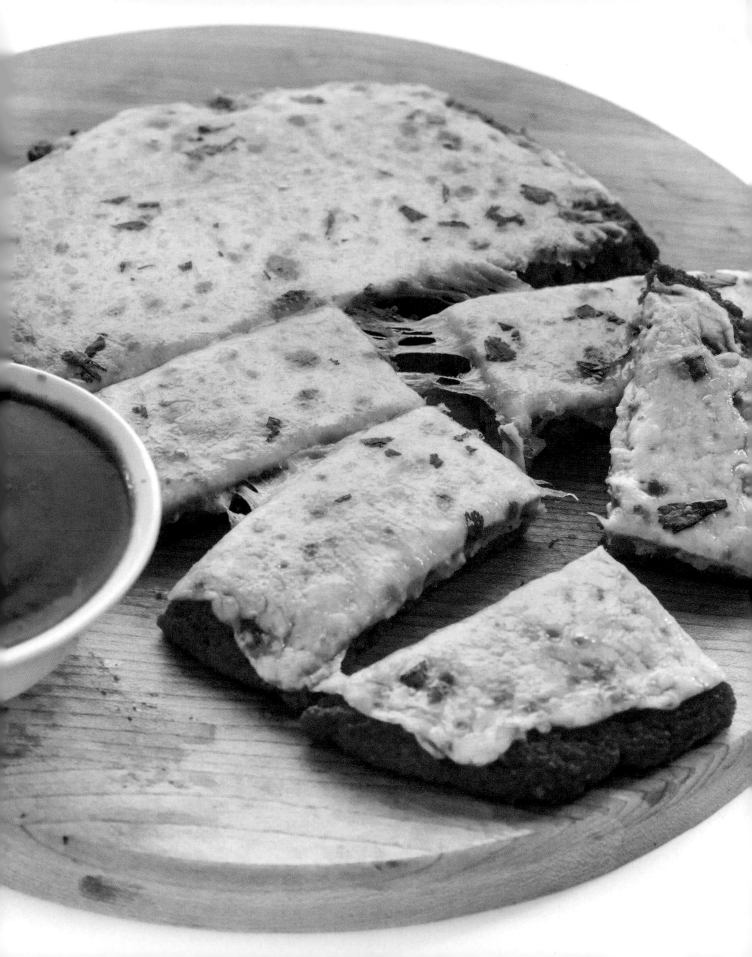

CRACKLIN' CORNBREAD

OPTION

Yield: 10 servings Prep Time: 15 minutes Cook Time: 45 minutes

---

As strange as it seems, coconut flour really can taste like cornbread, even without the addition of cornbread flavoring. Cooking it in a skillet gives you delightfully crispy edges with a tender and light center.

½ cup (1 stick) plus 1 tablespoon unsalted butter, divided

1 cup (110g) coconut flour

¾ cup ground pork rinds

2 medium jalapeño peppers, minced (optional)

1 tablespoon baking powder

½ teaspoon salt

6 large eggs, room temperature

1 cup water

½ teaspoon cornbread flavoring (optional; see tips)

DAIRY-FREE OPTION:

Use avocado oil or melted ghee in place of the butter. Coconut oil is not a great choice, as it would impart a stronger flavor.

1. Preheat the oven to 375°F. Place 1 tablespoon of the butter in a 10-inch cast-iron or other ovenproof skillet. Put the pan in the oven as it preheats.

2. Place the remaining ½ cup of butter in a microwave-safe bowl and heat on high in 30-second increments until melted.

3. In a large bowl, whisk together the coconut flour, ground pork rinds, jalapeños (if using), baking powder, and salt. Stir in the eggs, water, melted butter, and cornbread flavoring, if using, until well combined.

4. Remove the hot skillet from the oven and use a pastry brush to brush the melted butter over the bottom and up the sides. Spread the batter in the pan. Bake for 35 to 45 minutes, until the edges are golden and the center is firm to the touch.

5. Remove from the oven and let cool in the pan for 15 minutes before slicing.

TIPS: *You really want to use ground pork rinds here. I tried leaving in bigger pieces for more "cracklin'." Unfortunately, they soaked up moisture and became very chewy. You could sprinkle some bigger pieces on top, though.*

The cornbread flavoring is completely optional. I've been making "keto cornbread" without it for ages, but some of my readers really enjoy the flavor it gives this bread.

NUTRITIONAL INFORMATION
CALORIES: 214 | FAT: 15.5g | CARBS: 7.2g | FIBER: 4.1g | PROTEIN: 9g

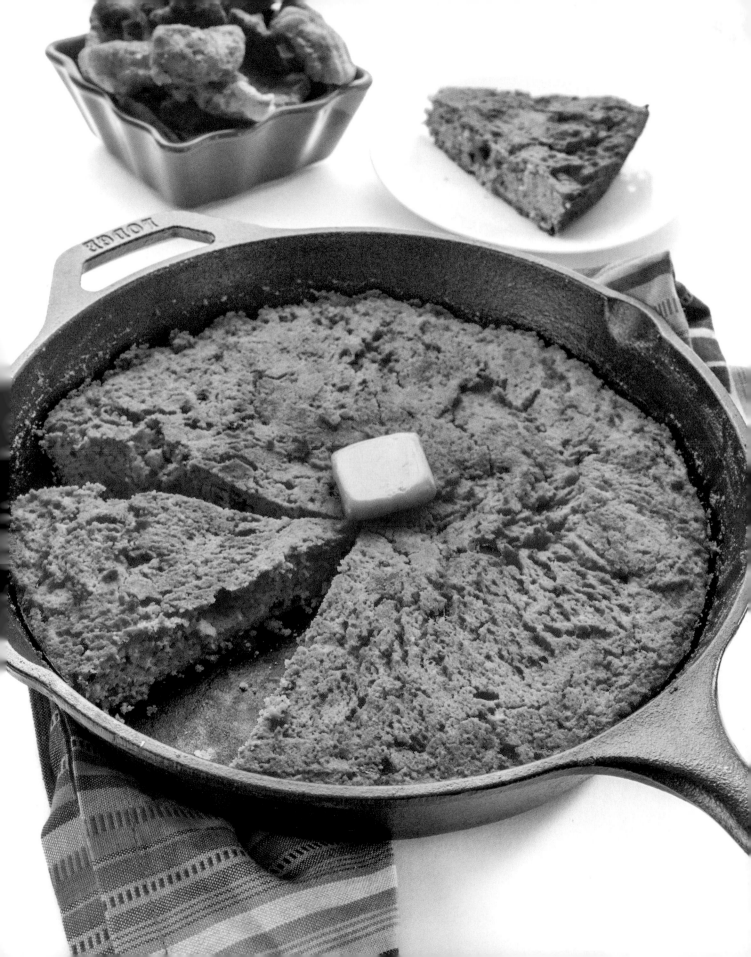

CHEWY KETO BAGELS

Yield: 8 bagels (1 per serving) Prep Time: 20 minutes (not including time to make dough) Cook Time: 20 minutes

These nut-free fathead bagels became an instant hit when I published them on my website. I knew I had to include them in a big book about keto baking.

1 teaspoon sesame seeds

1 teaspoon poppyseeds

1 teaspoon dried minced onions

½ teaspoon coarse sea salt

1 recipe Nut-Free Magic Mozzarella Dough (page 376)

1 tablespoon unsalted butter, melted

1. In a shallow dish, stir together the sesame seeds, poppyseeds, dried minced onions, and salt.

2. Preheat the oven to 350°F and line a baking sheet with a silicone baking mat or parchment paper.

3. Cut the prepared dough in half and divide each half into 4 equal portions so that you have 8 equal pieces of dough. Roll each piece into a log about 8 inches long. Pinch the ends of each log together to form a ring.

4. Brush the tops of the bagels with the melted butter and dip firmly into the seed mixture. Place on the prepared baking sheet and bake for 15 to 20 minutes, until the bagels have risen and are golden brown. Remove from the oven and let cool completely on the pan before slicing.

TIP: *I have tried making bagels with almond flour–based fathead dough, and it simply spreads too much. The bagels become almost as flat as pancakes. Coconut flour makes a much better keto bagel.*

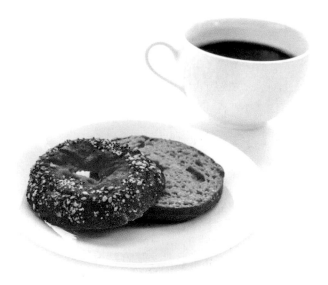

NUTRITIONAL INFORMATION

CALORIES: 190 | FAT: 12.3g | CARBS: 5.5g | FIBER: 2.6g | PROTEIN: 12.1g

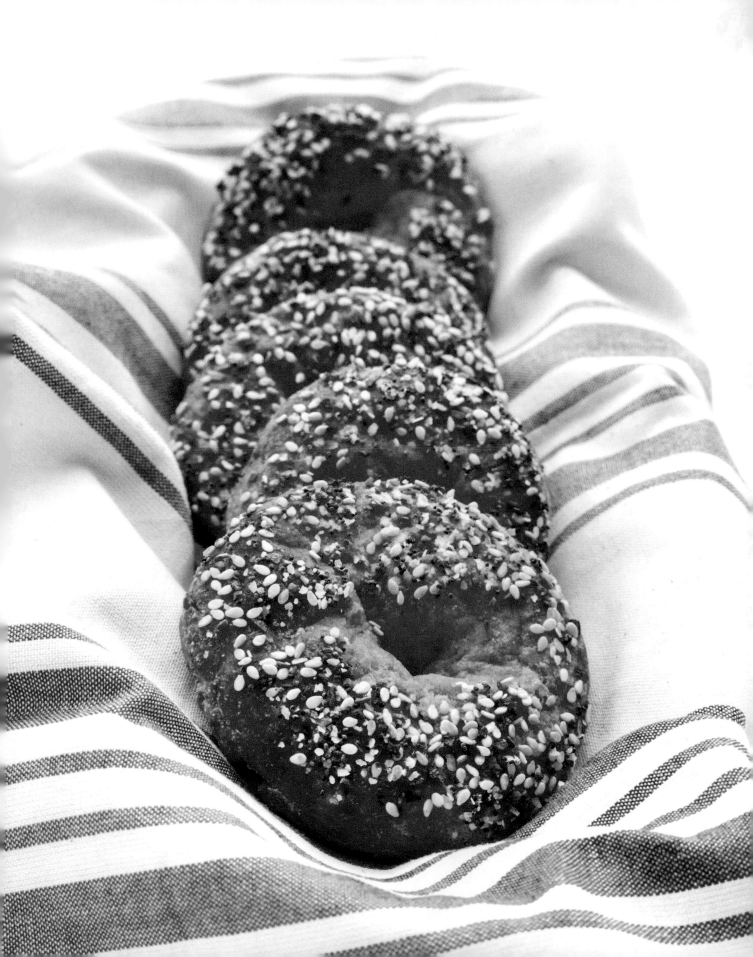

SPINACH FETA PINWHEELS

Yield: 16 rolls (1 per serving) **Prep Time:** 25 minutes (not including time to make dough) **Cook Time:** 22 minutes

These pretty pinwheels make a wonderful keto appetizer. I made some for a tapas party, and they were gone in the blink of an eye.

8 ounces frozen chopped spinach, thawed and drained

¾ cup crumbled feta cheese (about 3 ounces)

¼ ounce Parmesan cheese, grated (about ¼ cup)

2 cloves garlic, minced

½ teaspoon dried marjoram

½ teaspoon salt

½ teaspoon black pepper

1 recipe Nut-Free Magic Mozzarella Dough (page 376)

1 tablespoon unsalted butter, melted

Coarse sea salt, for sprinkling

1. Preheat the oven to 375°F and line a baking sheet with a silicone baking mat or parchment paper.

2. Squeeze out as much moisture from the spinach as possible and place the spinach in a medium bowl. Stir in the feta, Parmesan, garlic, marjoram, salt, and pepper until well combined.

3. Lightly grease another baking mat or large piece of parchment paper and transfer the prepared dough onto it. Pat into a rough square and top with another piece of parchment or waxed paper.

4. Roll out the dough to a 16-inch square. Spread the filling on top, leaving a ½-inch border. Roll up the dough tightly and pinch the seam to seal.

5. Use a very sharp knife to cut the dough into 1-inch slices and place the pinwheels cut side down on the prepared baking sheet. Brush with the butter and sprinkle with a little coarse salt.

6. Bake for 18 to 22 minutes, until the pinwheels are golden brown and just firm to the touch. Remove from the oven and let cool completely on the pan.

TIP: *Use frozen chopped spinach rather than whole leaf spinach. It's easier to cut through when slicing the rolls.*

NUTRITIONAL INFORMATION
CALORIES: 119 | FAT: 7.6g | CARBS: 3.7g | FIBER: 1.7g | PROTEIN: 7.7g

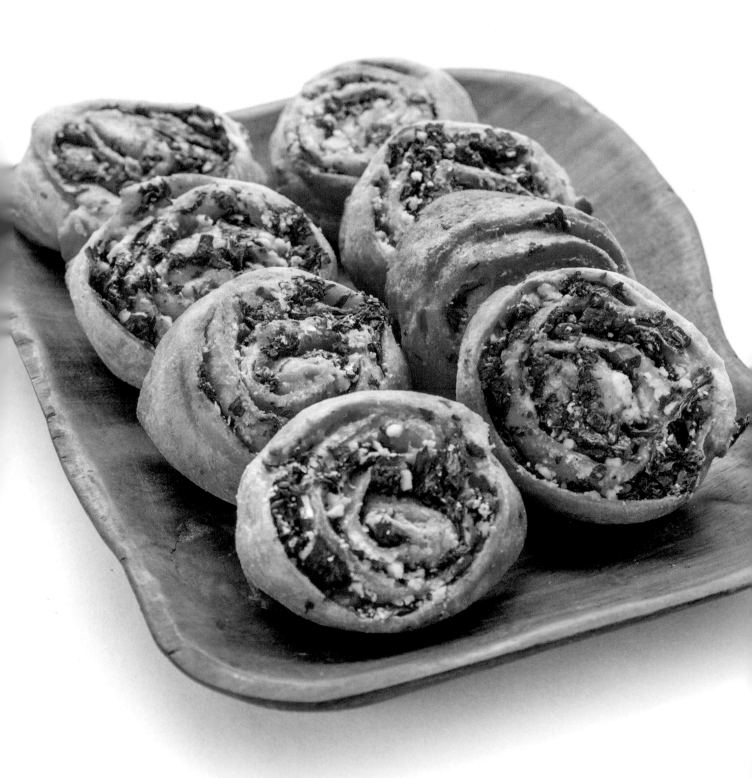

CLOVERLEAF DINNER ROLLS

Yield: 6 rolls (1 per serving) Prep Time: 20 minutes Cook Time: 25 minutes

These rolls are based on a dough similar to fathead dough, but made with cheddar cheese instead of mozzarella. They are buttery and rich, just as cloverleaf rolls should be.

1 cup shredded cheddar cheese (about 4 ounces)

3 tablespoons unsalted butter, divided

¼ cup (28g) coconut flour

2 tablespoons unflavored whey or egg white protein powder

2 teaspoons baking powder

½ teaspoon garlic powder

¼ teaspoon salt

2 large egg whites, room temperature

1 clove garlic, minced

1 teaspoon chopped fresh parsley

¼ teaspoon coarse sea salt

1. Preheat the oven to 350°F and grease 6 wells of a standard nonstick muffin pan very well.

2. Place the cheese and 2 tablespoons of the butter in a large microwave-safe bowl. Heat on high in 30-second increments until the cheese and butter are quite liquid and can be stirred together easily. Stir until combined.

3. Add the coconut flour, protein powder, baking powder, garlic powder, salt, and egg whites and stir to combine. Use a rubber spatula to knead the ingredients together against the sides of the bowl until the dough is uniform.

4. Roll the dough into ¾-inch balls and place 3 balls each in the prepared muffin cups. If the dough is very sticky, lightly oil your hands before rolling the balls.

5. In a small microwave-safe bowl, melt the remaining 1 tablespoon of butter. Stir in the garlic, parsley, and coarse salt. Brush half of this mixture over the rolls before baking.

6. Bake for 20 to 25 minutes, until puffed, golden brown, and just firm to the touch. Remove from the oven and let cool in the pan for 10 minutes before removing. Brush with the remaining garlic butter mixture and serve warm.

TIP: *Use a flexible spatula with a very thin blade to loosen the rolls from the pan. If you prefer, you can use parchment paper liners to keep them from sticking.*

NUTRITIONAL INFORMATION
CALORIES: 162 | FAT: 11.6g | CARBS: 4g | FIBER: 1.7g | PROTEIN: 8g

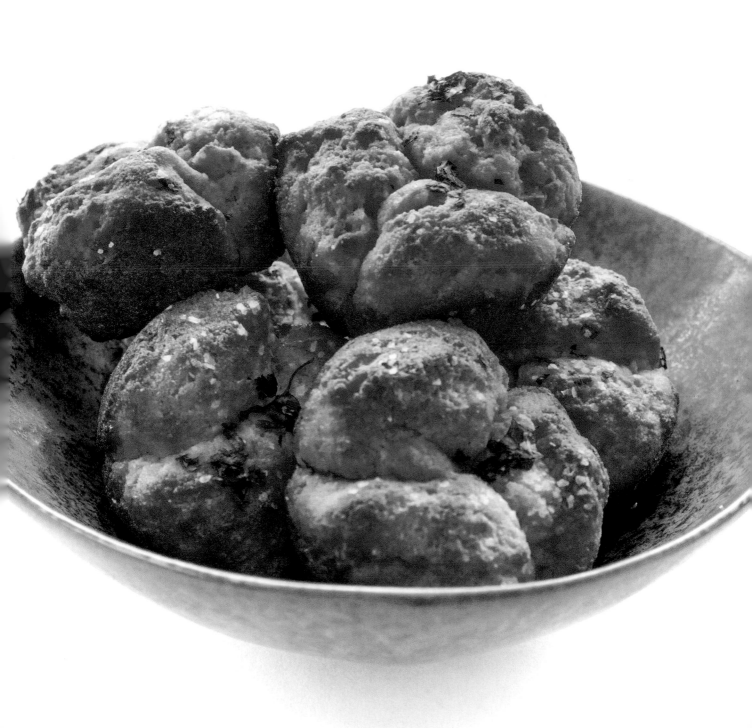

Chapter 12:
FLATBREADS, PIZZA & CRACKERS

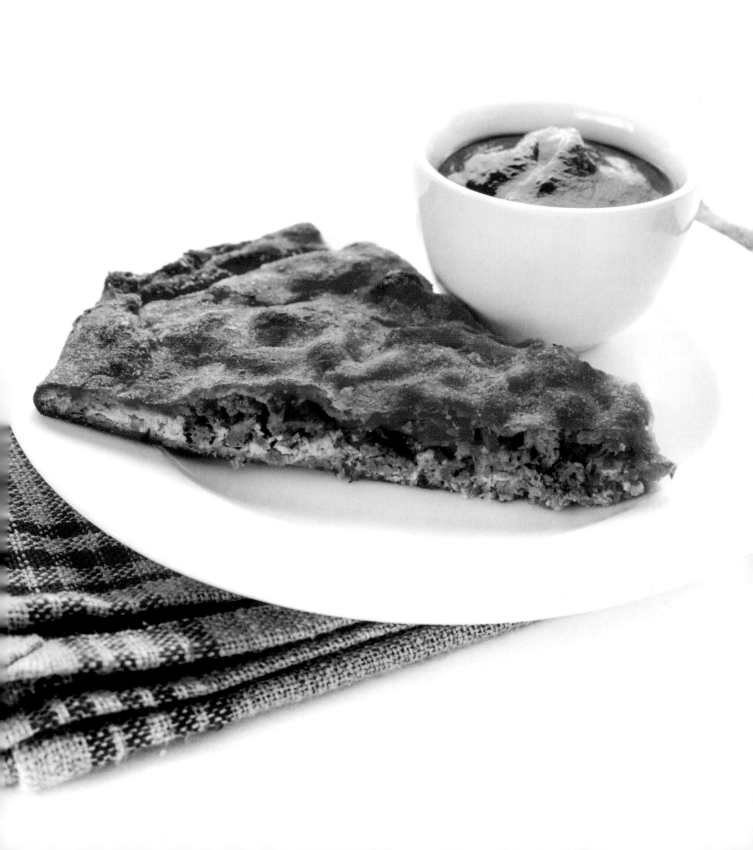

CLASSIC PEPPERONI PIZZA

Yield: 6 servings   Prep Time: 10 minutes (not including time to make dough)   Cook Time: 25 minutes

Fathead dough has changed the game for keto pizza lovers. This pizza is always a win with my family. Feel free to add your favorite toppings!

½ recipe Nut-Free Magic Mozzarella Dough (page 376)

¼ cup tomato paste

½ cup warm water

½ teaspoon garlic powder

½ teaspoon dried crushed oregano or basil

¼ teaspoon salt

¼ teaspoon black pepper

1 cup shredded mozzarella cheese (about 4 ounces)

2 ounces sliced pepperoni

½ ounce Parmesan cheese, grated (about ½ cup)

1. Preheat the oven to 350°F and line a work surface with a silicone baking mat or a large piece of parchment paper.

2. Place the prepared dough on the work surface. Cover with a piece of parchment paper and roll out to a 12-inch circle. Remove the top piece of parchment.

3. Transfer the baking mat or parchment paper with the pizza crust on it to a pizza stone or cookie sheet. Par-bake for 10 minutes, until just starting to brown and firm up.

4. In a medium bowl, whisk together the tomato paste, water, garlic powder, oregano, salt, and pepper. Spread the sauce mixture over the crust, leaving a ½-inch border.

5. Sprinkle with the mozzarella and top with the pepperoni, then sprinkle on the Parmesan.

6. Bake for another 12 to 15 minutes, until the cheese is melted and bubbly. Remove from the oven and let cool on the stone for 10 minutes before slicing and serving.

TIPS: *I prefer the consistency of the crust when it's baked on parchment paper on a pizza stone. However, I find it easier to roll out the crust on a silicone baking mat. You could simply transfer the untopped crust from the baking mat to a pizza stone or baking sheet lined with parchment.*

You can use the Magic Mozzarella Dough made with almond flour (page 375) for this recipe if you prefer.

NUTRITIONAL INFORMATION

CALORIES: 240 | FAT: 15g | CARBS: 6.7g | FIBER: 2.1g | PROTEIN: 15.6g

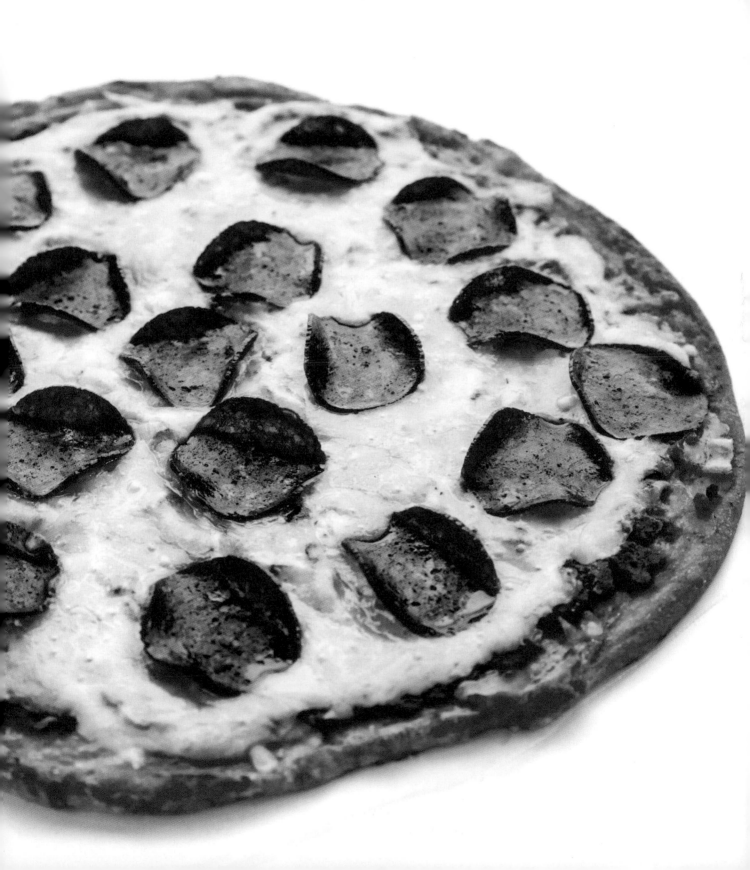

JALAPEÑO POPPER PIZZA

OPTION

Yield: 8 servings Prep Time: 15 minutes (not including time to make dough) Cook Time: 27 minutes

This is a fun take on pizza, and my husband declared it to be the best pizza he's ever had. Not just the best keto pizza, but the best pizza ever!

4 slices bacon, chopped

1 recipe Magic Mozzarella Dough (page 375)

4 ounces cream cheese, softened

1 cup shredded mozzarella cheese (about 4 ounces)

½ cup shredded cheddar cheese (about 2 ounces)

1 large jalapeño pepper, thinly sliced

NUT-FREE OPTION:

Use a half recipe of the Nut-Free Magic Mozzarella Dough (page 376).

1. In a medium skillet over medium heat, cook the chopped bacon until crisp, about 5 minutes. Transfer to a paper towel–lined plate to drain.

2. Preheat the oven to 350°F and line a work surface with a silicone baking mat or a large piece of parchment paper.

3. Place the prepared dough on the work surface. Cover with a piece of parchment paper and roll out to a 12-inch circle. Remove the top piece of parchment.

4. Transfer the baking mat or parchment paper with the pizza crust on it to a pizza stone or cookie sheet. Par-bake for 10 minutes, until just starting to brown and firm up.

5. Remove from the oven and spread with the cream cheese. Top with the mozzarella and cheddar, then sprinkle with the chopped bacon and sliced jalapeño.

6. Bake for another 10 to 12 minutes, until the cheese is melted and bubbly. Remove from the oven and let cool on the stone for 10 minutes before slicing and serving.

TIP: *Never try to bake the pizza dough directly on a pizza stone or baking sheet. It would stick like the dickens!*

NUTRITIONAL INFORMATION
CALORIES: 364 | FAT: 29.4g | CARBS: 5.7g | FIBER: 2.1g | PROTEIN: 14.7g

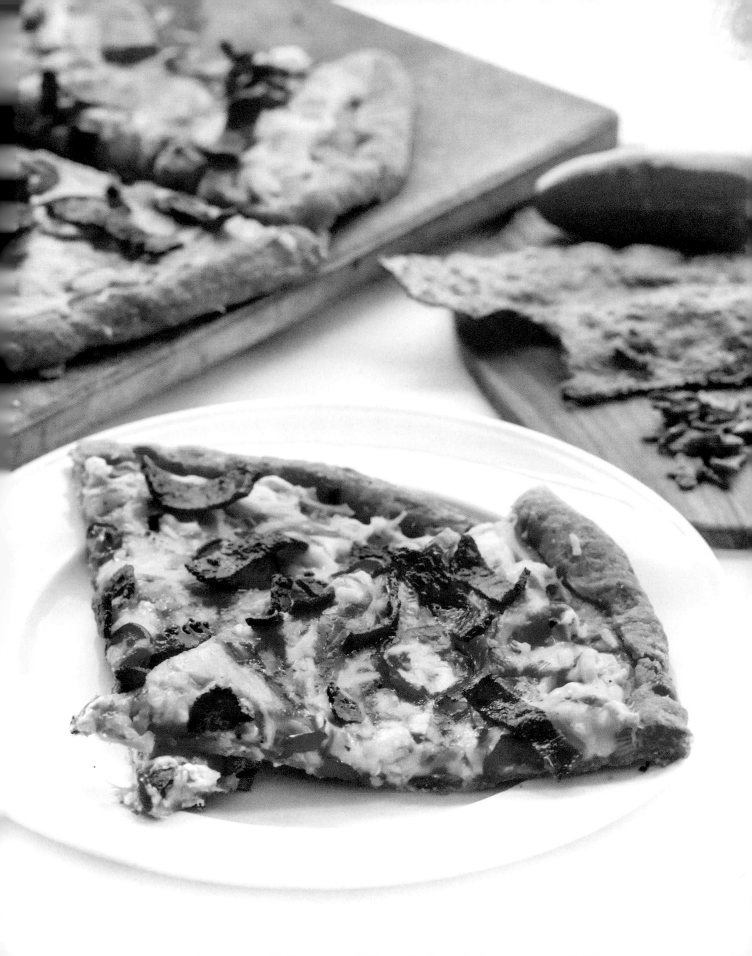

SAUSAGE AND BROCCOLI CALZONE

Yield: 4 servings   Prep Time: 20 minutes (not including time to make dough)   Cook Time: 30 minutes

A calzone is really just pizza folded over on itself and stuffed with delicious fillings, like sausage, broccoli, and cheese, of course.

4 ounces bulk Italian sausage

½ cup whole-milk ricotta cheese

2 tablespoons chopped fresh basil

1 clove garlic, minced

½ teaspoon salt

¼ teaspoon black pepper

½ recipe Nut-Free Magic Mozzarella Dough (page 376)

½ cup frozen broccoli, thawed and coarsely chopped

½ cup shredded mozzarella cheese (about 2 ounces)

1. In a medium skillet over medium heat, cook the sausage until no longer pink, about 5 minutes, breaking up any clumps with the back of a wooden spoon.

2. In a medium bowl, mix together the ricotta, basil, garlic, salt, and pepper.

3. Place the prepared dough on a silicone baking mat or a large piece of parchment paper. Top with a large piece of parchment and roll out to a 10-inch circle.

4. Spread the ricotta mixture over half of the dough, leaving a 1-inch border. Layer on the sausage and broccoli, then sprinkle with the mozzarella.

5. Use an offset spatula or a sharp knife to loosen the other half of the dough from the baking mat or parchment, then fold it over the filling. Crimp the edges of the calzone to seal well. Use a sharp knife to create 3 slits in the top to allow steam to escape.

6. Transfer the baking mat or parchment paper to a rimmed baking sheet and bake for 20 to 25 minutes, until golden brown. Let cool for 10 minutes before serving.

TIPS: *If you have one, I highly recommend prepping and baking this calzone on a silicone baking mat. It is really stuffed full, and a silicone mat will make it easier to transfer the calzone onto a baking sheet.*

Frozen broccoli is ideal here because it's softer once thawed and doesn't require any precooking before being added to the calzone.

SERVING SUGGESTION: *Serve with some low-carb marinara sauce for dipping.*

NUTRITIONAL INFORMATION

CALORIES: 339 | FAT: 21.9g | CARBS: 7.7g | FIBER: 2.9g | PROTEIN: 23.4g

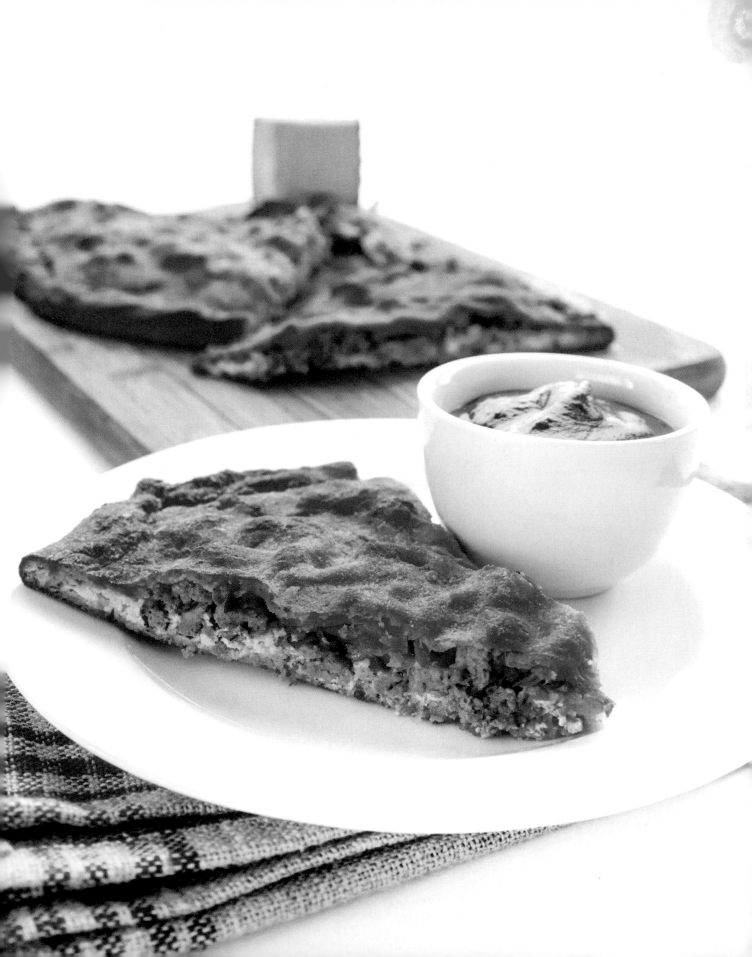

SMOKED SALMON FLATBREAD

Yield: 6 servings Prep Time: 25 minutes Cook Time: 30 minutes

Because I like playing and experimenting all the time, I took the coconut flour–based fathead dough and modified it a little for this flatbread. This version is a bit more buttery and rises less, so it's a true flatbread. This is an elegant appetizer to serve at parties.

Crust:

6 ounces shredded mozzarella cheese

2 tablespoons unsalted butter

¼ cup plus 1 tablespoon (34g) coconut flour

½ teaspoon garlic powder

½ teaspoon baking powder

¼ teaspoon salt

1 large egg, room temperature

Toppings:

2 ounces cream cheese, softened

¼ cup sour cream

4 ounces thinly sliced cold smoked salmon

2 thin slices red onion, cut in half

2 tablespoons coarsely chopped fresh dill

1 tablespoon capers, drained

Coarse sea salt

Cracked black pepper

TO MAKE THE CRUST:

1. Preheat the oven to 350°F and line a work surface with a silicone baking mat or a large piece of parchment paper. Lightly grease the mat or parchment.

2. In a large microwave-safe bowl, heat the cheese and butter on high in 30-second increments until they are well melted and can be stirred together.

3. All at once, add the coconut flour, garlic powder, baking powder, salt, and egg and stir together using a rubber spatula. Knead the dough up against the sides of the bowl with the spatula.

4. Turn the dough out onto the prepared work surface and continue to knead until cohesive. Cover with a piece of parchment paper and roll out to a 12 by 10-inch rectangle. Remove the top piece of parchment.

5. Transfer the baking mat or parchment paper to a cookie sheet and bake for 20 to 25 minutes, until lightly browned and firm to the touch. Remove from the oven and let cool on the pan.

TO TOP THE FLATBREAD:

6. In a medium bowl, beat the cream cheese and sour cream with an electric mixer until smooth. Spread this mixture over the cooled crust, leaving a ½-inch border.

7. Arrange the salmon, onion, dill, and capers over the cream cheese mixture. Sprinkle lightly with coarse salt and pepper.

8. Use a sharp knife or a pizza wheel to cut into pieces.

TIPS: *I always weigh the mozzarella for this recipe. Shredded mozzarella can get packed down and pressed together, and measuring by volume rather than weight can affect the outcome of the dough.*

This dough gets a bit sticky. Greasing the mat or parchment helps it release more easily after baking.

NUTRITIONAL INFORMATION

CALORIES: 231 | FAT: 16.1g | CARBS: 5.5g | FIBER: 2.2g | PROTEIN: 12.6g

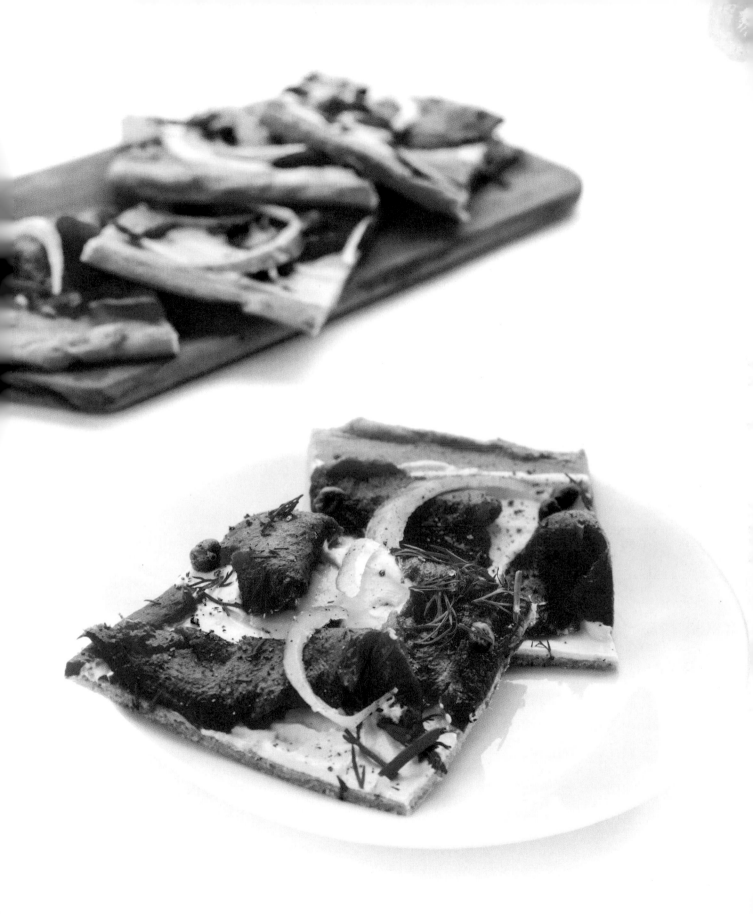

SOCCA FLATBREAD

OPTION

Yield: 8 servings Prep Time: 15 minutes, plus 15 minutes to rest batter Cook Time: 17 minutes

Socca is a flatbread from the South of France, and it is typically made with chickpea flour. Because lupin flour is also made from legumes, I decided to swap it in here. It was my first foray into baking with lupin flour, and it was highly successful.

1 cup lupin flour

½ teaspoon salt

½ teaspoon ground cumin

½ teaspoon garlic powder

1 cup lukewarm water

2 tablespoons avocado or coconut oil

1 tablespoon extra-virgin olive oil

½ teaspoon za'atar (see tip)

Coarse sea salt, for sprinkling

COCONUT-FREE OPTION:

Use avocado oil rather than coconut oil.

1. In a large bowl, whisk together the lupin flour, salt, cumin, and garlic powder. Slowly add the water, whisking continuously, until well combined and no lumps remain. Let sit for 15 minutes.

2. Set an oven rack in the center position and preheat the oven to 450°F. Place a 10-inch ovenproof skillet in the oven to heat.

3. Once the oven is preheated, remove the skillet and pour in the avocado oil. Swirl the pan to coat the bottom and sides with the oil.

4. Pour the batter into the hot skillet and use an offset spatula to spread to the edges. Place the pan on the center rack and bake for 12 to 15 minutes, until the top of the bread is dry and firm to the touch.

5. Turn on the broiler and broil until a few brown spots appear on the top, about 2 minutes.

6. Remove from the oven and brush with the olive oil, then sprinkle with the za'atar and coarse salt. Enjoy warm.

TIP: *Za'atar is a Middle Eastern spice blend made up of sesame seeds, sumac, and thyme. It's delicious on this flatbread, but you could also use Italian seasoning or herbs de Provence, or 1 teaspoon of any chopped fresh herb you might have.*

NUTRITIONAL INFORMATION

CALORIES: 69 | FAT: 6.2g | CARBS: 6.2g | FIBER: 5.5g | PROTEIN: 6.1g

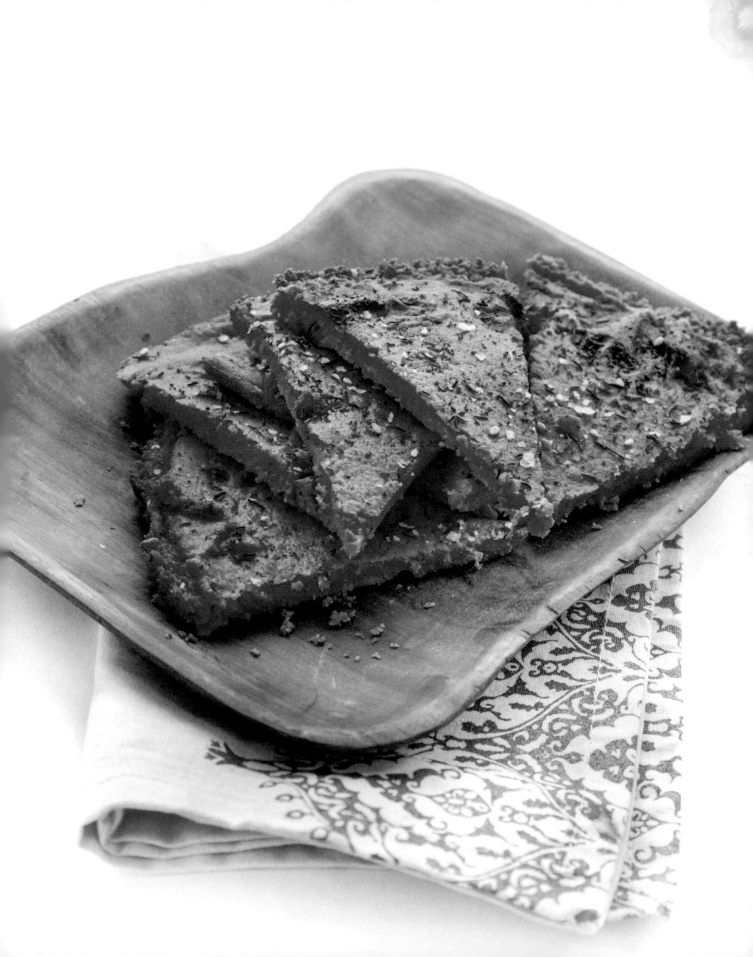

ROSEMARY PECAN CRACKERS

Yield: About 40 crackers (4 per serving)   Prep Time: 20 minutes   Cook Time: 40 minutes

These delicious crackers go with everything! If you don't need to be dairy-free, they are divine with a little Brie.

2 cups pecan meal (see tips)

2 tablespoons chopped fresh rosemary

1 tablespoon granulated erythritol sweetener

½ teaspoon garlic powder

½ teaspoon baking powder

½ teaspoon salt

1 large egg

1½ tablespoons avocado oil

Coarse sea salt, for sprinkling

1. Preheat the oven to 300°F. Line a work surface with a silicone baking mat or a large piece of parchment paper.

2. In a large bowl, combine the pecan meal, rosemary, sweetener, garlic powder, baking powder, and salt.

3. Stir in the egg and avocado oil until the dough comes together. Turn the dough out onto the prepared work surface and pat into a rough rectangle. Cover with a piece of parchment paper and roll out to about an ⅛-inch thickness, as evenly as you can. Remove the top piece of parchment.

4. Using a sharp knife or a pizza cutter, cut the dough into 2-inch squares. Sprinkle with coarse salt, pressing lightly to adhere. Transfer the baking mat or parchment paper to a cookie sheet.

5. Bake for 35 to 40 minutes, until the crackers are golden brown on the edges and firm to the touch. Remove from the oven and let cool completely before breaking apart. They will continue to crisp up as they cool.

TIPS: *You can purchase preground pecan meal (see page 401) or grind your own. The latter may be quite a bit more coarse, and the resulting crackers will be more fragile, but it does work. As always, measure out the meal after grinding the pecans.*

You can leave out the sweetener if you prefer, but there is something about bringing out the natural sweetness of the pecans that makes these crackers extra special.

NUTRITIONAL INFORMATION

CALORIES: 208 | FAT: 21.3g | CARBS: 4.4g | FIBER: 2.9g | PROTEIN: 13.2g

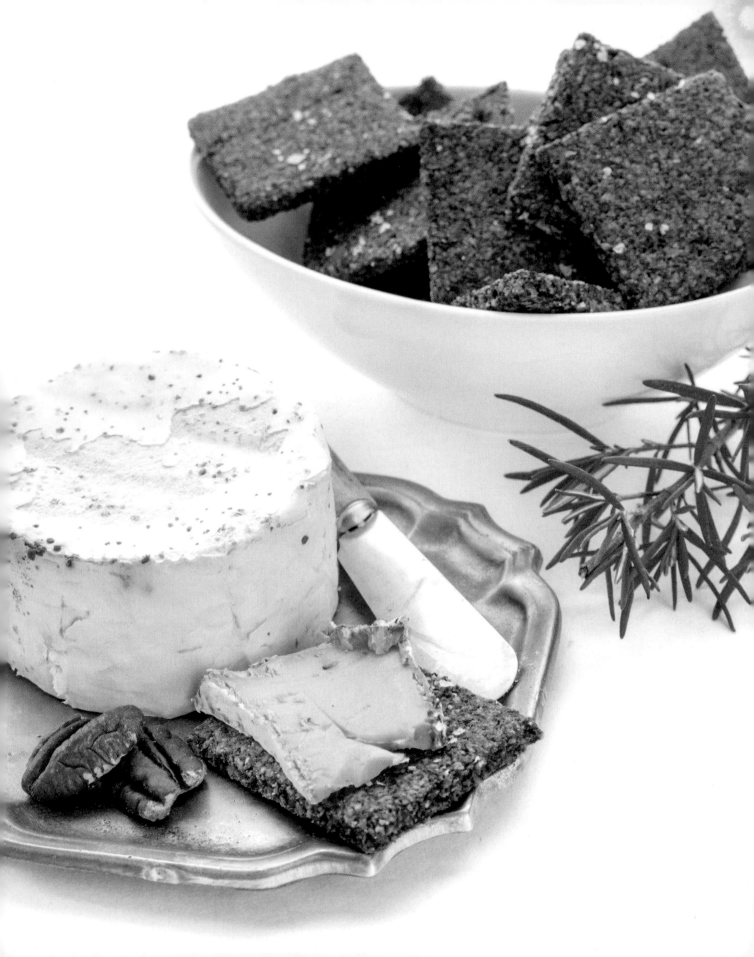

TOASTED SESAME CRACKERS

Yield: 32 crackers (4 per serving) Prep Time: 20 minutes Cook Time: 45 minutes

I was always a cheese and crackers girl, and I loved crackers with toasted sesame seeds. This is my keto version, and I no longer miss the old high-carb kind.

¼ cup sesame seeds

1 cup (100g) blanched almond flour

¼ cup sesame flour (see tip)

½ teaspoon baking powder

½ teaspoon salt

1 large egg

2 tablespoons sesame oil (untoasted)

1 tablespoon water

1. Preheat the oven to 300°F.

2. Spread the sesame seeds in a medium skillet over medium heat. Stir frequently until lightly toasted, about 4 minutes. Pour the seeds into a medium bowl.

3. To the sesame seeds, add the almond flour, sesame flour, baking powder, and salt and whisk to combine. Stir in the egg, sesame oil, and water until the dough comes together.

4. Gather the dough into a ball and transfer to a silicone baking mat or a large piece of parchment paper. Top with a piece of parchment. Roll out the dough to a 12-inch square, as even in thickness as possible. Remove the top piece of parchment.

5. Use a sharp knife or a pizza cutter to cut the dough into squares or diamonds, about 2 inches each. Transfer the baking mat or parchment paper to a cookie sheet.

6. Bake for 30 to 40 minutes, until the crackers are firm to the touch and the edges are golden brown.

7. Remove from the oven and let cool completely before breaking apart.

TIP: *Sesame flour is very fine and powdery, similar to coconut flour. It's very dense and absorbent and has a strong sesame flavor. If you prefer, you can replace the sesame flour with a full cup of almond flour and then skip the water.*

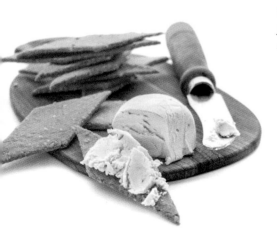

NUTRITIONAL INFORMATION

CALORIES: 168 | FAT: 14g | CARBS: 5.7g | FIBER: 3g | PROTEIN: 6.7g

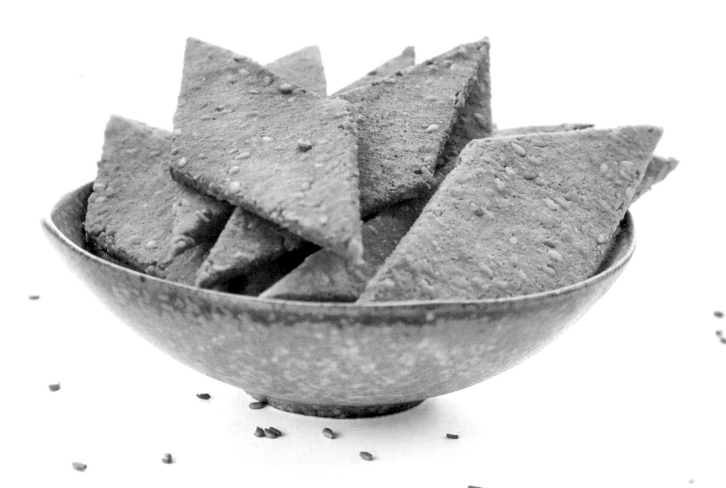

GRAHAM CRACKERS

OPTION

Yield: About 30 crackers (3 per serving) **Prep Time:** 15 minutes, plus 30 minutes to cool **Cook Time:** 1 hour

This recipe is featured in my first cookbook, *The Everyday Ketogenic Kitchen.* But I wanted to include it again because these crackers are the base for the Cannoli Icebox Cake (page 118). They are also rockin' good on their own!

2 cups (200g) blanched almond flour

⅓ cup brown sugar substitute

1 teaspoon ground cinnamon

1 teaspoon baking powder

⅛ teaspoon salt

1 large egg

2 tablespoons unsalted butter, melted but not hot

1 teaspoon vanilla extract

DAIRY-FREE OPTION:

Use avocado oil in place of the melted butter. I don't suggest coconut oil, as it keeps the crackers from crisping up properly.

1. Preheat the oven to 300°F.

2. In a large bowl, whisk together the almond flour, sweetener, cinnamon, baking powder, and salt. Stir in the egg, melted butter, and vanilla until the dough comes together.

3. Turn the dough out onto a silicone baking mat or a large piece of parchment paper and pat into a rough rectangle. Top with a piece of parchment. Roll out the dough as evenly as possible to a thickness of ⅛ to ¼ inch.

4. Remove the top piece of parchment and use a sharp knife or a pizza wheel to cut the dough into 2-inch squares. Prick each cracker two or three times with a fork to make decorative indentations. Transfer the baking mat or parchment paper to a cookie sheet.

5. Bake for 20 to 30 minutes, until just beginning to brown and firm up. Remove the crackers and turn off the oven. Let cool for 30 minutes, then break apart along the score marks.

6. Return the crackers to the warm oven with the oven off. If your oven has cooled down too much, set the temperature to no higher than 200°F. Let the crackers sit inside for another 30 minutes, then remove from the oven and let cool completely.

TIP: *The brown sugar substitute can make these a little softer than other crackers. I found that the best way to get them to crisp up completely is to return them to a warm oven and let them sit inside.*

NUTRITIONAL INFORMATION

CALORIES: 156 | FAT: 13.4g | CARBS: 6.2g | FIBER: 2.7g | PROTEIN: 5.2g

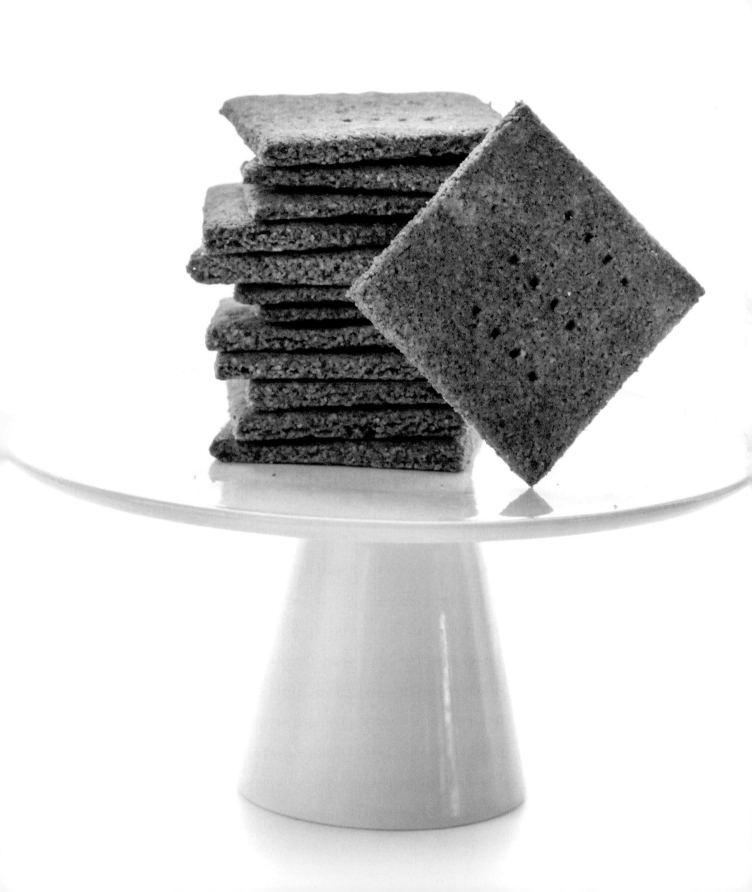

BUTTERY CHEESE CRACKERS

Yield: 60 crackers (6 per serving) Prep Time: 20 minutes Cook Time: 70 minutes

Another little twist on coconut flour fathead dough. My son declared that these crackers taste just like Cheez-Its.

6 ounces cheddar cheese, shredded

¼ cup (28g) coconut flour, plus more if needed

½ teaspoon baking powder

½ teaspoon salt

1 large egg white

1 tablespoon unsalted butter, melted but not hot

Coarse sea salt, for sprinkling

1. Preheat the oven to 300°F and line a work surface with a silicone baking mat or a large piece of parchment paper. Lightly grease the mat or parchment.

2. In a large microwave-safe bowl, heat the cheese on high in 30-second increments until it is well melted and can be stirred to a smooth consistency.

3. Add the coconut flour, baking powder, salt, and egg white and stir to combine. Work together well with a rubber spatula, kneading the dough up against the sides of the bowl. If the dough is very sticky, add another tablespoon of flour.

4. Turn the dough out onto the prepared work surface and top with a piece of parchment or waxed paper. Roll out as thinly as you can, no more than about ⅛ inch thick. Remove the top piece of parchment.

5. With a sharp knife or a pizza cutter, score the dough into 1-inch squares. Brush with the melted butter and sprinkle with the coarse salt, pressing lightly to adhere. Transfer the baking mat or parchment paper to a cookie sheet.

6. Bake for 20 to 25 minutes, until the crackers are golden brown and beginning to crisp up on the edges, then turn off the oven and leave the crackers inside until firm to the touch, 30 to 40 more minutes. If the crackers around the edges are browning too fast, simply remove them and let the remaining crackers sit in the warm oven. They will continue to crisp up as they cool.

TIPS: *I always weigh the mozzarella for this recipe. Shredded mozzarella can get packed down and pressed together, and measuring by volume rather than weight can affect the outcome of the dough.*

The more thinly and evenly you roll out the dough, the crisper the crackers will be. But keep an eye on them when they sit inside the warm oven, as they can brown quickly and unexpectedly. I always find myself breaking off the edge pieces early and returning the rest to the oven.

NUTRITIONAL INFORMATION

CALORIES: 92 | FAT: 6.4g | CARBS: 1.9g | FIBER: 1g | PROTEIN: 4.9g

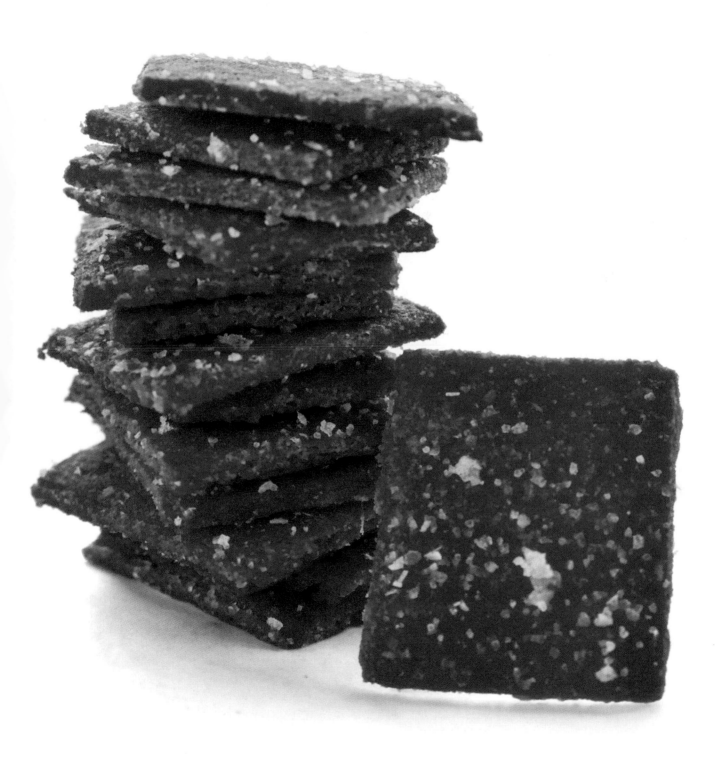

PARMESAN SAGE SHORTBREAD

Yield: 20 crackers (2 per serving) **Prep Time:** 30 minutes **Cook Time:** 45 minutes

Shortbread can be savory, too, you know! Feel free to change up the herbs here. Rosemary or thyme would be lovely.

2¼ cups (225g) blanched almond flour, plus more for dusting

1 ounce Parmesan cheese, grated (about 1 cup)

5 large fresh sage leaves, finely chopped

½ teaspoon xanthan gum

½ teaspoon salt

¼ teaspoon coarsely ground black pepper

6 tablespoons unsalted butter, diced, softened

Small fresh sage leaves, for garnish (optional)

Coarse sea salt, for sprinkling

1. Preheat the oven to 300°F and line a baking sheet with a silicone baking mat or a large piece of parchment paper.

2. Place the almond flour, Parmesan, chopped sage, xanthan gum, salt, and pepper in a food processor and pulse a few times to combine.

3. Scatter the butter over the top and process on high until the dough clumps together. Gather the dough into a ball.

4. Dust a work surface lightly with almond flour and transfer the dough to the surface. Top with a piece of parchment or waxed paper and roll out to ¼ inch thick. Remove the top piece of parchment and cut the dough into circles using a 2-inch round cookie cutter.

5. Using a sharp knife or an offset spatula, carefully lift and transfer the circles to the prepared baking sheet. Reroll the dough scraps and cut more circles until no more can be cut.

6. Decorate some of the crackers with small sage leaves, if desired, pressing into the dough. Sprinkle with coarse salt and press lightly to adhere.

7. Bake for 25 minutes, then turn off the oven and leave the crackers inside until golden and firm to the touch, about 20 more minutes. Remove from the oven and let cool completely.

TIPS: *These are very tender, fragile crackers, but they are melt-in-your-mouth delicious. I wouldn't recommend skipping the xanthan gum, as they need the extra structure to hold together.*

Watch the crackers carefully while they are in the warm oven. Depending on how well your oven holds its heat, they can darken quickly.

NUTRITIONAL INFORMATION

CALORIES: 216 | FAT: 19.7g | CARBS: 5.6g | FIBER: 2.8g | PROTEIN: 6.5g

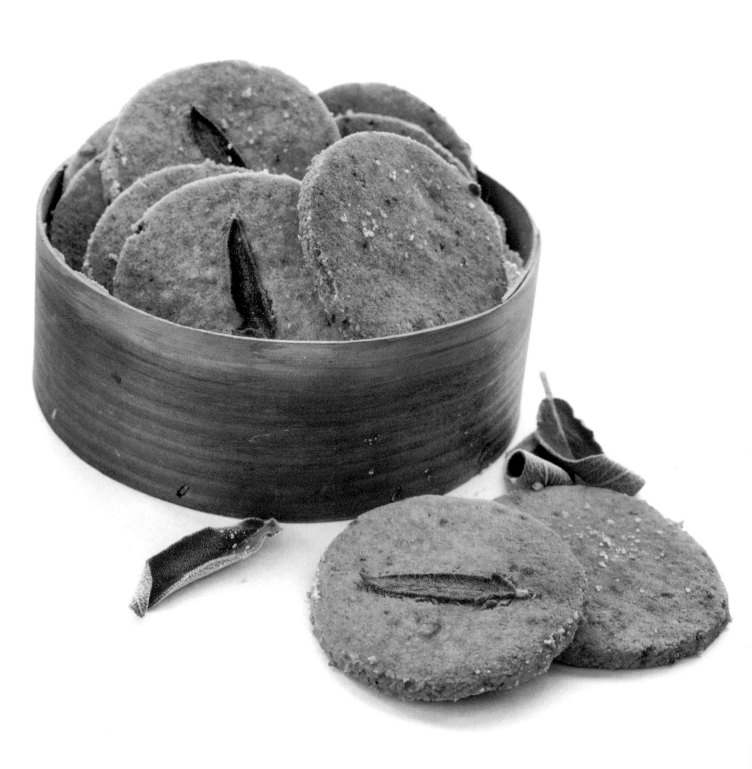

Chapter 13:
PIES & TARTS

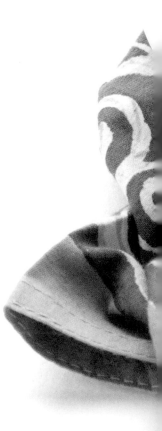

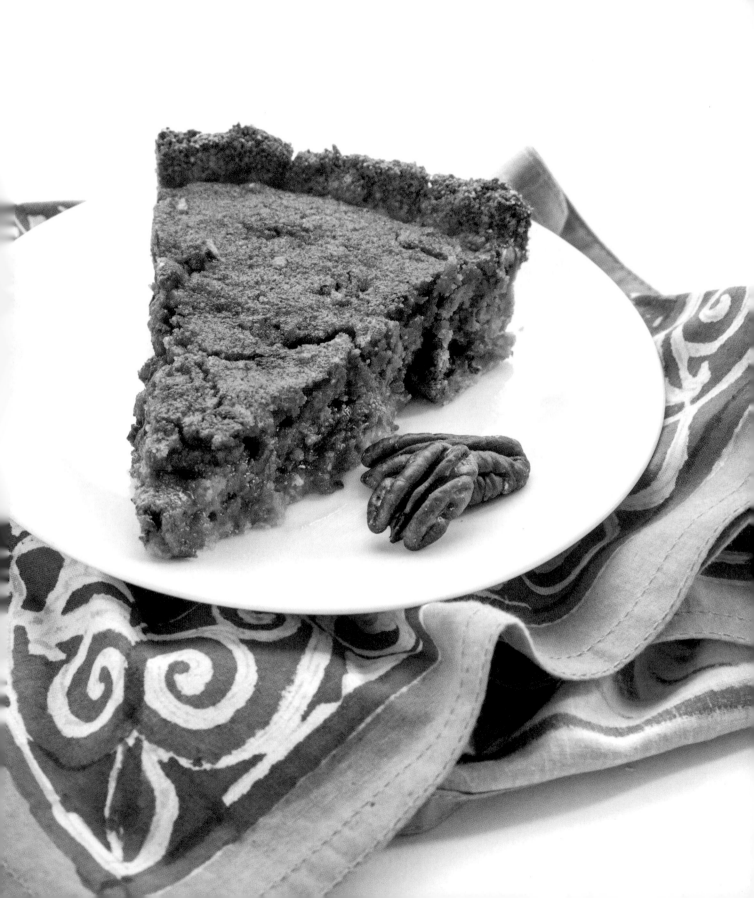

GERMAN CHOCOLATE BROWNIE PIE

Yield: 10 servings **Prep Time:** 15 minutes **Cook Time:** 40 minutes

When is a pie not a pie? When it's really brownies in disguise. But somehow, serving it in a pie plate just seems more elegant.

Brownie Base:

6 tablespoons unsalted butter, melted but not hot

½ cup granulated sweetener of choice

2 large eggs, room temperature

½ teaspoon vanilla extract

½ cup (50g) blanched almond flour

¼ cup cocoa powder

¼ teaspoon baking powder

⅛ teaspoon salt

1 tablespoon cold coffee or water

Topping:

½ cup heavy whipping cream

2 large egg yolks

¼ cup powdered erythritol sweetener

2 tablespoons Bocha Sweet or allulose (see tips)

2 tablespoons unsalted butter

½ cup unsweetened flaked or shredded coconut

½ cup chopped pecans, lightly toasted

½ teaspoon vanilla extract

Pecan halves, for garnish (optional)

TO MAKE THE BASE:

1. Preheat the oven to 350°F and grease a 9-inch glass or ceramic pie plate.

2. In a large bowl, whisk together the melted butter, sweetener, eggs, and vanilla. Stir in the almond flour, cocoa powder, baking powder, and salt, then stir in the coffee.

3. Spread the batter in the prepared pan and bake for 20 to 30 minutes, until the edges are puffed and the middle is just barely set. Remove from the oven and let cool completely.

TO MAKE THE TOPPING:

4. In a medium saucepan over medium heat, whisk together the cream, egg yolks, sweeteners, and butter. Cook, whisking frequently, until thickened, about 8 minutes.

5. Remove the pan from the heat and stir in the coconut, pecans, and vanilla. Spread over the cooled brownie base and garnish with pecan halves, if desired. Let sit for 20 minutes before slicing.

TIPS: *You can use all erythritol-based sweeteners here, but a little Bocha Sweet or allulose will keep the topping more moist, like a traditional German chocolate cake.*

The time range here is wide because how quickly the pie bakes can depend a lot on the type of pie plate you use. My recipe testers found that it baked faster in their glass pie plates, whereas it took a bit longer in my white ceramic pie plate.

NUTRITIONAL INFORMATION

CALORIES: 247 | FAT: 23.3g | CARBS: 4.6g | FIBER: 2.3g | PROTEIN: 4.5g

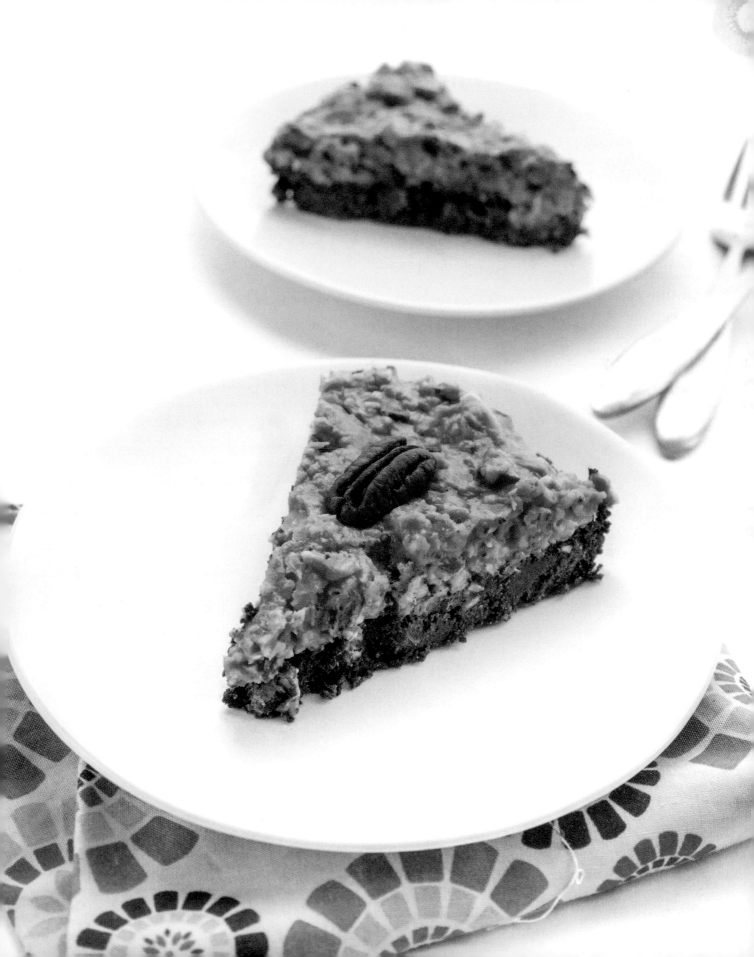

MASCARPONE BERRY TART

OPTION

Yield: 10 servings Prep Time: 30 minutes, plus 30 minutes to chill Cook Time: 20 minutes

Mascarpone cheese has a lovely sweet flavor on its own, and I find that I need to add very little sweetener to enhance it, especially when it is paired with the natural sweetness of fresh berries. This creamy tart is fresh and delicious.

1 recipe Coconut Flour Pie Crust (page 368)

8 ounces mascarpone cheese, softened

4 ounces cream cheese, softened

¼ cup plus 2 tablespoons powdered erythritol sweetener

¼ cup heavy whipping cream, room temperature

1 teaspoon grated lemon zest

1 teaspoon vanilla extract

½ cup fresh raspberries

½ cup fresh blueberries

½ cup sliced fresh strawberries

Thin strips of lemon zest, for garnish

1. Preheat the oven to 350°F and grease a 9-inch glass or ceramic tart pan.

2. Prepare the crust according to the directions and press into the bottom and up the sides of the prepared pan. Prick the bottom all over with a fork.

3. Bake for 20 minutes, until the edges are golden brown and the center is firm to the touch. Remove from the oven and let cool completely.

4. In a large bowl, beat the mascarpone, cream cheese, and sweetener with an electric mixer until well combined. Beat in the cream, grated lemon zest, and vanilla until smooth.

5. Spread the mascarpone mixture in the cooled tart crust and top with the fresh berries and strips of lemon zest. Refrigerate for 30 minutes to firm up before serving.

COCONUT-FREE OPTION:

I used the Coconut Flour Pie Crust here to keep the tart nut-free, but you could swap it with any nut-based crust if you prefer.

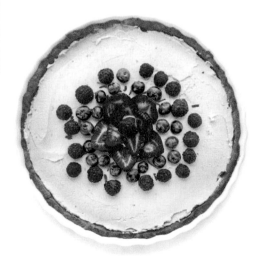

NUTRITIONAL INFORMATION

CALORIES: 270 | FAT: 21.2g | CARBS: 7.6g | FIBER: 3.3g | PROTEIN: 5g

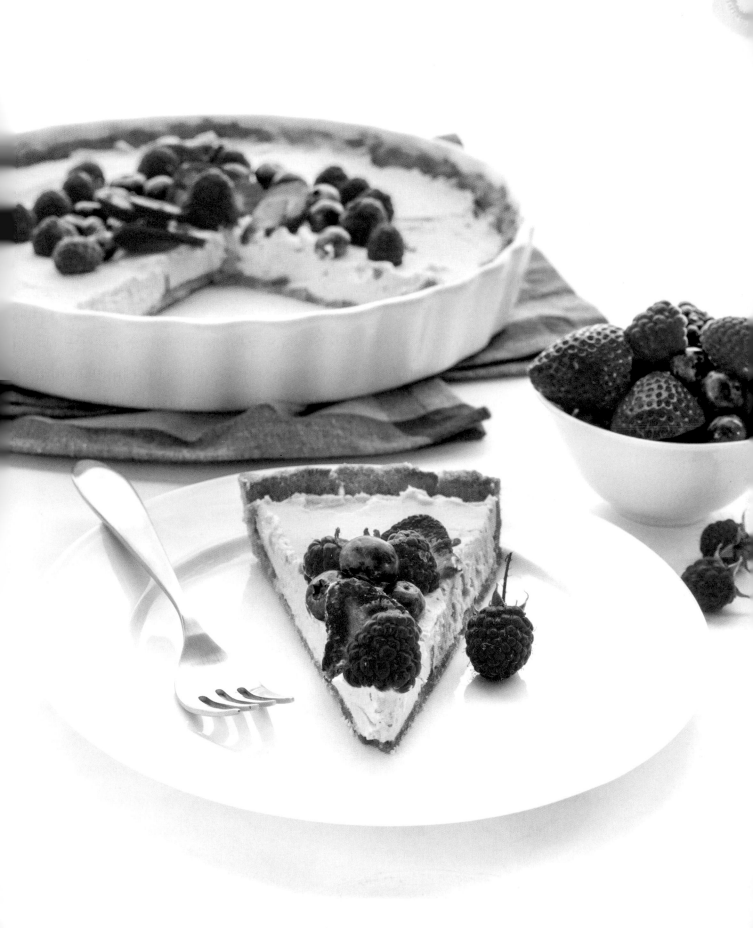

KENTUCKY CHOCOLATE CHIP COOKIE PIE

OPTION

Yield: 10 servings   Prep Time: 20 minutes, plus 1 hour to freeze crust   Cook Time: 50 minutes

This is my keto take on the famous Kentucky Derby Pie. It's a brilliant concept, filling a pie crust with what amounts to extra gooey chocolate chip cookie dough and pecans. You just can't go wrong!

1 recipe Easy Almond Flour Pie Crust (page 366)

½ cup (1 stick) unsalted butter, melted

½ cup brown sugar substitute

½ cup Bocha Sweet or allulose (see tips)

2 large eggs, room temperature

1 teaspoon vanilla extract

½ teaspoon salt

¼ cup (28g) coconut flour

¼ teaspoon baking powder

1 cup chopped pecans

⅓ cup sugar-free chocolate chips

1. Prepare the crust according to the directions and press firmly into the bottom and up the sides of a 9-inch glass or ceramic pie plate. Prick the bottom all over with a fork. Crimp the edges decoratively, if desired. Freeze for 1 hour.

2. Preheat the oven to 325°F.

3. In a large bowl, whisk together the melted butter, sweeteners, eggs, vanilla, and salt until well combined.

4. Stir in the coconut flour and baking powder until smooth. Fold in the pecans and chocolate chips.

5. Spread the batter in the frozen pie crust and bake for 40 to 50 minutes, until the crust is golden brown and the filling is just barely set.

6. Remove from the oven and let cool for 30 minutes, then serve immediately if you want to enjoy it warm and gooey. If you prefer a more solid filling, allow to cool completely.

NUT-FREE OPTION:

Use the Coconut Flour Pie Crust on page 368 and skip the pecans. If using the coconut flour crust, be sure to grease the pie plate first.

TIPS: *The sweetener in this recipe can be all erythritol based, but the filling will be less gooey and may recrystallize a bit.*

Once again, your bakeware matters. Glass works well here, but metal may overbrown the crust. You can always cover a pie that's browning too quickly with foil. Put the matte side toward the pie and the shiny side up to help deflect the heat.

SERVING SUGGESTION: *Oh so good with a scoop of Keto Vanilla Ice Cream (page 394).*

NUTRITIONAL INFORMATION
CALORIES: 281 | FAT: 24.6g | CARBS: 8g | FIBER: 4.9g | PROTEIN: 5.9g

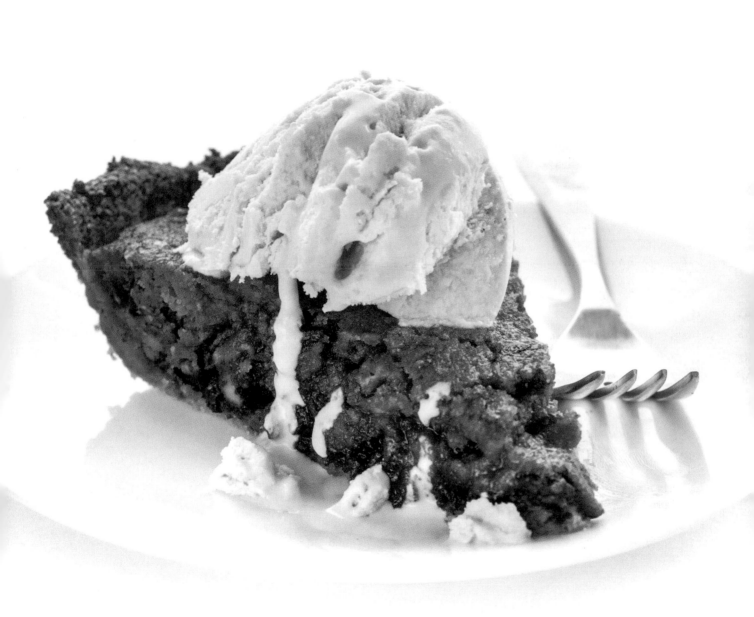

BLUEBERRY SOUR CREAM PIE

Yield: 10 servings   Prep Time: 20 minutes, plus 1 hour to set   Cook Time: 45 minutes

A taste of summer! Fruit pies can be pretty high in carbs, but turn it into a custard pie and you can still enjoy that great berry flavor.

1 recipe Coconut Flour Pie Crust (page 368)

⅓ cup powdered erythritol sweetener

⅓ cup granulated sweetener of choice

2 tablespoons coconut flour

½ teaspoon glucomannan or xanthan gum

1 cup sour cream

2 large eggs, room temperature

1 teaspoon grated lemon zest

½ teaspoon vanilla extract

1 cup fresh blueberries, divided

1. Preheat the oven to 350°F and grease a 9-inch glass or ceramic pie plate.

2. Prepare the crust according to the directions and press into the bottom and up the sides of the prepared pan. Prick the bottom all over with a fork.

3. Par-bake the crust for 10 minutes, until just a tiny bit golden around the edges. Remove from the oven and let cool while you prepare the filling.

4. Increase the oven temperature to 400°F.

5. In a large bowl, whisk together the sweeteners, coconut flour, and glucomannan. Whisk in the sour cream, eggs, lemon zest, and vanilla until well combined and smooth.

6. Gently fold in ¾ cup of the blueberries, then pour the mixture into the cooled crust. Sprinkle the remaining berries on top.

7. Bake for 20 minutes, then remove the pie and cover the whole thing with foil, shiny side up. Reduce the oven temperature to 350°F and bake for another 10 to 15 minutes, until the edges are set but the center still jiggles slightly.

8. Let cool completely in the pan, then refrigerate for 1 hour to set before slicing.

TIP: *Custard pies are easy to cook, but they are also easy to overcook. You really want the center to still jiggle while the sides are set. The middle will continue to cook for a while after the pie comes out of the oven.*

NUTRITIONAL INFORMATION

CALORIES: 153 | FAT: 10.8g | CARBS: 7.1g | FIBER: 2.9g | PROTEIN: 3.8g

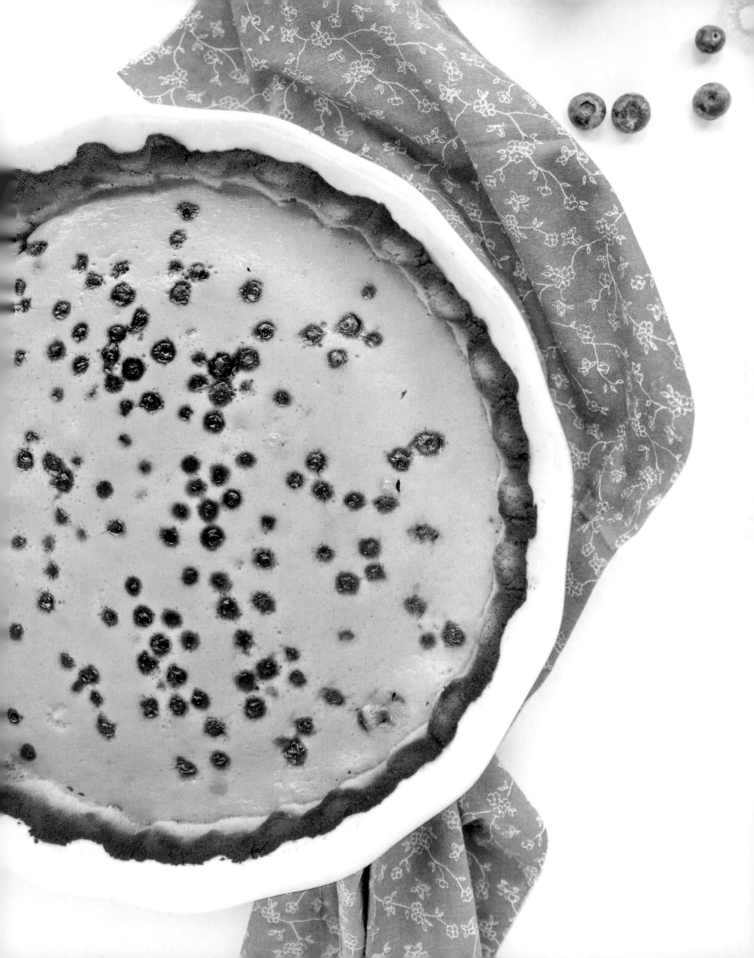

STRAWBERRY RHUBARB GALETTE

Yield: 8 servings   Prep Time: 20 minutes (not including time to make crust)   Cook Time: 35 minutes

I'm a strawberry rhubarb fanatic. I can't get enough of that tart-sweet combination!

2 cups chopped rhubarb

1½ cups sliced fresh strawberries

½ cup powdered erythritol sweetener

1 tablespoon coconut flour

½ teaspoon glucomannan or xanthan gum

½ recipe Sweet Nut-Free Magic Mozzarella Dough (page 376)

1 large egg yolk, lightly beaten

1. Preheat the oven to 350°F.

2. In a large bowl, toss together the rhubarb and strawberries. Sprinkle with the sweetener, coconut flour, and glucomannan and toss well to combine. Set aside.

3. Cover a work surface with a silicone baking mat or a large piece of parchment paper. Lightly grease the mat or paper.

4. Turn the prepared dough out onto the work surface and roll out evenly to a 12-inch circle. Transfer the baking mat or parchment to a rimmed baking sheet.

5. Top the with the rhubarb mixture, leaving a 2-inch border. Fold the edges of the crust over the filling and brush with the beaten egg yolk.

6. Bake for 25 to 35 minutes, until the crust is golden brown and the filling is bubbly. Remove from the oven and let cool in the pan for 20 minutes before slicing.

TIP: *The berries and rhubarb release quite a bit of moisture as they bake, and it sometimes leaks out a bit at the edges, so it's important to use a rimmed baking sheet. Use paper towels or a clean rag to blot up some of the juices during baking or after the galette comes out of the oven so it doesn't get soggy. It will firm up as it cools.*

SERVING SUGGESTION: *Top with lightly sweetened whipped cream for an extra-special dessert.*

NUTRITIONAL INFORMATION
CALORIES: 116 | FAT: 6.2g | CARBS: 6.8g | FIBER: 2.7g | PROTEIN: 6.9g

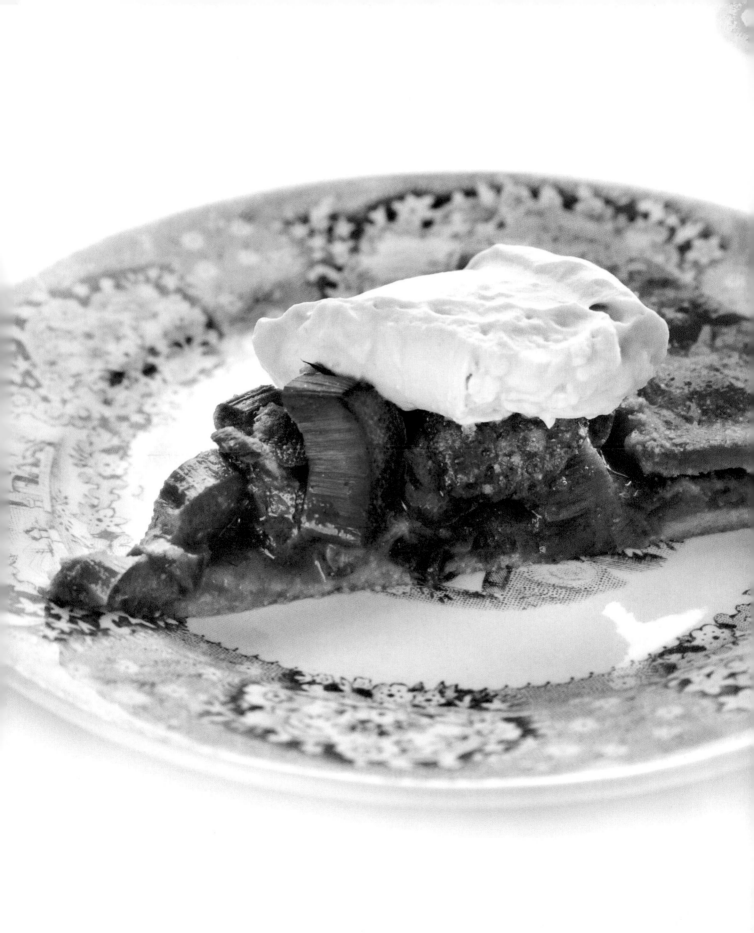

MINI CRUSTLESS PUMPKIN PIES

OPTION

Yield: 4 mini pies (1 per serving) Prep Time: 5 minutes, plus 1 hour to chill Cook Time: 40 minutes

---

Get your pumpkin pie fix with these mini custards. No crust, just sweet pumpkin pie filling.

½ cup pumpkin puree

⅓ cup heavy whipping cream

⅓ cup brown sugar substitute

1 large egg

1 large egg yolk

½ teaspoon vanilla extract

½ teaspoon pumpkin pie spice

DAIRY-FREE OPTION:

Use coconut cream from the top of a can of full-fat coconut milk in place of the heavy whipping cream.

1. Preheat the oven to 350°F and set four 4-ounce ramekins on a rimmed baking sheet.

2. Place all of the ingredients in a blender and blend until smooth. Alternatively, you can whisk them together in a large bowl until well combined.

3. Divide the pumpkin mixture among the ramekins and place the baking sheet in the oven. Bake for 30 to 40 minutes, until the pies are mostly set but still jiggle slightly in the very middle.

4. Remove from the oven and let cool on the baking sheet, then refrigerate for at least 1 hour before serving.

SERVING SUGGESTION: *Top the pies with lightly sweetened whipped cream and a sprinkle of cinnamon.*

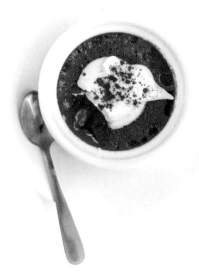

NUTRITIONAL INFORMATION

CALORIES: 116 | FAT: 9.2g | CARBS: 3.5g | FIBER: 0.9g | PROTEIN: 3g

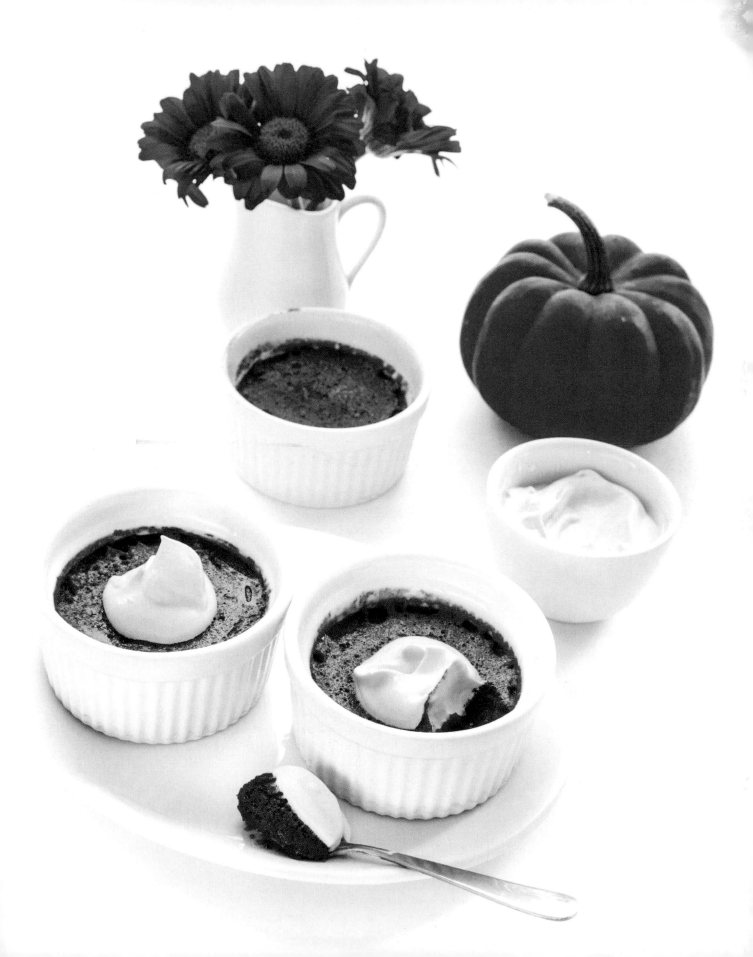

RASPBERRY TRUFFLE TART

OPTION

Yield: 10 servings   **Prep Time:** 20 minutes, plus 3 hours to chill   **Cook Time:** 45 minutes

Heavenly chocolate truffle filling with a hint of raspberries. This is a chocolate lover's dream!

1 recipe Keto Chocolate Pie Crust (page 370)

½ cup (1 stick) unsalted butter

4 ounces unsweetened chocolate, chopped

2 large eggs, room temperature

½ cup heavy whipping cream, room temperature

6 tablespoons powdered erythritol sweetener

6 tablespoons Bocha Sweet or allulose (see tips)

1 teaspoon raspberry extract

½ teaspoon vanilla extract

¼ teaspoon salt

1 cup fresh raspberries

Powdered erythritol sweetener, for sprinkling (optional)

NUT-FREE OPTION:

Use sunflower seed meal to prepare the chocolate pie crust.

1. Preheat the oven to 350°F and grease a 9-inch metal tart pan with a removable bottom.

2. Prepare the crust according to the directions and press into the bottom and up the sides of the prepared pan.

3. Set the tart pan on a rimmed baking sheet and par-bake for 10 minutes, then remove from the oven and let cool while you prepare the filling.

4. In a medium saucepan over low heat, melt the butter and chocolate, stirring until smooth. Remove the pan from the heat and let cool for 5 minutes.

5. In a large bowl, whisk together the eggs, cream, sweeteners, extracts, and salt. Whisk in the chocolate mixture until well combined.

6. Pour the filling into the cooled crust and bake until the filling 1 inch from the edge of the crust is set but the center still jiggles slightly, 30 to 35 minutes.

7. Remove from the oven and let cool completely, then gently loosen the crust with a knife and remove the sides of the pan. Refrigerate until the filling is firm, about 3 hours.

8. Decorate the top with the fresh raspberries and perhaps a sprinkling of powdered sweetener.

TIPS: *You can use all erythritol-based sweeteners in this recipe, but you may find that the filling recrystallizes once refrigerated.*

Placing the tart pan on a rimmed baking sheet is important. The removable bottom of a metal tart pan makes it easy to present and serve the pie, but it can push up easily when you're moving the tart in and out of the oven. The baking sheet will keep you from accidentally pushing up on the bottom and loosening the tart too soon.

NUTRITIONAL INFORMATION

CALORIES: 251 | FAT: 22.2g | CARBS: 7.8g | FIBER: 4.2g | PROTEIN: 5.7g

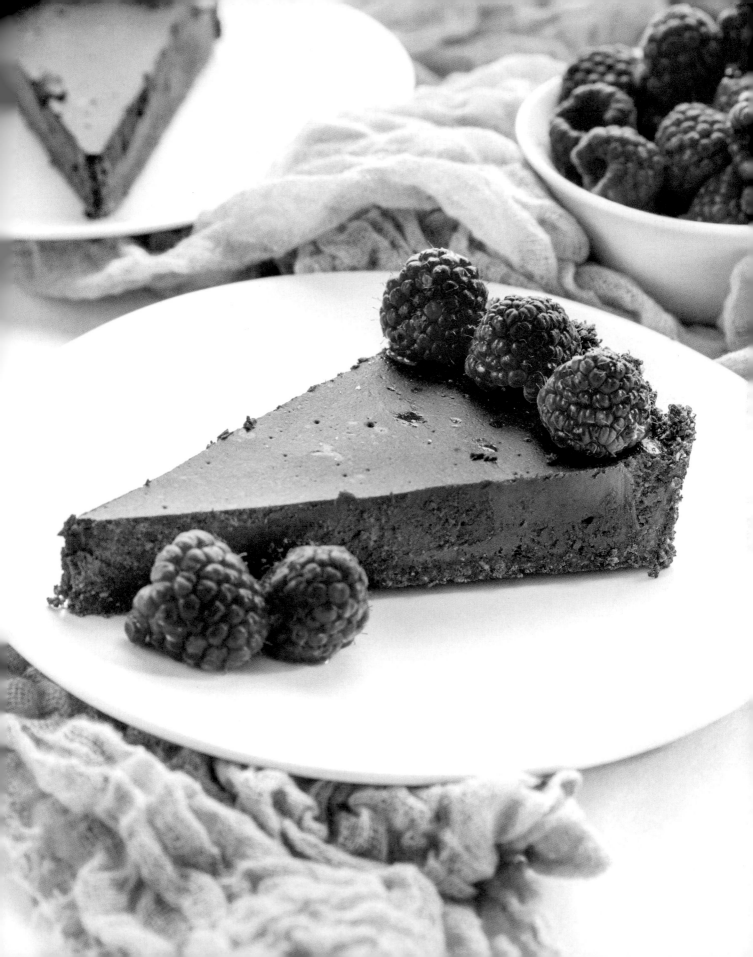

SALTED CARAMEL TART WITH CHOCOLATE GLAZE

Yield: 12 servings   **Prep Time:** 20 minutes, plus 1 hour to set (not including time to make glaze)   **Cook Time:** 28 minutes

Combining a caramel and chocolate filling with a pecan-based crust is like making a giant turtle candy!

1 recipe Easy Pecan Meal Pie Crust (page 366)

6 tablespoons brown sugar substitute

3 tablespoons Bocha Sweet (see tips)

¼ cup (½ stick) unsalted butter

½ cup heavy whipping cream

¼ teaspoon xanthan gum

½ teaspoon coarse sea salt, plus more for sprinkling

1 recipe Easy Chocolate Glaze (page 390)

1. Preheat the oven to 350°F and grease a 9-inch round tart pan or a 14 by 4½-inch rectangular tart pan (see tips). If the pan has a removable bottom, be sure to place the pan on a rimmed baking sheet.

2. Prepare the crust according to the directions, then press firmly into the bottom and up the sides of the prepared pan. Bake for 15 to 18 minutes, until golden brown and firm to the touch. Remove from the oven and let cool completely.

3. Bring the sweeteners and butter to a boil in a large saucepan over medium heat. Continue to boil for 3 to 5 minutes, watching carefully so it doesn't burn. It should turn a deep amber color and bubble thickly.

4. Remove the pan from the heat and stir in the cream. The mixture will bubble vigorously.

5. Return the pan to the heat and bring back to a boil. Boil for 3 minutes, watching carefully. Sprinkle the surface with the xanthan gum and whisk to combine. Whisk in the coarse salt.

6. Pour the caramel into the cooled crust and let sit until it's room temperature, then freeze for 1 hour to set the caramel.

7. Spread the chocolate glaze over the caramel filling. Sprinkle lightly with additional coarse salt.

TIPS: *Rectangular tart pans are fun and interesting and look beautiful, but you need to figure out the area of the pan before you use it. A 14 by 4½-inch tart pan has a total area of 63 inches. A 9-inch round tart pan has an area of 63 inches as well, so they can be swapped.*

If the crust mixture sticks to your fingers as you press it into the pan, simply cover the pan with a sheet of waxed or parchment paper and then use the paper to press the crust into the pan.

I do not recommend using allulose for this caramel filling. It makes the filling far too goopy and soft, and it takes more than 24 hours to set properly. You can use all erythritol-based sweeteners, but the filling will recrystallize.

NUTRITIONAL INFORMATION
CALORIES: 283 | FAT: 27.4g | CARBS: 4.1g | FIBER: 2.3g | PROTEIN: 2.6g

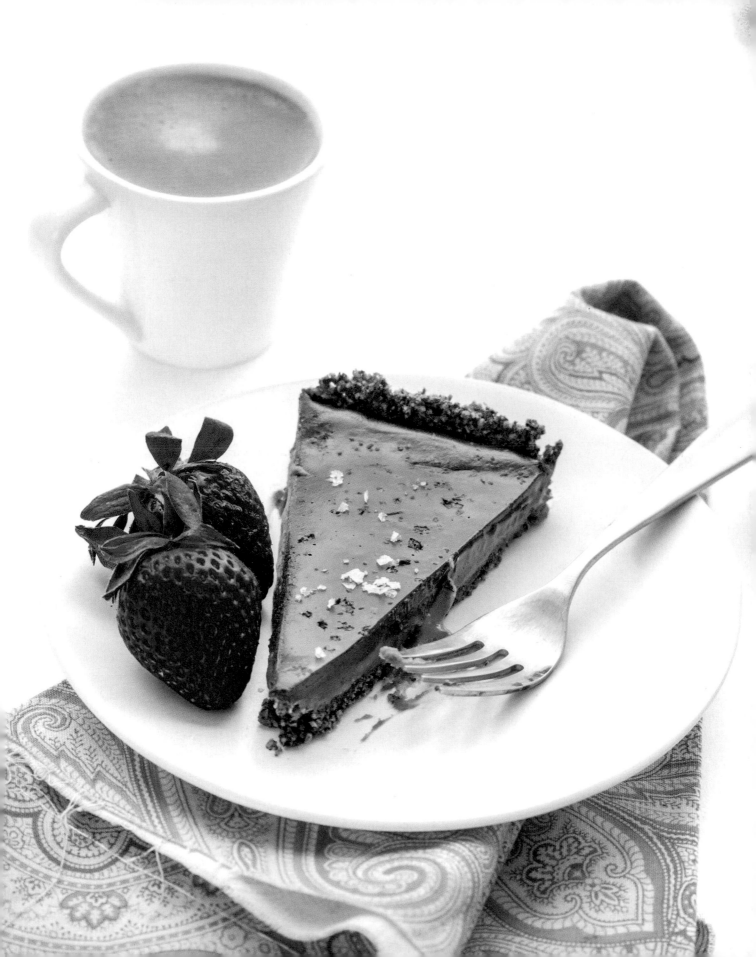

DAIRY-FREE COCONUT CREAM TARTS

Yield: 2 tarts (½ tart per serving) Prep Time: 20 minutes, plus 2 hours to chill Cook Time: 30 minutes

I have a slight obsession with macadamia nuts. Making a tart crust with them takes this tropical dessert to a whole new level.

Crust:

¾ cup macadamia nuts

2 tablespoons powdered erythritol sweetener

⅛ teaspoon salt

1½ tablespoons coconut oil, melted

Filling:

½ cup full-fat coconut milk

2 large egg yolks

3 tablespoons granulated sweetener of choice

⅛ teaspoon salt

¼ teaspoon glucomannan or xanthan gum

½ teaspoon coconut extract

¼ cup unsweetened shredded coconut

Topping:

⅓ cup chilled coconut cream (see tips)

2 tablespoons powdered erythritol sweetener

½ teaspoon vanilla extract

Unsweetened flaked coconut, for garnish

TO MAKE THE CRUST:

1. Preheat the oven to 325°F and lightly grease two 4-inch metal tart pans with removable bottoms. Set the pans on a rimmed baking sheet.

2. Place the macadamia nuts, sweetener, and salt in a food processor and grind into a fine meal. Do not overprocess or the nuts will turn into butter.

3. Transfer the nut mixture to a bowl and stir in the melted coconut oil. Divide the mixture between the prepared pans and press into the bottoms and up the sides.

4. Bake for 18 to 22 minutes, until just beginning to brown. Remove from the oven and let cool completely.

TO MAKE THE FILLING:

5. Bring the coconut milk to a simmer in a small saucepan over medium heat.

6. In a medium bowl, whisk the egg yolks with the sweetener and salt. Slowly add the hot coconut milk to the yolks, whisking continuously.

7. Pour the filling mixture back into the saucepan and set over low heat. Cook, whisking continuously, until the mixture thickens. Because it's such a small amount, this should take only 2 to 3 minutes.

8. Remove the pan from the heat. Whisk in the glucomannan and coconut extract until well combined, then stir in the shredded coconut. Let cool for 10 minutes, then divide the filling between the cooled crusts and spread to the edges. Chill for at least 2 hours.

NUTRITIONAL INFORMATION

CALORIES: 387 | FAT: 38.4g | CARBS: 6.6g | FIBER: 2.8g | PROTEIN: 4.6g

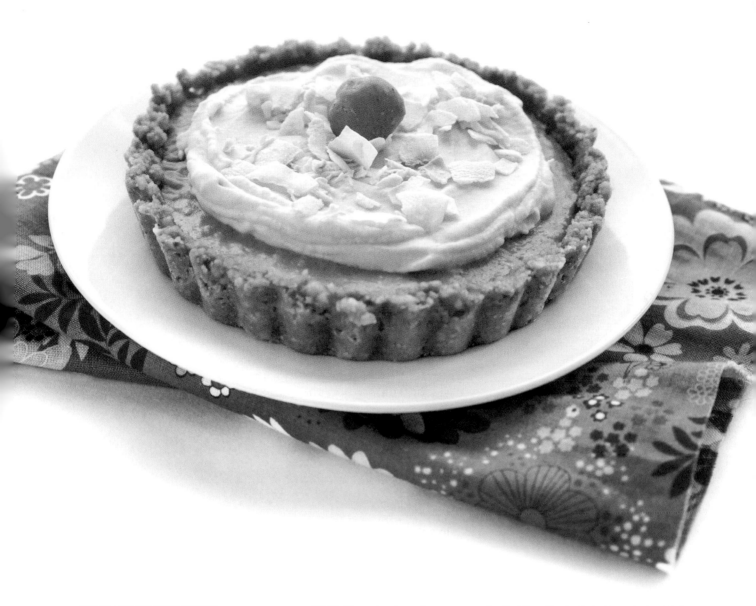

TO MAKE THE TOPPING:

9. In a medium bowl, whip the chilled coconut cream, sweetener, and vanilla with an electric mixer.

10. Top the chilled tarts with the whipped cream and garnish with flaked coconut.

TIPS: *Macadamia nuts are very oily. Setting the tart pans on a rimmed baking sheet will help catch any oils that leak out through the seams. Saves you the trouble of cleaning your oven!*

It is important to chill the coconut cream before whipping it. Refrigerate the unopened can for at least 12 hours, then scoop out the thickened cream when you are ready to make the topping.

These tarts are very calorie dense and filling. A serving is half a tart, but you may find even that too much to eat in one sitting.

Want to turn this into a full-sized tart or pie? Each 4-inch tart pan has an area of 12½ square inches, which means that this recipe has a total area of 25 inches. A 9-inch pie plate has an area of 63½ inches, which means that you need to scale up this recipe by 2.5 times.

BACON SPINACH ARTICHOKE QUICHE

Yield: 8 servings Prep Time: 25 minutes Cook Time: 1 hour

I love a good quiche for dinner or brunch. This one is full of great flavor from the spinach, artichokes, and bacon.

1 recipe Savory Almond Flour Pie Crust (page 366) (see tip)

6 ounces marinated artichoke hearts, drained and chopped

2 ounces fresh spinach, chopped

6 pieces bacon, cooked crisp and chopped

7 large eggs

½ cup heavy whipping cream

1 ounce Parmesan cheese, grated (about 1 cup)

2 cloves garlic, minced

¾ teaspoon salt

½ teaspoon black pepper

1. Preheat the oven to 325°F.

2. Prepare the crust according to the directions and press into the bottom and up the sides of a 9-inch glass or ceramic pie plate. Prick the bottom all over with a fork.

3. Par-bake for 10 minutes, then remove from the oven and let cool for at least 20 minutes.

4. Increase the oven temperature to 350°F. Sprinkle the cooled crust with the artichokes, spinach, and bacon.

5. In a large bowl, whisk together the eggs, cream, Parmesan, garlic, salt, and pepper. Pour this mixture over the fillings in the crust.

6. Bake for another 45 to 50 minutes, until the quiche is just set in the middle. If the edges of the crust are browning too quickly, cover with thin strips of foil.

7. Remove from the oven and let cool for 15 minutes before slicing and serving.

TIP: *Try using the bacon grease from the cooked bacon in place of the butter in this crust. It's absolutely delicious for a savory pie!*

NUTRITIONAL INFORMATION

CALORIES: 322 | FAT: 27.5g | CARBS: 6.2g | FIBER: 2.6g | PROTEIN: 11.6g

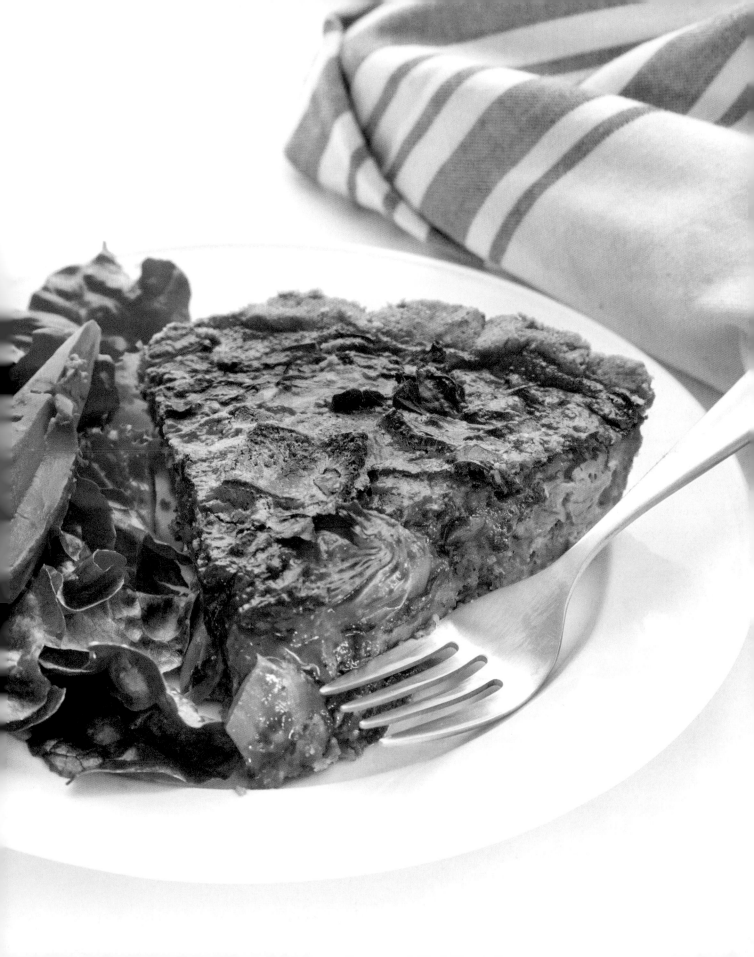

SAUSAGE AND MUSHROOM TART

Yield: 10 servings   Prep Time: 30 minutes   Cook Time: 50 minutes

We tend to think of tarts as being sweet desserts, but savory tarts are delicious, too. This one makes a great dinner and can be cut into smaller pieces for an appetizer.

1 recipe Savory Coconut Flour Pie Crust (page 368)

12 ounces bulk Italian sausage, hot or mild

2 tablespoons unsalted butter

8 ounces button mushrooms, chopped

¼ cup chopped onions

1 tablespoon chopped fresh rosemary

1 teaspoon fresh thyme leaves

1 cup shredded Gruyère or fontina cheese

1. Preheat the oven to 350°F and grease a 9-inch round tart pan or a 14 by 4½-inch rectangular tart pan. If the pan has a removable bottom, be sure to place it on a rimmed baking sheet.

2. Prepare the crust according to the directions and press into the bottom and up the sides of the prepared pan. Prick the bottom all over with a fork. Par-bake for 10 minutes. Remove from the oven and let cool while you prepare the filling.

3. In a large skillet over medium heat, cook the sausage until well browned, about 7 minutes, breaking up any clumps with the back of a wooden spoon. Use a slotted spoon to transfer the sausage to a large bowl, leaving any fat in the pan behind.

4. Add the butter to the pan and let melt, then add the mushrooms and onions. Sauté until the mushrooms are golden, about 4 minutes. Stir in the rosemary and thyme and cook for another minute. Transfer everything, including any juices, to the bowl with the sausage and mix to combine.

5. Spread the mixture in the cooled tart crust and sprinkle with the shredded cheese. Bake for 20 to 25 minutes, until the filling is bubbling and the cheese is melted.

6. Remove from the oven and let cool for 15 minutes before slicing and serving.

TIP: *You may have noticed that I specify a greased pan for the coconut flour crust but not for the almond flour crust. Nuts tend to have such a high fat content that I haven't found greasing to be necessary. But if you're worried that the crust may stick to your tart pan or pie plate, go ahead and grease your pan every time.*

NUTRITIONAL INFORMATION

CALORIES: 339 | FAT: 25.5g | CARBS: 7.4g | FIBER: 3g | PROTEIN: 16.4g

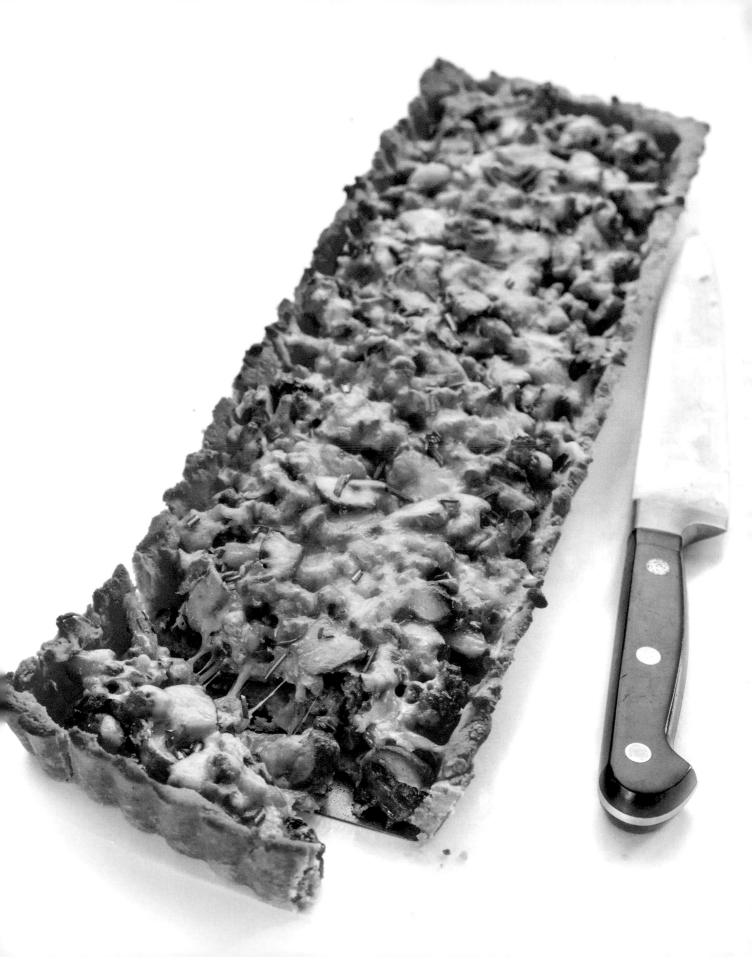

TOMATO RICOTTA TART

Yield: 10 servings   Prep Time: 30 minutes, plus 1 hour to freeze pie dough   Cook Time: 65 minutes

A delicious summer savory tart with fresh tomatoes and basil.

1 recipe Savory Almond Flour Pie Crust (page 366)

1 cup whole-milk ricotta cheese

½ cup shredded mozzarella cheese (about 2 ounces)

½ ounce Parmesan cheese, grated (about ½ cup)

¼ cup fresh basil leaves, chopped

1 large egg

2 cloves garlic, minced

¾ teaspoon salt

½ teaspoon black pepper

8 ounces fresh tomatoes, thinly sliced

Small basil leaves, for garnish

Coarse sea salt, for garnish

1. Prepare the crust according to the directions and press firmly into the bottom and partway up the sides of a 9-inch round ceramic tart pan. Freeze for 1 hour.

2. Preheat the oven to 350°F and lightly grease a large piece of parchment paper. Press the greased side of the parchment into the frozen crust, making sure it also covers the edges, and add pie weights to hold down the parchment (see tips).

3. Par-bake for 20 minutes, then remove from the oven and let cool for at least 20 minutes. Do not remove the pie weights or parchment until cooled.

4. Return the oven heat to 350°F. In a medium bowl, whisk together the ricotta, mozzarella, Parmesan, basil, egg, garlic, salt, and pepper until well combined. Spread over the cooled crust.

5. Arrange the tomato slices on top and bake for 40 to 45 minutes, until the filling is mostly set. Remove from the oven and let cool completely, then garnish with a few fresh basil leaves and some coarse salt.

TIPS: *Using pie weights to hold the crust in place as it bakes is useful for very liquidy fillings such as this. Both the ricotta and the tomatoes release liquid during baking, and the crust can disintegrate if not firmly baked ahead.*

Pie weights are little ceramic or metal balls that hold down a crust as it bakes. They help keep a crust from puffing up or shrinking. If you don't have any, you can nest another pie plate inside the first one, on top of the parchment paper.

NUTRITIONAL INFORMATION

CALORIES: 219 | FAT: 18g | CARBS: 5.8g | FIBER: 2.1g | PROTEIN: 9.6g

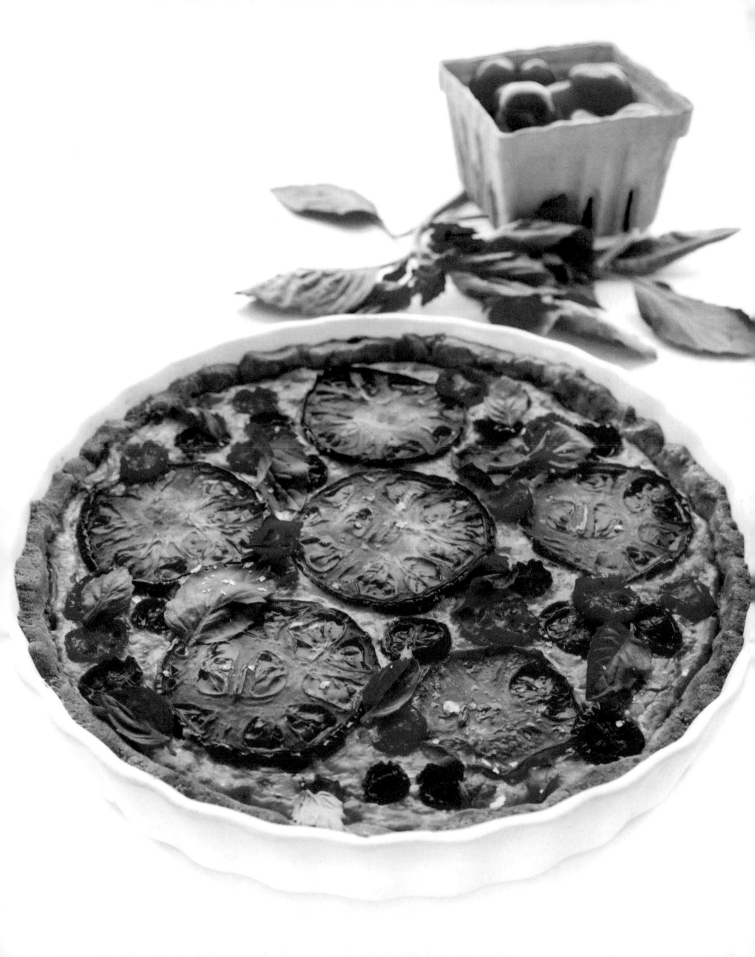

TOURTIERE

Yield: 10 servings Prep Time: 25 minutes Cook Time: 50 minutes

Tourtiere is a traditional French Canadian meat pie, and my mum and I made it every Christmas growing up. It's one of my fondest memories, so making a keto tourtiere was truly meaningful to me. The cloves in the meat filling are what gives tourtiere its distinctive flavor.

1 pound ground beef

1 pound ground pork

½ cup chopped onions

2 cloves garlic, minced

¼ cup water

1 teaspoon salt

½ teaspoon black pepper

½ teaspoon dried thyme leaves

¼ teaspoon ground dried sage

¼ teaspoon ground cloves

½ recipe Nut-Free Magic Mozzarella Dough (page 376)

1 large egg yolk

1 tablespoon water

1. In a 10-inch ovenproof skillet over medium heat, cook the beef and pork until nicely browned but not cooked through, 8 to 10 minutes, breaking up any clumps with the back of a wooden spoon. Add the onions and garlic and sauté until the onions are translucent, another 4 minutes.

2. Stir in the water, salt, pepper, thyme, sage, and cloves and bring to a boil. Reduce the heat to low and simmer until the meat is fully cooked, another 5 minutes. Remove from the heat while you prepare the crust.

3. Preheat the oven to 350°F. Prepare a work surface with a silicone baking mat or a large piece of parchment paper. Lightly grease the mat or parchment.

4. Prepare the dough according to the directions and transfer to the prepared work surface. Cover with another piece of parchment paper.

5. Roll out the dough to a 12-inch circle and carefully loosen and lift off the work surface. Place over the filling, then trim and crimp the edges to fit the pan. Cut a few slits in the top to allow steam to escape.

6. In a small bowl, whisk the egg yolk with the water until well combined. Brush the egg wash over the crust.

7. Bake until the crust is golden and firm to the touch, 25 to 30 minutes. Remove from the oven and let cool for 20 minutes before serving.

TIPS: *Reserve the trimmed pieces of dough and then roll them out again. Use cookie cutters or a sharp knife to cut out pretty decorative shapes for the top of the pie.*

The tourtiere I remember had only a top crust, so that's how I made this one. The filling was almost scooped onto your plate, with a lovely piece of pastry on top. If you really want a bottom crust, try making the full amount of the coconut flour–based fathead dough. You will want to par-bake it for at least 10 minutes and then let it cool before filling it.

NUTRITIONAL INFORMATION

CALORIES: 372 | FAT: 24.3g | CARBS: 4.1g | FIBER: 1.6g | PROTEIN: 30.3g

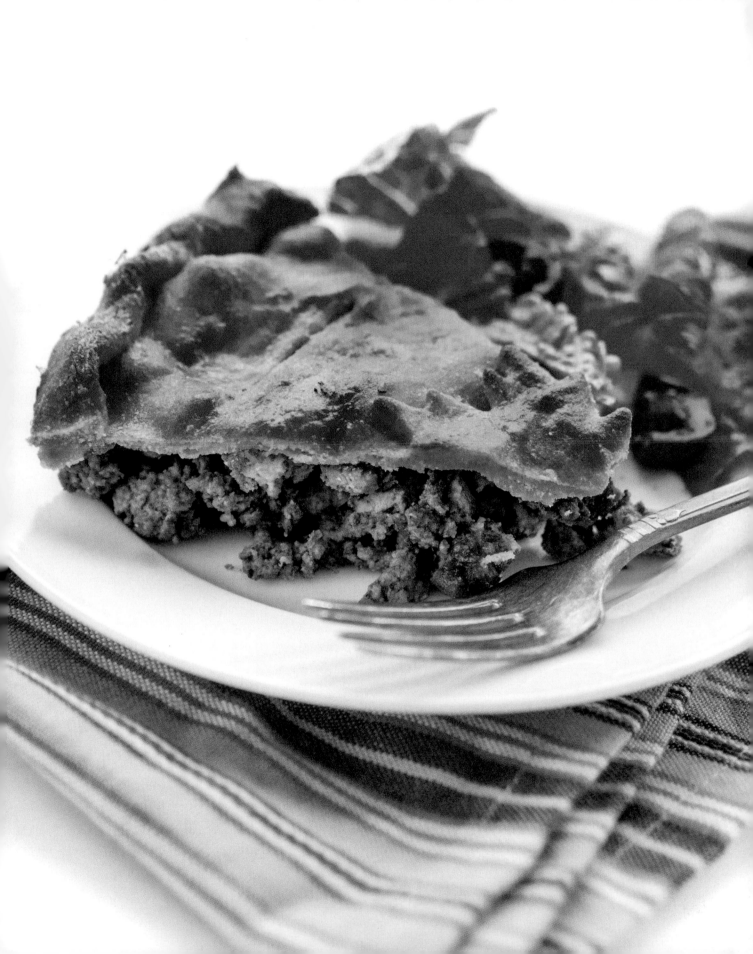

LINZERTORTE

Yield: 10 servings Prep Time: 40 minutes, plus 30 minutes to chill pastry Cook Time: 47 minutes

Is linzertorte a cake or a tart? I am calling it a tart because it has a distinct crust with a filling. This classic Austrian dessert may need a category all its own.

Crust:

1 cup (100g) blanched almond flour, plus more for the work surface

1 cup hazelnut meal

½ cup granulated erythritol sweetener

¼ cup (28g) coconut flour

1 teaspoon ground cinnamon

½ teaspoon salt

¼ teaspoon ground cloves

½ cup (1 stick) unsalted butter, cut into small pieces, softened

1 large egg

Filling:

1 cup fresh raspberries

¼ cup water

⅓ cup powdered erythritol sweetener

¼ teaspoon glucomannan or xanthan gum

Powdered erythritol sweetener, for garnish

TO MAKE THE CRUST:

1. Lightly grease a 9-inch springform pan and line the bottom with parchment paper.

2. Place the almond flour, hazelnut meal, sweetener, coconut flour, cinnamon, salt, and cloves in a food processor. Pulse a few times to combine. Sprinkle the butter pieces over the top and pulse until the mixture resembles coarse crumbs.

3. Add the egg and process until the dough comes together. Press about two-thirds of the dough into the bottom of the prepared pan, making the sides just a little higher. Refrigerate for 30 minutes.

4. Lay a sheet of waxed paper or parchment paper on a work surface and lightly dust with almond flour. Gather the remaining dough into a ball and place on the paper. Top with another piece of paper and roll out to a 9-inch circle. Refrigerate this as well, with the parchment in place.

TO MAKE THE FILLING:

5. In a medium saucepan over medium heat, bring the raspberries and water to a boil. Cook until the berries can be mashed easily, about 5 minutes. Remove the pan from the heat.

6. Stir in the sweetener and sprinkle the surface with the glucomannan, whisking quickly to combine. Let sit for about 10 minutes to thicken.

TO ASSEMBLE:

7. Preheat the oven to 325°F. Par-bake the bottom crust for 12 minutes, then remove from the oven and let cool for 15 minutes. Spread with the filling.

8. Carefully cut the pastry circle into 10 strips and gently loosen from the paper with an offset spatula. Place 5 strips at evenly spaced intervals on top of the filling, then place the other 5 strips crosswise over the top to create a lattice.

NUTRITIONAL INFORMATION

CALORIES: 174 | FAT: 15g | CARBS: 5.7g | FIBER: 2.8g | PROTEIN: 3.7g

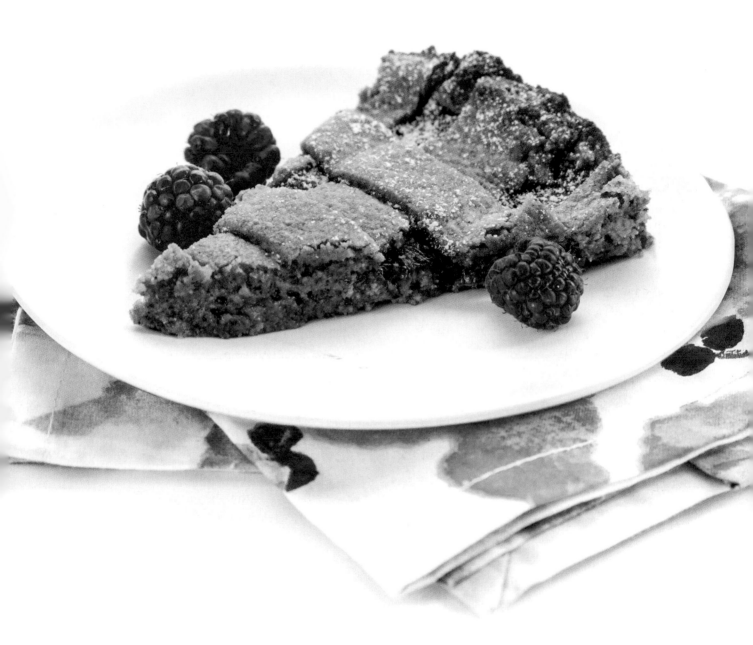

9. Set the springform pan on a rimmed baking sheet to catch any oil that may leak out. Bake for about 30 minutes, until the top crust is golden brown. Let cool completely, then dust with powdered sweetener.

TIP: *When arranging the lattice, be sure to use the longest strips for the center of the lattice in both directions. If any of the strips are too long for the tart, just break them off and save them. Roll them into a ball and then press it into a cookie to bake alongside the tart.*

RASPBERRY CREAM CHEESE TURNOVERS

Yield: 9 turnovers (1 per serving) Prep Time: 25 minutes (not including time to make dough) Cook Time: 20 minutes

When I was a kid, my mum would make turnovers whenever she had leftover pastry crust. She would just roll it into a square, fill it with jam, and fold it over. Those were the best little treats in the world.

Pastries:

1 recipe Sweet Coconut-Free Magic Mozzarella Dough (page 375)

4 ounces cream cheese, softened

3 tablespoons powdered erythritol sweetener

1 tablespoon heavy whipping cream, room temperature

¼ teaspoon vanilla extract

½ cup fresh raspberries

Glaze (Optional):

¼ cup powdered erythritol sweetener

¼ teaspoon vanilla extract

1½ tablespoons water

> **VARIATION: RASPBERRY CREAM CHEESE DANISH.**
>
> *Instead of filling the dough and folding it over, simply roll the sides up a bit and spread the cream cheese in the center. Top with berries and bake. The danishes will take about the same amount of time to bake as the turnovers.*

1. Preheat the oven to 350°F and line a rimmed baking sheet with a silicone baking mat or parchment paper.

2. Place the prepared dough on another silicone baking mat or large piece of parchment paper and cover with parchment or waxed paper. Roll out to a 15-inch square. Remove the top piece of parchment.

3. Using a sharp knife or a pizza cutter, cut the dough into 9 even squares, each about 5 inches.

4. In a medium bowl, beat the cream cheese, sweetener, cream, and vanilla with an electric mixer until smooth. Spread about 1 tablespoon of the cream cheese mixture over one triangular half of each square, leaving a ½-inch border. Top with 4 or 5 fresh raspberries.

5. Fold the uncovered half of each pastry over the filling, matching up the corners to create a triangle. Pinch the seams together and place on the prepared baking sheet. Bake for about 20 minutes, until golden brown and just firm to the touch. Remove from the oven and let cool completely on the pan.

6. Whisk all of the glaze ingredients in a small bowl and drizzle lightly over the cooled turnovers.

TIPS: *I wanted to make these turnovers coconut-free, so I used an almond flour–only version of Magic Mozzarella Dough. It took a lot of extra almond flour to make up for the coconut flour. This adds some carbs and makes each of these turnovers quite filling. You could do regular mozzarella dough or even coconut flour dough if you prefer. You would need only a half recipe of the coconut flour dough.*

You could also make the turnovers smaller, cutting the dough into 16 squares, about 4 inches.

NUTRITIONAL INFORMATION

CALORIES: 304 | FAT: 25.5g | CARBS: 7.3g | FIBER: 3g | PROTEIN: 10.5g

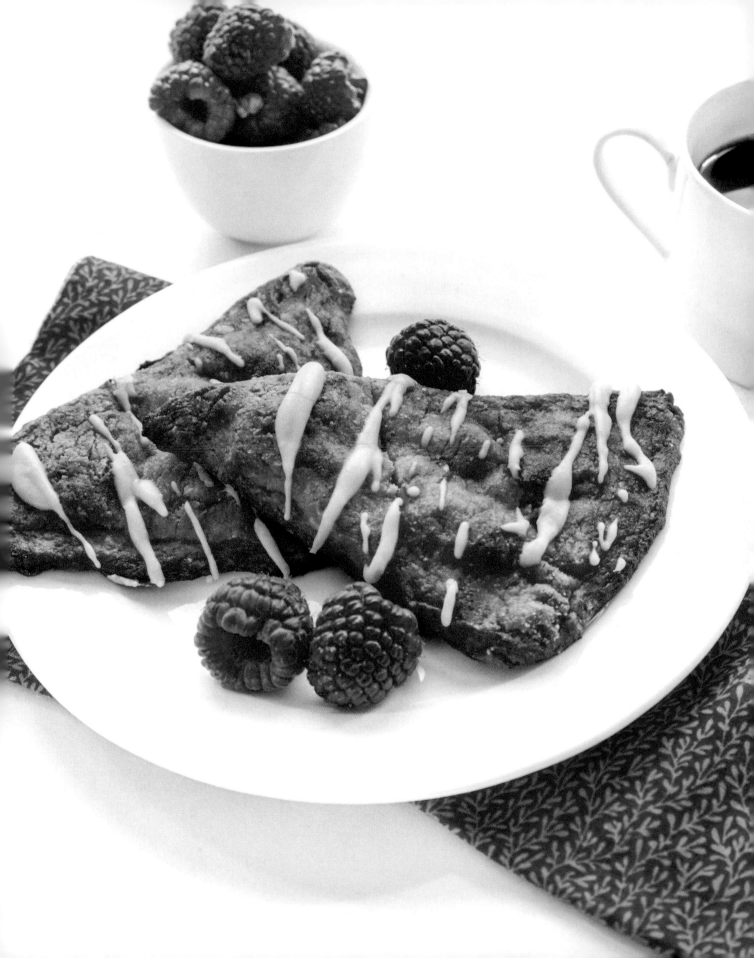

ZUCCHINI CRISP

Yield: 9 servings Prep Time: 35 minutes Cook Time: 45 minutes

Let's face it, a crisp is really just a pie without a bottom crust. I don't pretend that zucchini are apples, so I refuse to call this recipe "Mock Apple Crisp." I love real apple crisp, and if I could eat it and still be low-carb, I would! But zucchini is pretty special in its own way, and this crisp has a wonderful sweet caramel flavor. So good with a dollop of keto vanilla ice cream on top.

Topping:

¾ cup (75g) blanched almond flour

6 tablespoons granulated erythritol sweetener

¼ cup unsweetened shredded coconut

¼ cup finely chopped pecans

½ teaspoon ground cinnamon

¼ teaspoon salt

3½ tablespoons unsalted butter, chilled and cut into small cubes

Filling:

2 pounds zucchini (about 2 large)

½ cup brown sugar substitute

¼ cup granulated erythritol sweetener

2 tablespoons fresh lemon juice

1 teaspoon ground cinnamon

¼ teaspoon ground nutmeg

¼ teaspoon glucomannan or xanthan gum

SERVING SUGGESTION: *Top with Keto Vanilla Ice Cream (page 394) or lightly sweetened whipped cream.*

TO MAKE THE TOPPING:

1. Preheat the oven to 300°F and line a rimmed baking sheet with parchment paper.

2. Place the almond flour, sweetener, coconut, pecans, cinnamon, and salt in a food processor. Pulse a few times to combine. Scatter the butter pieces over the top and process on high until the mixture resembles coarse crumbs.

3. Transfer the topping mixture to the prepared baking sheet and spread into an even layer. Press down firmly with your hands to help it clump together.

4. Bake for 20 to 25 minutes, until the edges are golden brown. Remove from the oven and let cool completely to crisp up. Meanwhile, prepare the filling.

TO MAKE THE FILLING:

5. Peel the zucchini and slice them in half lengthwise. Use a sharp knife or a spoon to remove the seeds in the center, then cut each half crosswise in ¼-inch-thick slices. You should get about 6 cups of slices.

6. Place the slices in a pot and add the sweeteners, lemon juice, cinnamon, and nutmeg. Stir to combine. Cook over low heat, stirring frequently, until the zucchini is very tender, about 20 minutes.

7. Remove the pan from the heat. Using a slotted spoon, spoon the zucchini into an 8-inch square glass or ceramic baking dish, leaving the liquid behind in the pan.

8. Sprinkle the surface of the liquid with the glucomannan and whisk vigorously to combine. Pour over the zucchini in the baking dish. Let sit for 10 minutes to thicken.

NUTRITIONAL INFORMATION

CALORIES: 153 | FAT: 13.2g | CARBS: 6.3g | FIBER: 2.8g | PROTEIN: 3.7g

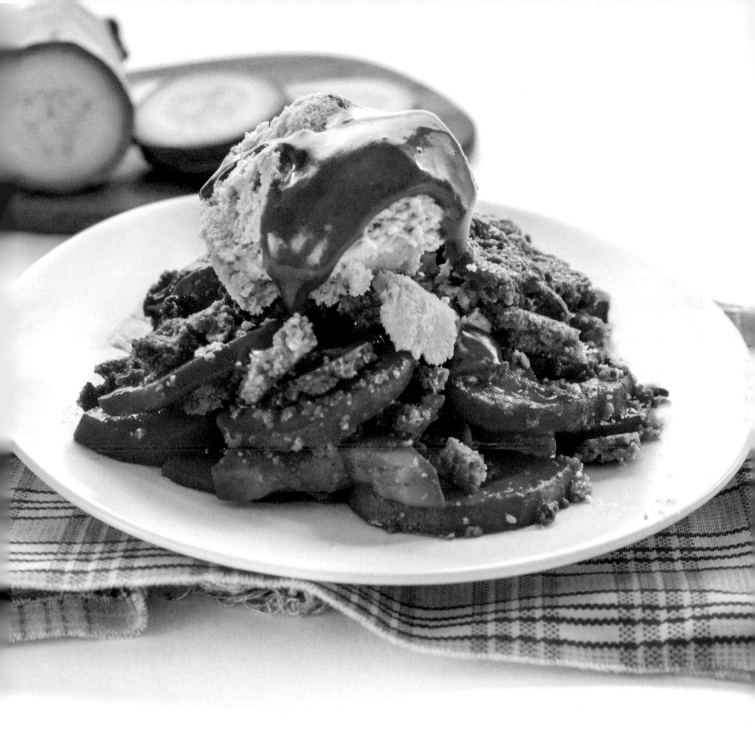

TO ASSEMBLE:

9. Crumble the topping with your fingers and sprinkle over the zucchini filling. You can break up the pieces finely or coarsely, as desired.

10. Place the zucchini crisp in the still-warm oven for 10 minutes before serving.

TIP: *This recipe may involve a fair bit of prep and cook time, but you can be prepping the filling while the topping cooks, so the total time is misleading.*

Chapter 14:
CUSTARDS, SOUFFLÉS & OTHER BAKED DESSERTS

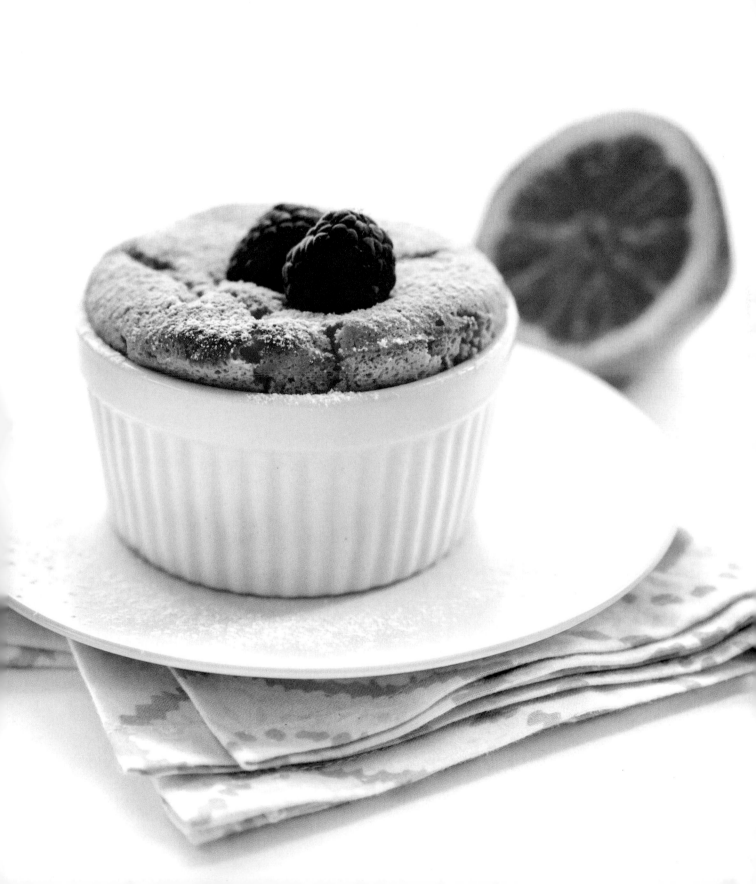

OLD-FASHIONED BAKED CUSTARD

Yield: 4 servings Prep Time: 15 minutes Cook Time: 40 minutes

Custard always seems so plain and uninteresting—until you taste it and realize that the rich creaminess is heavenly and needs no dressing up. This custard would even be good for breakfast.

1½ cups heavy whipping cream

2 large eggs

6 tablespoons granulated sweetener of choice

⅛ teaspoon salt

½ teaspoon vanilla extract

Ground nutmeg or cinnamon, for sprinkling

1. Preheat the oven to 350°F and set four 4-ounce ramekins in a large baking dish.

2. In a large saucepan over medium heat, scald the cream by bringing it to a full boil. Watch it carefully so it doesn't boil over.

3. In a large bowl, whisk the eggs with the sweetener and salt. Slowly pour the hot cream into the eggs, whisking continuously until well combined. Whisk in the vanilla.

4. Divide the mixture among the ramekins and sprinkle with nutmeg or cinnamon. Pour hot or boiling water into the baking dish until it comes about halfway up the sides of the ramekins. Be sure not to get any water into the custards themselves. Transfer the baking dish to the oven.

5. Bake for 30 to 40 minutes, until a knife inserted in the center comes out clean but the custard still jiggles slightly when shaken. Remove the dish from the oven and carefully remove the ramekins from the water bath. Let cool completely.

TIP: *A bain marie, or water bath, is critical to achieving the right consistency for desserts like this one. Out of curiosity, I tried one of the custards without the bain marie, and it was quite hilarious. It puffed up alarmingly and then sank dramatically when removed from the oven. It also tasted more eggy and had a bit of a curdled consistency.*

SERVING SUGGESTION: *The custard can be served at room temperature or chilled. It really doesn't need much else, but a few fresh berries are a delicious addition.*

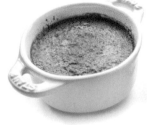 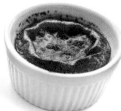

NUTRITIONAL INFORMATION

CALORIES: 350 | FAT: 33.5g | CARBS: 2.8g | PROTEIN: 5g

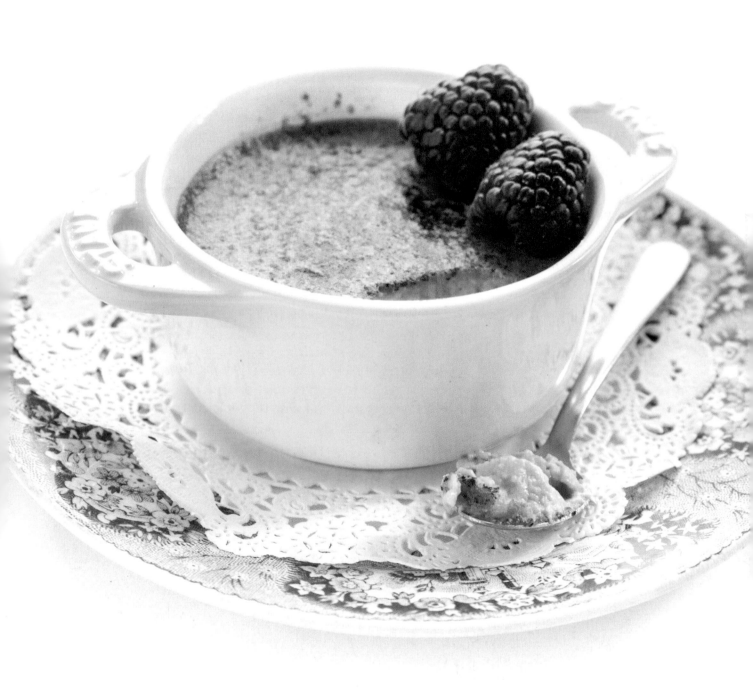

CRÈME BRÛLÉE

Yield: 6 servings **Prep Time:** 15 minutes, plus 2 hours to chill **Cook Time:** 50 minutes

One of my all-time favorite desserts!

1¾ cups heavy whipping cream

4 large egg yolks

⅓ cup granulated sweetener of choice

½ teaspoon vanilla extract

2 tablespoons granulated erythritol sweetener

Special equipment: Kitchen torch (optional)

TIPS: *Crème brûlée takes only egg yolks and cooks at a lower temperature than custard. It is amazingly creamy but has a looser consistency.*

How long the crème brûlée takes to set depends on the depth of your ramekins. I have deeper 4-ounce ramekins as well as shallow fluted ones. Crème brûlée may take as little as 30 minutes to bake in shallow dishes, depending on your oven. Be sure to watch it carefully.

For the topping, the only sweetener that will really caramelize and harden properly is an erythritol-based sweetener such as Swerve. Allulose may caramelize, but it will take quite a bit of cooking to harden up properly.

1. Preheat the oven to 300°F and set six 4-ounce ramekins in a large baking dish.

2. In a medium saucepan over medium-low heat, heat the cream until just hot and steam rises from the surface. Do not allow to simmer or boil. Remove the pan from the heat.

3. In a large bowl, beat the egg yolks and sweetener with an electric mixer until pale yellow and thickened, about 3 minutes. Slowly add the hot cream, whisking continuously. Whisk in the vanilla.

4. Divide the mixture among the ramekins. Pour hot or boiling water into the baking dish until it comes about halfway up the sides of the ramekins. Be sure not to get any water into the ramekins themselves. Transfer the baking dish to the oven.

5. Bake until the custard is just set but still slightly wobbly in the middle, 30 to 45 minutes. Remove the baking dish from the oven and carefully remove the ramekins from the water bath. Let cool to room temperature, then wrap each ramekin tightly in plastic wrap and chill for at least 2 hours.

6. Before serving, remove the ramekins from the fridge and lightly blot the tops with a paper towel. Sprinkle each with 1 heaping teaspoon of the erythritol sweetener.

7. Ignite a kitchen torch and run it back and forth over each custard until the sweetener caramelizes. Let set for a few moments to harden. Alternatively, you can brown the topping under the broiler for 1 to 2 minutes.

NUTRITIONAL INFORMATION

| CALORIES: | 280 | FAT: | 27.2g | CARBS: | 2.4g | PROTEIN: | 3.2g |

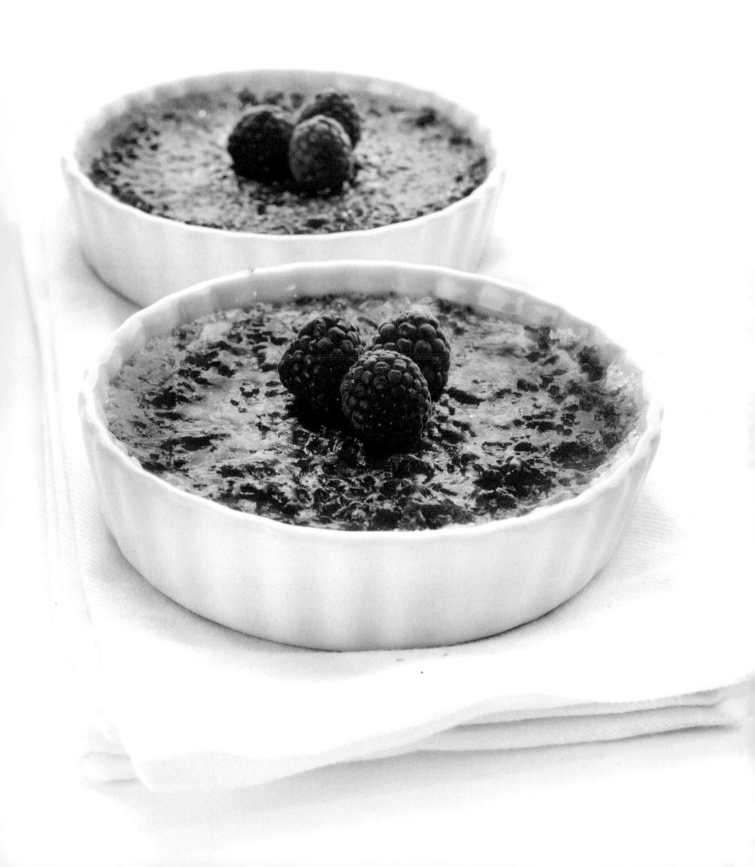

DAIRY-FREE CARAMEL FLAN

Yield: 6 servings **Prep Time:** 20 minutes **Cook Time:** 55 minutes

Whether you call this crème caramel or flan, it's truly an amazing and impressive dairy-free dessert.

¼ cup brown sugar substitute

¼ cup Bocha Sweet or allulose

2 teaspoons water

1 (13.5-ounce) can full-fat coconut milk

2 large eggs

2 large egg yolks

½ cup powdered erythritol sweetener

1 teaspoon vanilla extract

TIPS: *The flan can be refrigerated after baking, but let it come to room temperature before serving.*

The best ramekins for a flan like this are the small 4-ounce steep-sided ones. The flan looks extra impressive when you flip it over, with the gorgeous caramel on top.

A mix of sweeteners is really important for the caramel topping. The brown sugar substitute gives it a beautiful caramel color, and the Bocha Sweet or allulose keeps it softer, even after being refrigerated.

1. Preheat the oven to 350°F and lightly grease six 4-ounce ramekins. Set the ramekins in a large baking dish.

2. In a medium saucepan over medium heat, whisk together the brown sugar substitute, Bocha Sweet, and water. Cook, whisking frequently, until the sweeteners have dissolved. Divide the mixture among the prepared ramekins.

3. Place the coconut milk in the same pan and set over low heat, whisking until the coconut cream and coconut water are well combined. Remove the pan from the heat and set aside.

4. In a large bowl, whisk the whole eggs, egg yolks, powdered sweetener, and vanilla until smooth. Slowly whisk in the coconut milk, trying not to froth the mixture.

5. Divide the coconut milk mixture among the ramekins. Pour hot or boiling water into the baking dish until it comes come about halfway up the sides of the ramekins. Be sure not to get any water into the ramekins themselves. Transfer the baking dish to the oven.

6. Bake for 30 to 50 minutes, until the flan is almost set. It shouldn't really jiggle in the middle when shaken but shouldn't be puffed up, either.

7. Remove the dish from the oven and carefully remove the ramekins from the water bath. Let cool completely.

8. To serve, run a sharp knife around the edge of each ramekin. Cover with a small serving plate and flip the whole thing over, then give the ramekin a good shake to loosen the flan.

NUTRITIONAL INFORMATION

CALORIES: 178 | FAT: 15.7g | CARBS: 2.2g | PROTEIN: 4.3g

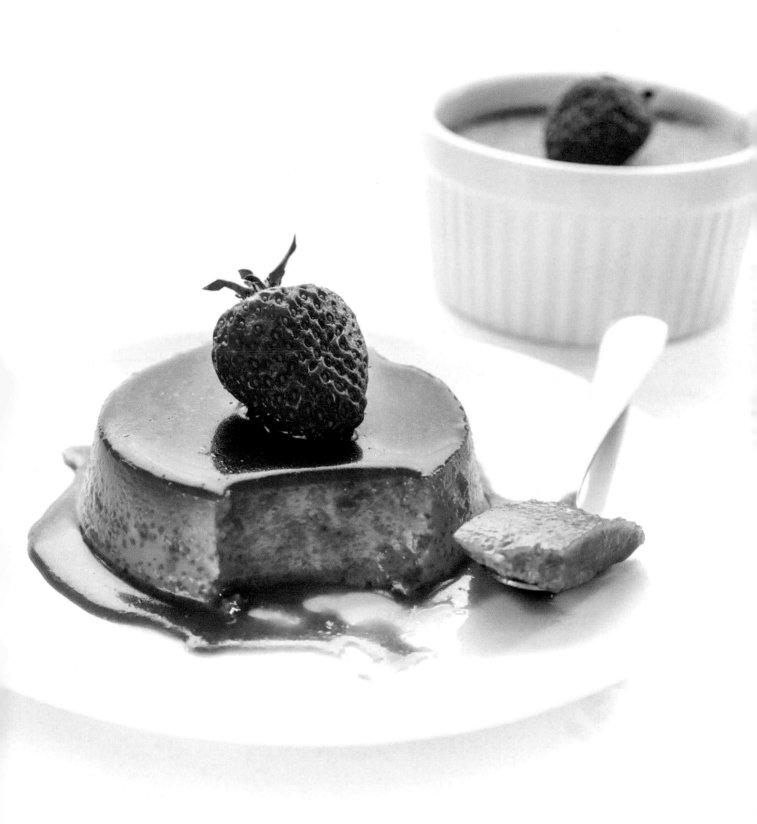

DAIRY-FREE CHOCOLATE POTS DE CRÈME

Yield: 5 servings   Prep Time: 20 minutes, plus 3 to 4 hours to chill   Cook Time: 55 minutes

Pot de crème is a little thicker than traditional custard, but so rich and creamy that a little goes a long way.

1 (13.5-ounce) can full-fat coconut milk

¼ cup powdered erythritol sweetener

2 tablespoons Bocha Sweet

2½ ounces unsweetened chocolate, chopped

1 teaspoon vanilla extract

3 large egg yolks

¼ teaspoon salt

SERVING SUGGESTION: *Top with a little whipped coconut cream and some fresh berries, if desired.*

1. Preheat the oven to 300°F and set five 4-ounce ramekins in a large baking dish.

2. In a medium saucepan over medium heat, bring the coconut milk and sweeteners to a simmer, whisking frequently to dissolve the sweeteners. Remove the pan from the heat and add the chopped chocolate. Let sit for 3 to 4 minutes to melt. Add the vanilla and whisk until smooth.

3. In a medium bowl, whisk together the egg yolks and salt. Slowly add about 1 cup of the chocolate mixture, whisking continuously, to temper the yolks. Then whisk the chocolate/egg yolk mixture back into the pan.

4. Return the pan to low heat and cook, whisking continuously, until the mixture has thickened, about 3 minutes.

5. Divide the mixture among the prepared ramekins. Pour hot or boiling water into the baking dish until it comes about halfway up the sides of the ramekins. Be sure not to get any water into the ramekins themselves. Loosely cover the whole baking dish with foil.

6. Transfer the dish to the oven and bake for 35 to 45 minutes, until the pots de crème are set around the edges but still jiggle slightly in the center. Remove the dish from the oven and carefully remove the ramekins from the water bath. Let cool completely, then refrigerate until set, 3 to 4 hours.

TIPS: *A mix of sweeteners works best here to keep the pot de crème from recrystallizing too much. But if you have only erythritol, that will work.*

I admit, five is an awkward number of servings. But I found my mixture to be a little too much for four small ramekins. And hey, I have five people in my family, so for once, this works out well for us—no fighting over who gets what!

NUTRITIONAL INFORMATION

CALORIES: 263 | FAT: 23.3g | CARBS: 6.4g | FIBER: 2.4g | PROTEIN: 5g

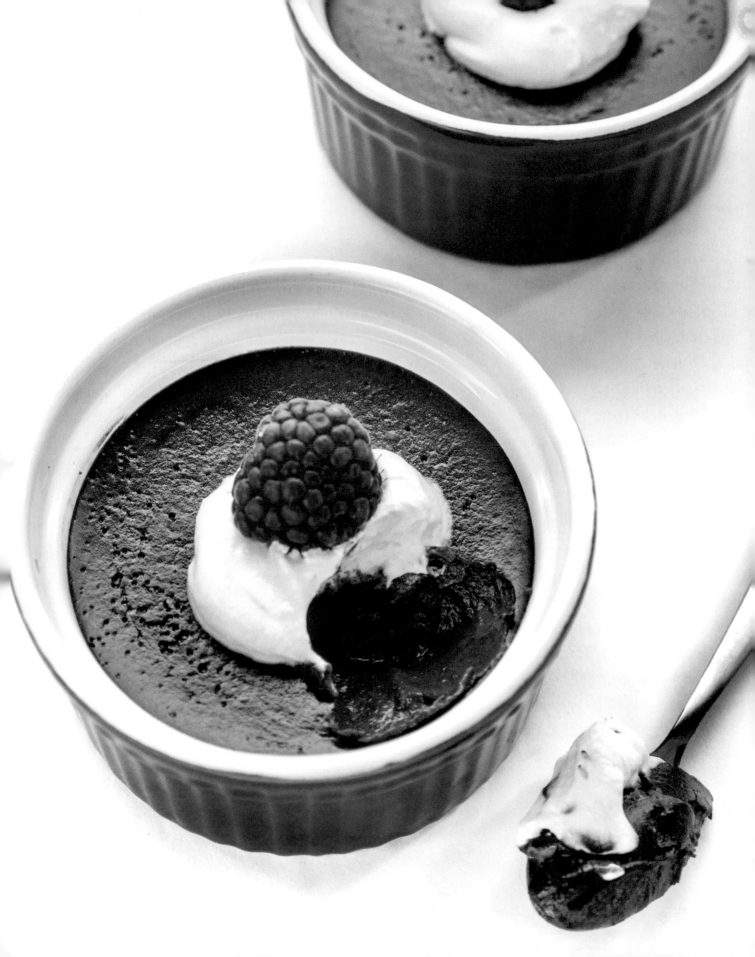

CLASSIC CHOCOLATE SOUFFLÉS

Yield: 4 soufflés (1 per serving)   Prep Time: 30 minutes   Cook Time: 23 minutes

Nothing looks more impressive than a chocolate soufflé rising delightfully above the rim of a baking dish.

Granulated sweetener of choice, for the ramekins

½ cup heavy whipping cream

2 tablespoons powdered erythritol sweetener

⅛ teaspoon glucomannan or xanthan gum

2 ounces unsweetened chocolate, chopped

2 large eggs, separated, room temperature

2 tablespoons water

½ teaspoon vanilla extract

⅛ teaspoon cream of tartar

Pinch of salt

2 tablespoons granulated erythritol sweetener

SERVING SUGGESTION: *Dust the soufflés with powdered sweetener or top them with a little lightly sweetened whipped cream. A red raspberry is a nice touch, too.*

1. Preheat the oven to 375°F and lightly grease four 4-ounce ramekins. Lightly coat the bottoms and sides of the ramekins with granulated sweetener (see tips). Set the ramekins on a rimmed baking sheet.

2. In a medium saucepan over medium heat, bring the cream and powdered sweetener to a boil, whisking frequently. Remove the pan from the heat, sprinkle with the glucomannan, and whisk to combine.

3. Add the chopped chocolate and let sit for a few minutes to melt, then whisk to combine. Let cool for a few more minutes.

4. Whisk in the egg yolks, then whisk in the water and vanilla.

5. In a large bowl, beat the egg whites, cream of tartar, and salt with an electric mixer until frothy. Add the granulated sweetener and beat until the whites are thick and glossy and hold stiff peaks.

6. Add about one-third of the egg whites to the chocolate and fold in to lighten, then carefully fold the chocolate mixture back into the remaining egg whites until just combined.

7. Divide among the prepared ramekins, filling them almost to the top. Transfer the baking sheet to the oven and bake for 12 to 18 minutes, until the soufflés are puffed well above the rim. Remove from the oven and serve immediately.

TIPS: *Sprinkling the greased ramekins with granulated sweetener helps the soufflés "climb" the sides and rise.*

Resist opening the oven door while the soufflés are baking. They will rise better if no drafts come into the oven.

Like any good soufflé, these stay puffed up for only 5 minutes or so. Then they begin to sink quite quickly. Get them to the table right after taking them out of the oven. They are a bit too hot to eat, but they look impressive!

NUTRITIONAL INFORMATION
CALORIES: 248 | FAT: 19.7g | CARBS: 5.1g | FIBER: 2.4g | PROTEIN: 5.8g

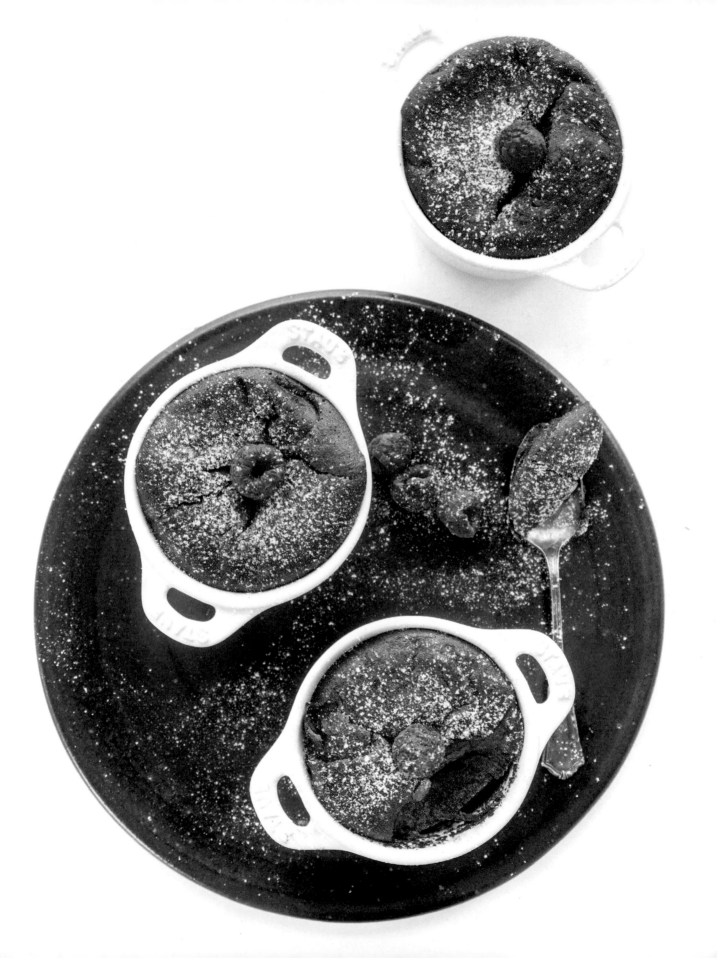

DAIRY-FREE LEMON SOUFFLÉS

Yield: 4 soufflés (1 per serving)   **Prep Time:** 30 minutes   **Cook Time:** 27 minutes

Soufflés come in a variety of flavors. This light and airy dessert is sure to be a hit with lemon lovers.

Granulated sweetener of choice, for the ramekins

2 large eggs, separated, room temperature

2 teaspoons grated lemon zest

2 tablespoons fresh lemon juice

2 tablespoons granulated erythritol sweetener

½ cup unsweetened almond milk

¼ cup (25g) blanched almond flour

½ teaspoon lemon extract

½ teaspoon vanilla extract

⅛ teaspoon salt

¼ cup powdered erythritol sweetener, plus more for dusting

SERVING SUGGESTION: *You can serve these soufflés in so many ways—with just a sprinkling of powdered sweetener, with some fresh berries, or with whipped cream. A few strands of lemon zest make for an elegant presentation.*

1. Preheat the oven to 400°F and grease four 4-ounce ramekins with coconut oil. Lightly coat the bottoms and sides of the ramekins with granulated sweetener. Set the ramekins on a rimmed baking sheet.

2. In a medium bowl, whisk together the egg yolks, lemon zest, lemon juice, and granulated sweetener.

3. In a medium saucepan over medium-low heat, bring the almond milk just to a simmer. Slowly add about half of the hot almond milk to the egg yolks, whisking continuously. Then slowly pour the yolk mixture back into the pan, whisking continuously. Continue to cook over medium-low heat until the mixture starts to thicken, whisking continuously.

4. Remove from the heat and whisk in the almond flour and extracts. Set aside to cool.

5. In a large bowl, beat the egg whites and salt with an electric mixer until foamy. Slowly add the powdered sweetener, beating until the whites hold stiff peaks.

6. Add about one-third of the whites to the almond milk mixture and gently fold in to lighten. Then gently fold this mixture back into the remaining egg whites until no streaks remain.

7. Divide the mixture among the prepared ramekins and bake for 18 to 22 minutes, until the soufflés are puffed and the edges are golden brown. They will still jiggle ever so slightly in the middle.

8. Remove from the oven and serve immediately with a dusting of powdered sweetener.

TIPS: *Setting the ramekins on a baking sheet isn't absolutely necessary, but it does help you get all of the soufflés into and out of the oven in one go.*

Resist opening the oven door while the soufflés are baking. They will rise better if no drafts come into the oven.

NUTRITIONAL INFORMATION

CALORIES: 87 | FAT: 6g | CARBS: 2.5g | FIBER: 1g | PROTEIN: 4.8g

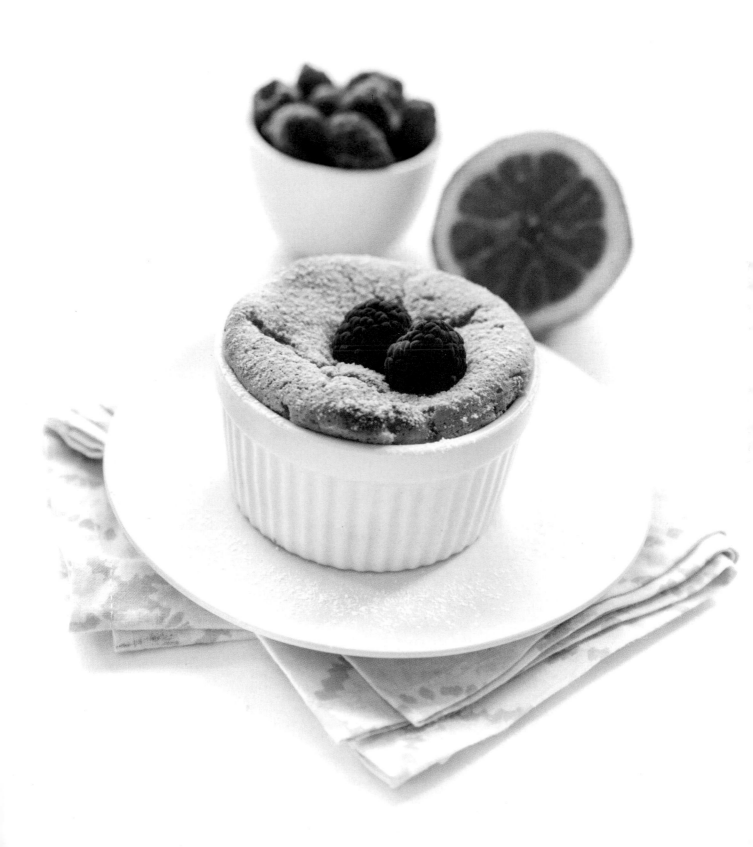

PAVLOVA

Yield: 8 servings Prep Time: 30 minutes Cook Time: 2½ hours

Pavlova is a dessert from Australia that features a crisp meringue shell filled with whipped cream and fruit. It's a little like eating a sweet cloud!

Meringue Shell:

4 large egg whites, room temperature

¼ teaspoon cream of tartar

¼ teaspoon salt

½ teaspoon vanilla extract

¼ cup granulated erythritol sweetener

¼ cup powdered erythritol sweetener

Filling:

1 cup heavy whipping cream

¼ cup powdered erythritol sweetener

½ teaspoon vanilla extract

½ cup quartered fresh strawberries

½ cup fresh raspberries

¼ cup fresh blueberries

¼ cup fresh blackberries

TO MAKE THE SHELL:

1. Preheat the oven to 200°F and line a rimmed baking sheet with parchment paper. Draw an 8-inch circle on the parchment with a pencil. Turn the paper upside down on the baking sheet so you can still see the circle but the pencil won't bleed onto the shell.

2. In a large bowl, beat the egg whites, cream of tartar, and salt with an electric mixer until frothy. With the mixer still running, add the vanilla. Then beat in the sweeteners 1 tablespoon at a time, until the egg whites are glossy and hold stiff peaks.

3. Transfer the egg whites onto the parchment and spread to the edges of the circle you drew. Build up the sides so that they are about an inch higher than the center. Bake for 70 to 90 minutes, until just firm to the touch and no longer sticky. Be sure to check the center of the meringue and not just the edges.

4. Turn off the heat and let the meringue sit inside the oven for another hour or so, until completely dry to the touch. Keep an eye on it, making sure it doesn't get too brown.

5. Remove from the oven and let cool completely on the pan, then gently slide a sharp knife or an offset spatula under the meringue to remove it from the parchment paper. Carefully lift and set on a serving plate.

TO MAKE THE FILLING:

6. In a large bowl, whip the cream with the sweetener and vanilla until it holds stiff peaks. Fill the cavity in the meringue with the whipped cream.

7. Arrange the berries over the top of the whipped cream. Serve immediately or chill for a few hours before serving.

NUTRITIONAL INFORMATION
CALORIES: 129 | FAT: 10.5g | CARBS: 3.9g | FIBER: 1.1g | PROTEIN: 2.7g

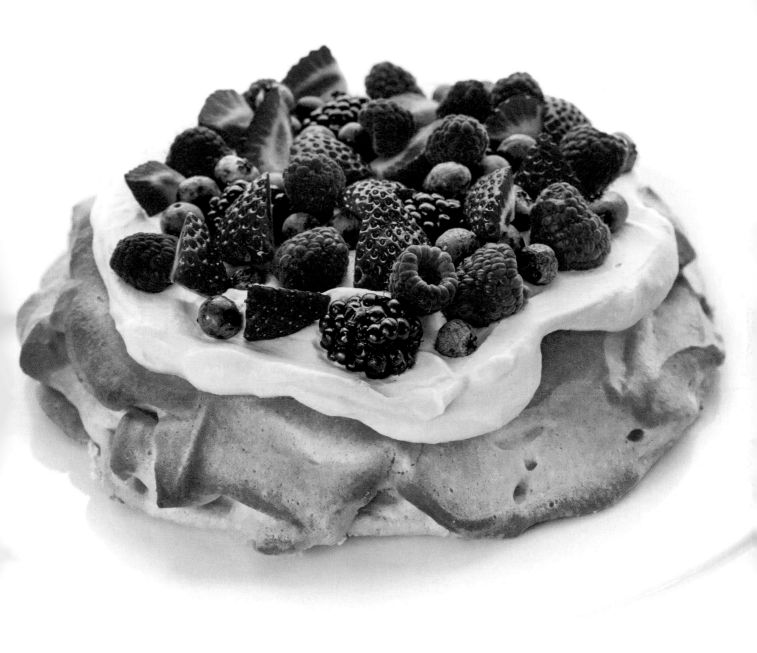

TIPS: *You can really only use erythritol sweeteners here, unless you want the meringue shell to be like marshmallow goo.*

Be sure your vanilla extract is alcohol based. Any drop of oil will keep the egg whites from beating properly.

It's hard to keep meringue snow white, so expect to see some browning. The meringue will take on a light tan color. Keep your eye on it while it sits in the warm oven.

SUMMER BERRY COBBLER

Yield: 8 servings Prep Time: 20 minutes Cook Time: 30 minutes

When I made the Cream Cheese Biscuits (page 240), I realized that the dough would be wonderful as a topping for a sweet summer cobbler. It needed only a few minor adjustments.

Filling:

1 cup fresh raspberries

1 cup quartered fresh strawberries

¼ cup fresh blueberries

¼ cup granulated sweetener of choice

½ teaspoon glucomannan or xanthan gum

Topping:

¾ cup plus 2 tablespoons (87.5g) blanched almond flour

¼ cup granulated sweetener of choice

2 tablespoons unflavored whey or egg white protein powder

1 teaspoon baking powder

¼ teaspoon salt

3 ounces cream cheese, cut into chunks

2 tablespoons heavy whipping cream

½ teaspoon vanilla extract

1. Preheat the oven to 350°F.

2. For the filling, place the raspberries, strawberries, and blueberries in a glass or ceramic pie plate. Sprinkle with the sweetener and glucomannan and toss to combine well. Spread out into a single layer.

3. For the topping, place the almond flour, sweetener, protein powder, baking powder, and salt in a food processor. Pulse a few times to combine. Add the cream cheese, cream, and vanilla and process until the dough begins to come together.

4. Break the dough into small pieces and scatter over the filling. Bake for 25 to 30 minutes, until the filling is bubbling and the topping is light golden brown.

5. Remove from the oven and let cool for 20 minutes before serving.

TIP: *If you prefer, you can skip the thickener in the filling. But it really does make the filling thicker and the juices more syrupy as they cool.*

SERVING SUGGESTION: *What else do you do with a warm cobbler besides topping it with Keto Vanilla Ice Cream (page 394)?*

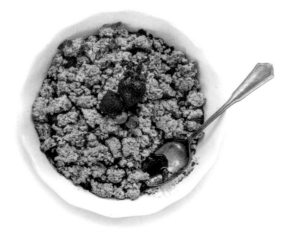

NUTRITIONAL INFORMATION

CALORIES: 145 | FAT: 10.7g | CARBS: 7.4g | FIBER: 2.8g | PROTEIN: 4.7g

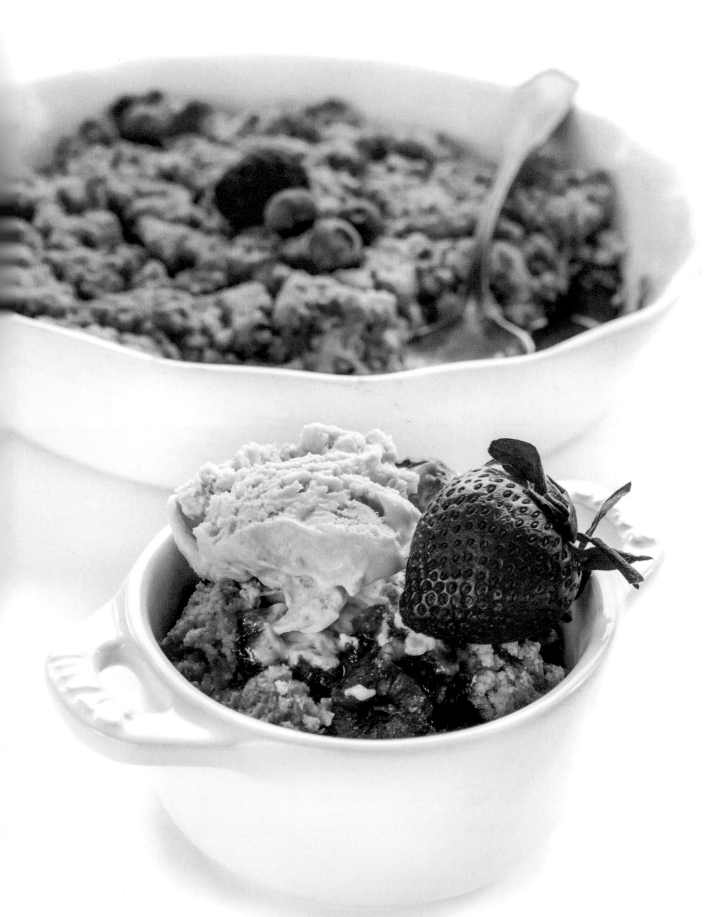

HOT FUDGE PUDDING CAKES

Yield: 6 cakes (1 per serving) Prep Time: 20 minutes Cook Time: 23 minutes

Somewhere between soufflé and pudding, there is a cake that's calling your name.

¼ cup (½ stick) unsalted butter

1½ ounces unsweetened chocolate, chopped

¼ cup plus 1 tablespoon cocoa powder, divided

1½ tablespoons brown sugar substitute

⅓ cup heavy whipping cream, room temperature

⅓ cup granulated sweetener of choice

2 large egg yolks, room temperature

2 teaspoons vanilla extract

¼ teaspoon salt

½ cup pumpkin seed meal or sunflower seed meal

2 teaspoons baking powder

1 to 2 tablespoons water

¼ cup plus 2 tablespoons lukewarm coffee

1. Preheat the oven to 375°F. Grease six 4-ounce ramekins and set them on a rimmed baking sheet.

2. In a heatproof bowl set over a pan of barely simmering water, melt the butter and chocolate, whisking frequently. Whisk in ¼ cup of the cocoa powder. Remove from the heat and let cool.

3. In a small bowl, whisk the remaining 1 tablespoon of cocoa powder with the brown sugar substitute, breaking up any clumps with a fork. Set aside.

4. In a large bowl, whisk together the cream, granulated sweetener, egg yolks, vanilla, and salt.

5. Whisk in the pumpkin seed meal and baking powder until combined, then add the melted chocolate mixture. The batter will get very thick, so stir in the water, 1 tablespoon at a time, until the batter has a scoopable consistency.

6. Divide the batter among the prepared ramekins and spread to the edges with a spoon. Sprinkle the tops with the cocoa powder/brown sugar substitute mixture. Then drizzle 1 tablespoon of coffee over each.

7. Bake for 15 to 18 minutes, until puffed but still a little wet-looking in the center. Remove from the oven and let cool for 10 minutes before serving. The cakes will fall, but the bottoms should have a gooey, liquidy consistency.

TIP: *Coffee enhances and amplifies chocolate flavors, but you can always use water if you prefer.*

SERVING SUGGESTION: *Top the cakes with ice cream or whipped cream for an extra-special dessert.*

NUTRITIONAL INFORMATION

CALORIES: 245 | FAT: 20.7g | CARBS: 7.5g | FIBER: 3.2g | PROTEIN: 5.5g

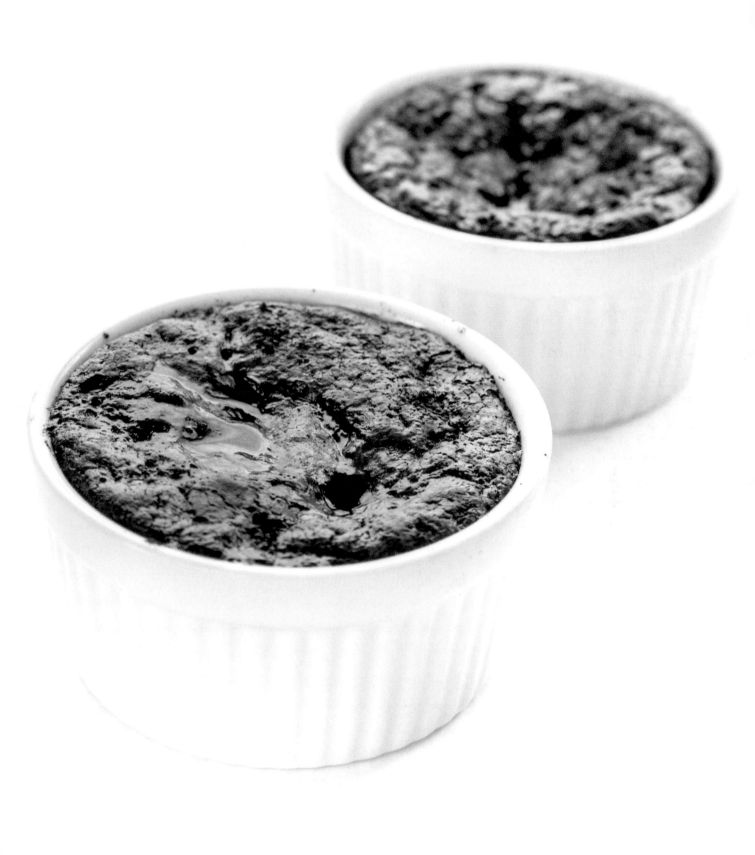

CLASSIC TIRAMISU

Yield: 12 servings Prep Time: 25 minutes, plus 4 hours to chill (not including time to make ladyfingers) Cook Time: 7 minutes

In the regular world, tiramisu would be a no-bake dessert. But since we have to make the keto ladyfingers ourselves, it's a baked recipe and deserves to be included in this book.

4 large egg yolks

⅓ cup granulated erythritol sweetener

⅓ cup Bocha Sweet or allulose

8 ounces mascarpone cheese, softened

1 cup heavy whipping cream

½ teaspoon vanilla extract

½ cup cold coffee

1 tablespoon rum (optional)

1 recipe Ladyfingers (page 174)

1 tablespoon cocoa powder

1. Place the egg yolks and sweeteners in a large heatproof bowl set over a pan of barely simmering water. Whisk continuously until the mixture is about doubled in volume and reaches 165°F on an instant-read thermometer, 5 to 7 minutes.

2. Remove the bowl from the pan. Add the mascarpone in small pieces while beating on low with an electric mixer until smooth.

3. In another large bowl, beat the cream with the vanilla until it holds stiff peaks. Gently fold the cream into the mascarpone mixture.

4. In a shallow bowl, mix together the coffee and rum, if using. Dip half of the ladyfingers briefly into the coffee mixture and place in an 8-inch square baking pan or dish. Break the ladyfingers as needed to cover any gaps.

5. Spread half of the mascarpone mixture over the ladyfingers, smoothing the top. Repeat the layers with the remaining ladyfingers and mascarpone mixture.

6. Dust the top thoroughly with the cocoa powder. Refrigerate for at least 4 hours or up to overnight before serving.

TIPS: *This is a good recipe to use up leftover egg yolks from making meringues or Pavlova (page 354).*

Gently cooking the yolks in a double boiler while whisking helps increase the volume of the mixture and makes the yolks safe to eat. I highly recommend an instant-read thermometer.

Mascarpone can be tricky to work with and can curdle easily. Adding it in chunks to the warm egg yolk mixture and beating on low speed can help prevent curdling.

NUTRITIONAL INFORMATION
CALORIES: 243 | FAT: 22.2g | CARBS: 2.7g | FIBER: 0.9g | PROTEIN: 5.7g

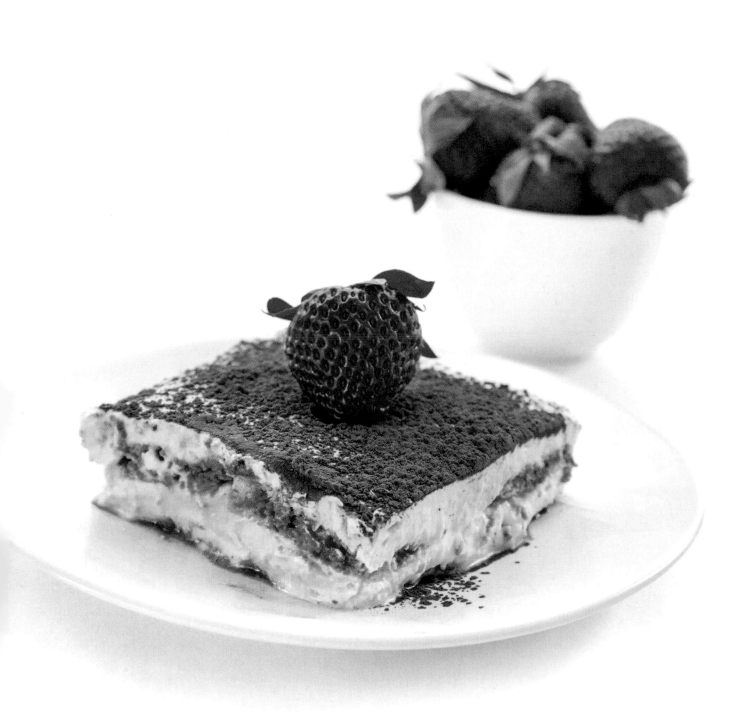

CHOCOLATE LASAGNA

Yield: 16 servings Prep Time: 30 minutes, plus 3 hours to chill Cook Time: 25 minutes

This layered chocolate dessert also goes by the name "Sex in a Pan." Some people find that a little crude; others find it amusing. Either way, this sweet treat truly is that good!

Chocolate Crust:

1¼ cups (125g) blanched almond flour

¼ cup cocoa powder

¼ cup powdered erythritol sweetener

¼ teaspoon salt

¼ cup (½ stick) unsalted butter, melted

1 tablespoon water

Cheesecake Layer:

1 (8-ounce) package cream cheese, softened

⅓ cup powdered erythritol sweetener

½ teaspoon vanilla extract

½ cup heavy whipping cream, room temperature

Chocolate Pudding Layer:

1 cup heavy whipping cream

1 cup unsweetened almond milk

½ cup powdered erythritol sweetener

4 large egg yolks

½ teaspoon glucomannan or xanthan gum

⅓ cup cocoa powder

3 tablespoons unsalted butter, cut into 3 pieces

½ teaspoon vanilla extract

Topping:

1 cup heavy whipping cream, chilled

3 tablespoons powdered erythritol sweetener

½ teaspoon vanilla extract

1 tablespoon cocoa powder

½ ounce sugar-free dark chocolate

TO MAKE THE CRUST:

1. Preheat the oven to 325°F and grease a 9-inch square baking pan.

2. In a medium bowl, whisk together the almond flour, cocoa powder, sweetener, and salt. Add the melted butter and water and stir until the mixture begins to clump together.

3. Press the mixture firmly and evenly into the bottom of the prepared pan and bake for about 15 minutes, until just firm to the touch. Remove from the oven and let cool.

TO MAKE THE CHEESECAKE LAYER:

4. In a large bowl, beat the cream cheese and sweetener with an electric mixer until smooth. Beat in the vanilla.

5. Add the cream and beat until smooth, then spread over the cooled crust and refrigerate while you prepare the chocolate pudding layer.

TO MAKE THE CHOCOLATE PUDDING LAYER:

6. Place the cream, almond milk, and sweetener in a medium saucepan over medium heat. Bring to a simmer, stirring to dissolve the sweetener.

7. In a medium bowl, whisk the egg yolks until smooth. Slowly whisk about ½ cup of the hot cream mixture into the yolks to temper them. Then slowly whisk the tempered yolks back into the saucepan.

NUTRITIONAL INFORMATION

CALORIES: 303 | FAT: 28.3g | CARBS: 6.3g | FIBER: 2.6g | PROTEIN: 5g

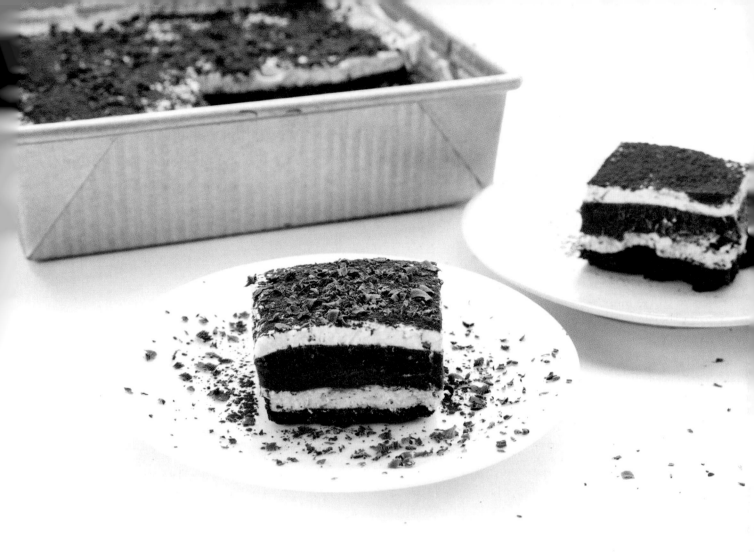

8. Reduce the heat to medium-low and sprinkle the surface with the glucomannan, whisking vigorously to combine. Whisk in the cocoa powder and cook until thickened, 3 to 4 minutes. Remove the pan from the heat and add the butter pieces and vanilla. Whisk until smooth.

9. Let cool for 15 minutes, then spread over the cheesecake layer. Refrigerate for at least 2 hours.

TO MAKE THE TOPPING:

10. Beat the cream, sweetener, and vanilla with the electric mixer until stiff peaks form. Spread over the chocolate pudding layer. Dust with the cocoa powder. Use a vegetable peeler or cheese slicer to shave the chocolate over the top.

11. Chill for another hour to set completely.

TIP: *This dessert really isn't that difficult to make, but it does have a lot of moving parts. It's best to devote a good chunk of time to it so that you can make all the layers properly. Trust me, it's worth the time and effort.*

Chapter 15:
EXTRAS

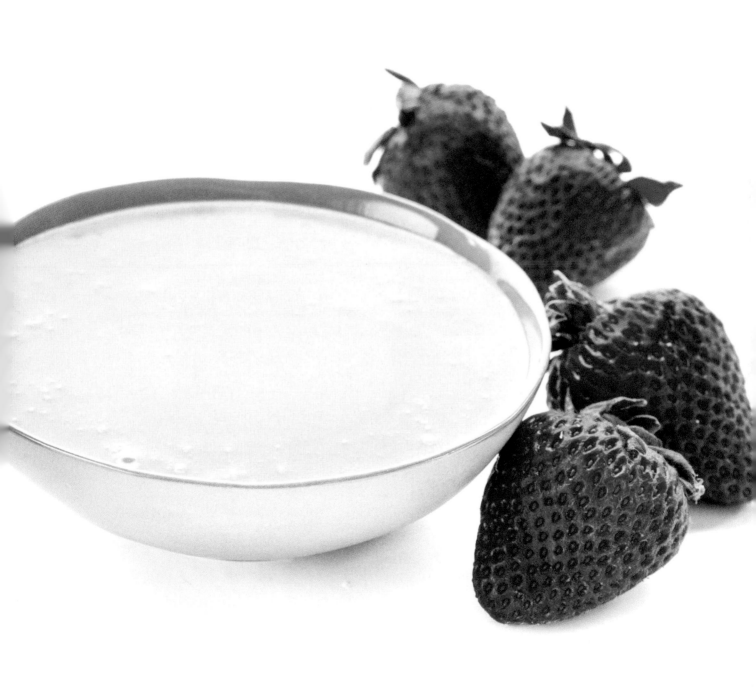

EASY ALMOND FLOUR PIE CRUST

OPTION

Yield: One 9-inch crust (10 servings) Prep Time: 10 minutes Cook Time: —

This is an amazingly versatile pie and tart crust that I use over and over, both in this book and on *All Day I Dream About Food*. The recipe below is for the raw pastry dough. Baking directions can be found in each recipe that calls for this crust.

1½ cups (150g) blanched almond flour

¼ cup granulated erythritol sweetener

¼ teaspoon salt

¼ cup (½ stick) unsalted butter, melted

In a medium bowl, whisk together the almond flour, sweetener, and salt. Stir in the melted butter until the dough comes together and resembles coarse crumbs. Use the dough as directed in the specific recipe.

TIPS: *I find that for glass and ceramic pans, I don't need to grease them. But metal tart pans heat the crust more during baking, so it's a good precaution to grease those.*

If you want to make this crust ahead of time, it's best to press it into the pan you plan to use and then store it. Wrap the whole pan in plastic wrap as tightly as you can, place in a resealable freezer bag, and refrigerate for up to a week or freeze for up to 2 months. Let it come to room temperature before baking.

DAIRY-FREE OPTION:

Use coconut oil in place of the butter. Ghee works as well.

VARIATIONS:

SAVORY ALMOND FLOUR PIE CRUST.

Skip the sweetener and add ½ teaspoon garlic powder for a savory crust.

EASY PECAN MEAL PIE CRUST (OR OTHER NUT PIE CRUST).

Follow the method above, but replace the almond flour with pecan meal. Note that you can use this same method with many other nut meals/flours and even some seed meals/flours. In addition to pecan meal, I've made this crust with hazelnut meal and pumpkin seed meal. They have slightly different textures.

If you are grinding your own nuts or seeds, be sure to measure the meal or flour after grinding. The nutritional counts will vary slightly depending on which nut or seed you use.

NUTRITIONAL INFORMATION

CALORIES: 137 | FAT: 12.7g | CARBS: 3.6g | FIBER: 1.8g | PROTEIN: 3.7g

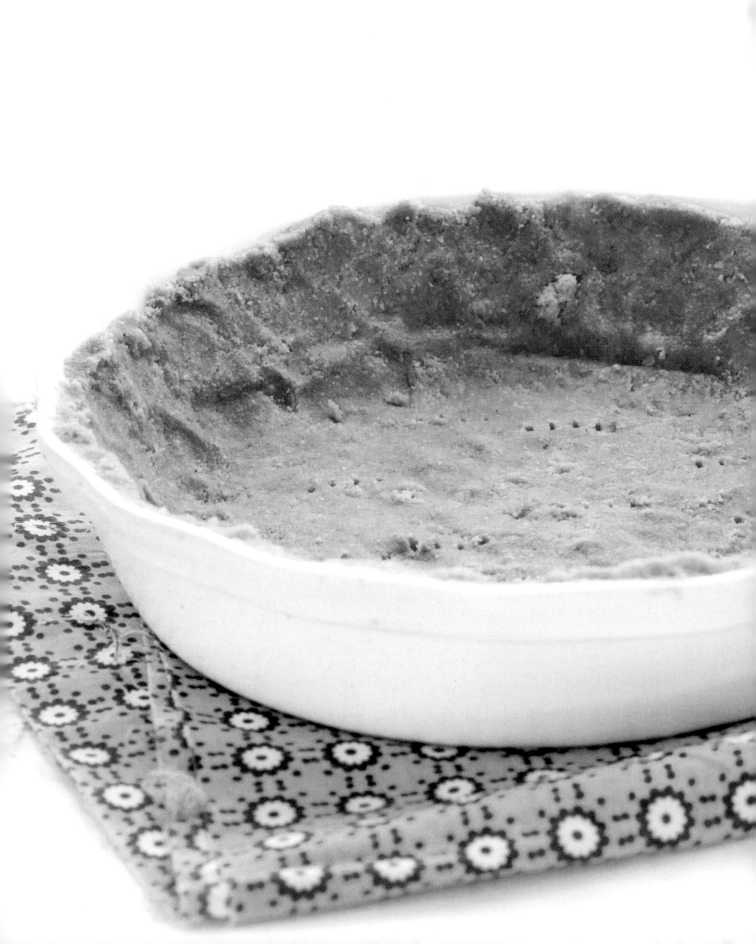

COCONUT FLOUR PIE CRUST

Yield: One 9-inch crust (10 servings) Prep Time: 15 minutes Cook Time: —

I tried so many ways to get a decent coconut flour pie crust. I didn't love any of them until I added some cream cheese. That made all the difference! Now it's tender but still stands up to the fillings. The recipe below is for the raw pastry dough. Baking directions can be found in each recipe that calls for this crust.

¼ cup (½ stick) unsalted butter

2 ounces cream cheese

1 large egg, room temperature

1 large egg white, room temperature

⅔ cup (73g) coconut flour

3 tablespoons powdered erythritol sweetener

½ teaspoon vanilla extract

¼ teaspoon salt

1. In a microwave-safe bowl, heat the butter and cream cheese on high for 20 to 30 seconds. They should be quite soft but not fully melted. Beat with an electric mixer until smooth and well combined.

2. Beat in the whole egg and egg white until well combined. Add the coconut flour, sweetener, vanilla, and salt and beat until the dough comes together.

3. Use the dough as directed in the specific recipe.

VARIATION: SAVORY COCONUT FLOUR PIE CRUST.

Skip the sweetener and vanilla extract and add ½ teaspoon garlic powder and an additional ¼ teaspoon salt.

TIPS: *Unlike the nut-based crusts, this crust requires you to grease the pie plate first. It is drier and has more of a tendency to stick to the pan.*

If you want to make this crust ahead of time, it's best to press it into the pan you plan to use and then store it. Wrap the whole pan in plastic wrap as tightly as you can, place in a resealable freezer bag, and refrigerate for up to a week or freeze for up to 2 months. Let it come to room temperature before baking.

NUTRITIONAL INFORMATION

CALORIES: 102 | FAT: 7.4g | CARBS: 4.6g | FIBER: 2.7g | PROTEIN: 2.4g

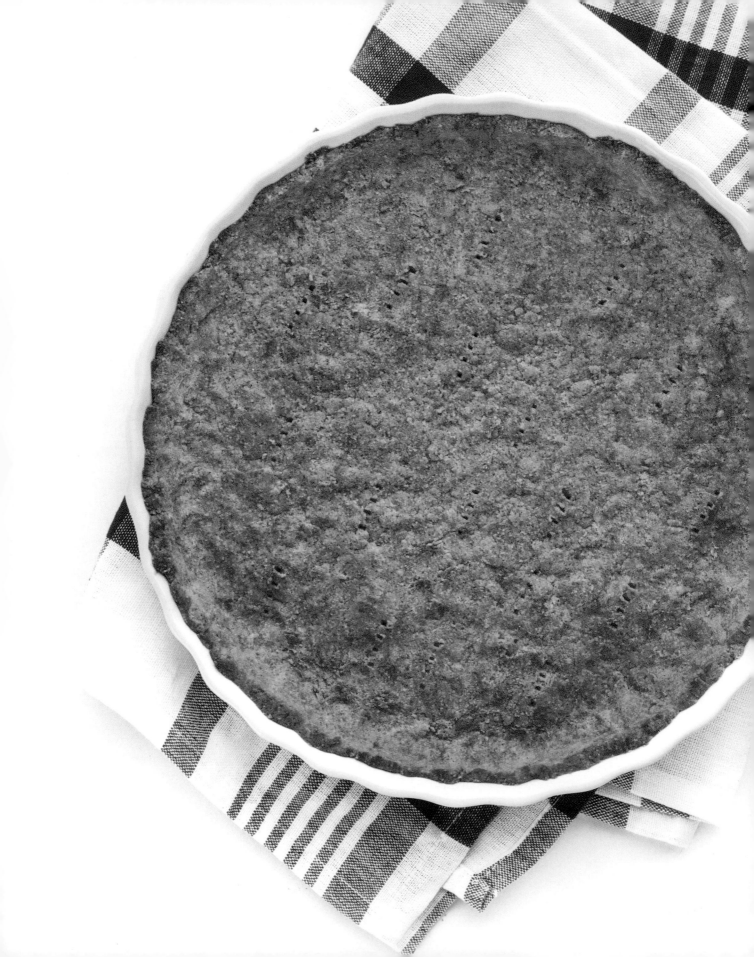

KETO CHOCOLATE PIE CRUST

   OPTION OPTION BEG

Yield: One 8- or 9-inch crust (10 servings) **Prep Time:** 10 minutes **Cook Time:** —

This delicious chocolate crust is useful for pies, tarts, bars, and cheesecake. It's wonderfully versatile and oh so tasty. Although I list it as 10 servings, it's divided into 12 to 16 servings for many of the desserts in this book. The recipe below is for the raw pastry dough. Baking directions can be found in each recipe that calls for this crust.

1¼ cups (125g) blanched almond flour

¼ cup cocoa powder

¼ cup powdered erythritol sweetener

¼ teaspoon salt

¼ cup (½ stick) unsalted butter, melted

In a medium bowl, whisk together the almond flour, cocoa powder, sweetener, and salt. Stir in the melted butter until the dough comes together and resembles coarse crumbs. Use the dough as directed in the specific recipe.

TIPS: *The consistency of this crust can vary somewhat depending on your cocoa powder. If you find it too crumbly to press into the pan, try adding an additional ½ to 1 tablespoon melted butter. Even a little water can help. You will know it's right when you can squeeze a ball of the dough and it holds together. Don't add too much water, though, or it may stick to the pan a bit more.*

I find that for glass and ceramic pans, I don't need to grease them. But metal tart pans heat the crust more during baking, so it's a good precaution to grease those.

If you want to make this crust ahead of time, it's best to press it into the pan you plan to use and then store it. Wrap the whole pan in plastic wrap as tightly as you can, place in a resealable freezer bag, and refrigerate for up to a week or freeze for up to 2 months. Let it come to room temperature before baking.

DAIRY-FREE OPTION:

Use coconut oil or ghee instead of butter.

NUT-FREE OPTION:

Use sunflower seed meal or pumpkin seed meal in place of the almond flour.

NUTRITIONAL INFORMATION

CALORIES: 126 | FAT: 11.6g | CARBS: 4.3g | FIBER: 2.3g | PROTEIN: 3.5g

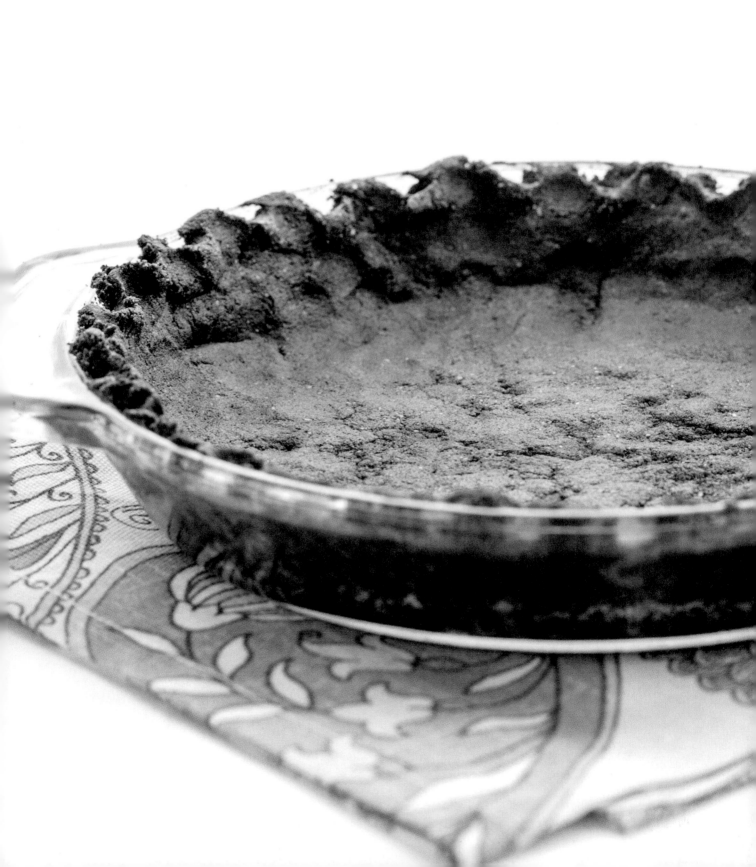

SHORTBREAD CRUST

OPTION   OPTION

Yield: One 8- or 9-inch square crust (16 servings) Prep Time: 10 minutes Cook Time: —

This is my favorite crust for bars, and you will see it used quite a few times in the recipes in this book. It's similar to the basic pie crust but contains a little less almond flour and uses chilled butter. I love its shortbreadlike consistency—it's slightly crumbly but still holds together once baked.

1¼ cups (125g) blanched almond flour

¼ cup powdered erythritol sweetener

¼ teaspoon salt

¼ cup (½ stick) unsalted butter, chilled and cut into small pieces

Place the almond flour, sweetener, and salt in the bowl of a food processor. Pulse a few times to combine. Scatter the butter pieces over the surface and pulse until the mixture resembles coarse crumbs. Use as directed in the specific recipe.

DAIRY-FREE OPTION:

Use room-temperature coconut oil or ghee and add it in small pieces to the food processor.

NUT-FREE OPTION:

Use sunflower seed meal or pumpkin seed meal in place of the almond flour. (Note that it will give the crust a grayish or greenish hue, depending on which one you use.)

TIPS: *You can also go old-fashioned and cut the butter into the pastry using a pastry cutter or two sharp knives. However, a food processor tends to distribute the butter more evenly.*

If you want to make this crust ahead of time, it's best to press it into the pan you plan to use and then store it. Wrap the whole pan in plastic wrap as tightly as you can, place in a resealable freezer bag, and refrigerate for up to a week or freeze for up to 2 months. Let it come to room temperature before baking.

NUTRITIONAL INFORMATION

CALORIES: 76 | FAT: 7.1g | CARBS: 1.9g | FIBER: 0.9g | PROTEIN: 1.9g

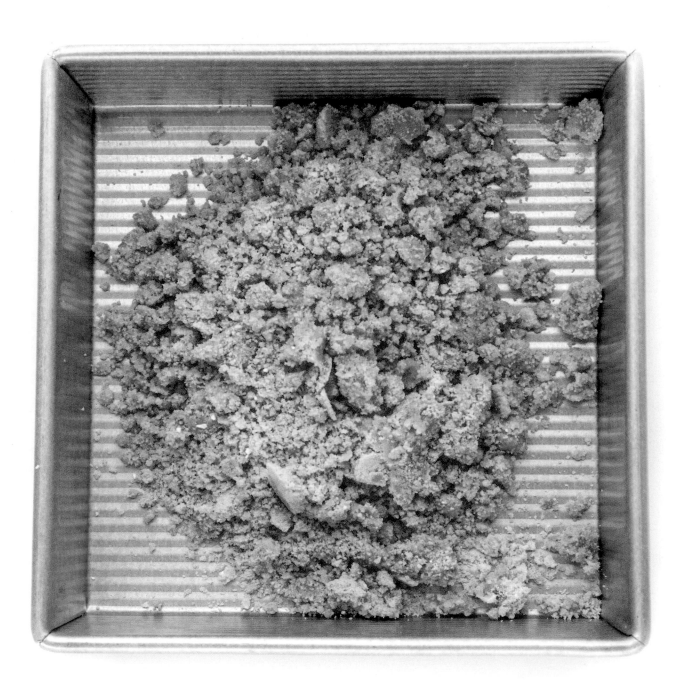

FATHEAD DOUGH TWO WAYS

So-called fathead dough, named after the folks behind the *Fat Head* movie, has changed the game when it comes to keto breads, pizzas, and other baked goods. The origins of the dough are a little unclear, but it may be a website called Cooky's Creations, which was discovered and made famous by Tom Naughton (the director of *Fat Head*) and his family.

Since then, every keto blogger and recipe developer has put their own spin on this dough, myself included. I played with it quite a bit and came up with two versions, both of which I love. One contains both almond flour and coconut flour for extra stability, but it can be made entirely with almond flour if needed. The other is made entirely with coconut flour for a nut-free option.

Both versions are incredibly versatile and useful, so I decided to include them both in this book. You can use them interchangeably for most recipes, although the coconut flour–only version is about twice as big as the one made with both flours. You can easily cut the coconut flour version in half or double the almond flour–based version, depending on the recipe for which you plan to use it.

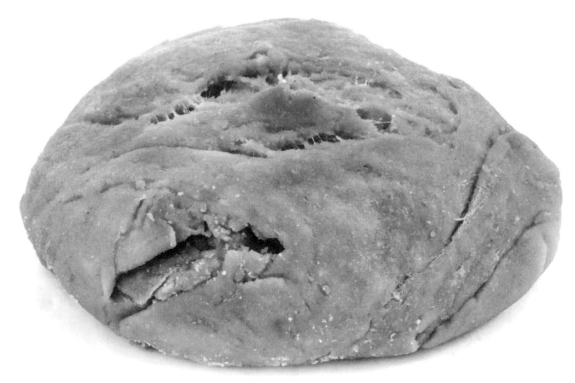

MAGIC MOZZARELLA DOUGH

OPTION

Yield: 6 servings (may vary depending on recipe for which it is used) **Prep Time:** 10 minutes **Cook Time:** 5 minutes

This was my first variation on fathead dough, and it is loved by many readers. It makes a great pizza crust, and it's wonderful in sweet recipes, too. Be sure to check out the Jalapeño Popper Pizza (page 288) and the Raspberry Cream Cheese Turnovers (page 336) to see how versatile it is.

6 ounces preshredded part-skim mozzarella cheese (see tips)

5 tablespoons unsalted butter

½ cup (50g) blanched almond flour, plus more for the work surface

¼ cup (28g) coconut flour

2 teaspoons baking powder

½ teaspoon garlic powder

¼ teaspoon salt

1 large egg

VARIATIONS:

SWEET MAGIC MOZZARELLA DOUGH.

Replace the garlic powder with 1 teaspoon vanilla extract. Add ¼ cup powdered erythritol sweetener along with the almond flour in Step 3.

COCONUT-FREE MAGIC MOZZARELLA DOUGH.

This dough can be made with all almond flour, but you need quite a bit more of it to replace the coconut flour. It can take almost 2 full cups of almond flour.

1. Sprinkle a silicone baking mat or a large piece of parchment paper with almond flour.

2. In a large saucepan, melt the cheese and butter over low heat until they are melted and can be stirred together.

3. Remove the pan from the heat, then add the almond flour, coconut flour, baking powder, garlic powder, salt, and egg. Stir everything together until a cohesive dough forms. Use a rubber spatula to really knead the dough in the pan. It may still contain some streaks of cheese.

4. Turn the dough out onto the prepared work surface and knead until uniform. This will take only a little kneading. If, after kneading for a minute or so, the dough is still very sticky, add a tablespoon or two more almond flour and work it in. Use the dough as directed in the specific recipe.

TIPS: *The best mozzarella for this dough is the preshredded part-skim type because it contains some anticoagulating agents that help with the consistency. Yes, it contains a tiny bit of starch, but it makes a difference and adds almost nothing to the overall carb count. I often use the Whole Foods brand because it contains potato starch rather than cornstarch.*

I always weigh the mozzarella for this recipe. Shredded mozzarella can get packed down and pressed together, and measuring by volume rather than weight can affect the outcome of the dough.

Fathead doughs are best made fresh because they lose their elasticity as they cool. If you really want to make the dough ahead for pizza, you can roll it out into a pizza crust and then freeze or refrigerate the crust.

NUT-FREE
MAGIC MOZZARELLA DOUGH

Yield: 8 servings (may vary depending on recipe for which it is used) **Prep Time:** 10 minutes **Cook Time:** 2 minutes

This version of fathead dough is great for the Chewy Keto Bagels (page 278) because it spreads less during baking and ends up chewier. For many recipes, such as the Sausage and Broccoli Calzone (page 290), I use only a half batch. It's great for pizza, too; a full batch would make two 12-inch pizza crusts.

½ cup (55g) coconut flour

2 teaspoons baking powder

¾ teaspoon xanthan gum

12 ounces preshredded part-skim mozzarella cheese (see tip)

2 large eggs

1. Cover a work surface with a silicone baking mat or a large piece of parchment paper. In a medium bowl, whisk together the coconut flour, baking powder, and xanthan gum. Set aside.

2. In a large microwave-safe bowl, heat the cheese on high in 30-second increments until almost liquid. Stir in the flour mixture and eggs and knead in the bowl using a rubber spatula.

3. Turn the dough out onto the prepared work surface and continue to knead until cohesive. Use the dough as directed in the specific recipe.

VARIATION: SWEET NUT-FREE MAGIC MOZZARELLA DOUGH.

Add ⅓ cup powdered erythritol sweetener along with the coconut flour in Step 1.

TIP: *The cheese you use can make or break this recipe. The best kind to use for magic mozzarella dough is preshredded part-skim mozzarella, although it does contain a little added starch to keep it from clumping.*

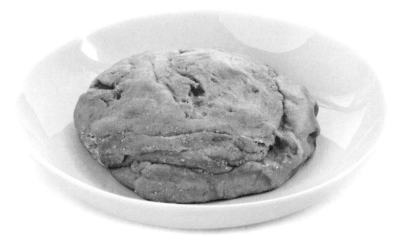

NUTRITIONAL INFORMATION

CALORIES: 190 | FAT: 12.3g | CARBS: 5.5g | FIBER: 2.6g | PROTEIN: 12.1g

WHIPPED CREAM FROSTING

Yield: About 4 cups (16 servings) Prep Time: 15 minutes Cook Time: —

Nothing is simpler than whipped cream frosting. To make it last and stay firm, you need something to help stabilize it. Otherwise, it softens too easily and can become runny. A little gelatin goes a long way here.

2 tablespoons water

2 teaspoons grass-fed gelatin

2 cups heavy whipping cream

⅓ cup powdered erythritol sweetener (or more if you like it sweeter)

½ teaspoon vanilla extract

TIPS: *Heavy cream or whipping cream typically doubles in volume when whipped, so this recipe makes about 4 cups of frosting, which is perfect for the Coconut Layer Cake (page 98). But it is easy to cut in half for smaller projects.*

Stabilized whipped cream is usually good for as long as your whipping cream is fresh. Keep it in an airtight container in the fridge.

1. Pour the water into a small microwave-safe bowl and sprinkle with the gelatin. Let sit for a few minutes to bloom.

2. Warm gently in the microwave for about 20 seconds, then whisk to dissolve the gelatin. Let cool to lukewarm.

3. In a large bowl, beat the cream, sweetener, and vanilla with an electric mixer until it begins to hold medium peaks.

4. Continue beating while slowly drizzling the gelatin mixture into the bowl. Beat until the frosting holds stiff peaks.

5. Spread or pipe on your favorite keto cakes and cupcakes.

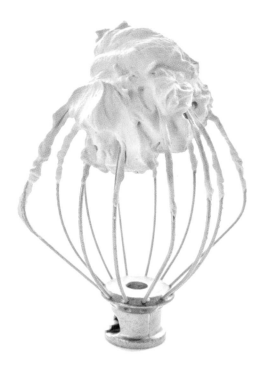

SWISS MERINGUE BUTTERCREAM

Yield: About 4 cups (16 servings) **Prep Time:** 20 minutes **Cook Time:** 10 minutes

Swiss meringue buttercream is the ultimate in frosting. Unlike American-style buttercream, which relies solely on butter and sweetener for structure, Swiss meringue incorporates beaten egg whites for a lighter consistency. It uses a lot less sweetener, and the end result is far less cloying. It's also more stable at room temperature, so cakes can sit out longer without the frosting melting.

It's hard to describe the silky, rich texture of this frosting. It spreads and pipes better than any butter-only frosting. Admittedly, it takes more effort to make, but it is worth it. This is the one recipe where I specify using a stand mixer because it makes beating Swiss meringue much easier. You can make it with a mixing bowl and a handheld mixer, but be prepared to stand there mixing for a full 10 minutes!

4 large egg whites

½ cup powdered erythritol sweetener

⅓ cup Bocha Sweet or allulose (see tips)

1 cup (2 sticks) unsalted butter, softened, cut into tablespoons

1 teaspoon vanilla extract

¼ teaspoon salt

1. Set the bowl of a stand mixer over a pan of barely simmering water. Place the egg whites and sweeteners in the bowl.

2. Whisk gently but constantly until the sweeteners have dissolved and the egg whites are hot and slightly frothy. They should reach about 150°F on an instant-read thermometer.

3. Transfer the bowl to the mixer and attach the whisk. Whip the egg whites at medium-high speed until they are thick and glossy and the bottom of the bowl is no longer warm, anywhere between 5 and 10 minutes. The temperature should be about 90°F on an instant-read thermometer.

4. Start adding the butter pieces one at a time until fully incorporated and the frosting is smooth and creamy. Reduce the mixer speed to medium-low, add the vanilla and salt, and whisk until combined.

5. Spread or pipe on your favorite keto cakes and cupcakes.

TIPS: *Swiss meringue buttercream holds up really well. It can be made ahead and refrigerated for up to a week or frozen for up to a month. Store it in an airtight container and let it come to room temperature. You can rewhip it a bit to make it light and fluffy again before using.*

The mix of sweeteners here is pretty important. You can make the buttercream with all erythritol, but it likely will recrystallize a bit, especially if refrigerated. A combination of an erythritol-based sweetener, such as Swerve, and one that keeps things softer, such as Bocha Sweet, xylitol, or possibly allulose, is necessary to achieve the correct consistency.

Making Swiss meringue is all about getting the temperature right, but it's easy to fix if you don't nail it at first:

NUTRITIONAL INFORMATION

| CALORIES: | 109 | FAT: | 10.7g | CARBS: | 0.1g | PROTEIN: | 1g |

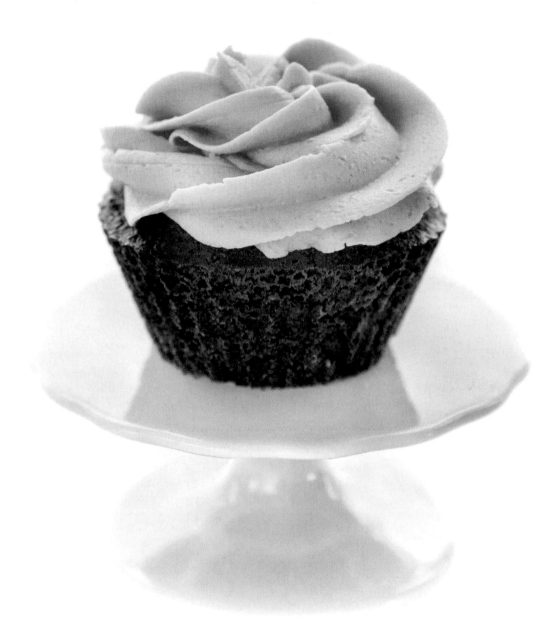

- *If it's too hot, the buttercream will become soupy and thin. Simply refrigerate it for 10 to 20 minutes, until it becomes hard around the edges but is still soupy in the middle. Begin whipping again until it firms and thickens.*

- *If it's too cold, the buttercream will curdle and become lumpy. In this case, you want to reheat it very gently over the pan of warm water. Once the edges look a bit melted, begin whipping again on low speed, then slowly increase the speed until the buttercream comes together.*

You can add other flavors to Swiss meringue buttercream quite easily. A little raspberry extract and natural red food coloring makes a beautiful pink frosting. A teaspoon of espresso powder whisked into the warm egg whites produces a lovely coffee-flavored frosting. You can even add melted chocolate slowly during the whipping process, but it can thicken considerably, so you may need to add a little heavy cream to thin it out.

CREAM CHEESE FROSTING

  OPTION   OPTION BEG

Yield: About 3 cups (12 servings) Prep Time: 10 minutes Cook Time: —

A classic cream cheese frosting is always delicious and goes with just about any dessert.

1 (8-ounce) package cream cheese, softened

6 tablespoons unsalted butter, softened

½ cup powdered erythritol sweetener

¾ teaspoon vanilla extract

⅓ cup heavy whipping cream, room temperature

1 to 2 tablespoons water or unsweetened almond milk, room temperature, if needed

1. In a large bowl, beat the cream cheese and butter with an electric mixer until smooth. Add the sweetener and vanilla and beat until well combined.

2. Beat in the cream until smooth. If the frosting is too thick, add a little room-temperature water or almond milk until a spreadable consistency is achieved.

3. Spread or pipe on your favorite keto cakes and cupcakes.

TIPS: *Although I like the flavor of heavy cream best, I sometimes find that it makes frostings a little too thick. Adding a tablespoon or two of a thin liquid, like water or almond milk, can make it easier to spread and pipe the frosting.*

This is another frosting recipe that is infinitely adaptable for other flavors. A little grated lemon zest and some lemon juice in place of the water makes a tangy and delicious frosting.

As long as you are using fresh ingredients that aren't about to expire, cream cheese frosting should be good for up to 5 days in the fridge. Store in an airtight container. Unfortunately, freezing tends to change the consistency of the frosting and make it clumpy. Sometimes it separates upon thawing.

DAIRY-FREE OPTION:

Use Kite Hill almond milk cream cheese in place of the regular cream cheese, softened coconut oil or ghee in place of the butter, and full-fat coconut milk or almond milk in place of the cream. Almond milk may make the frosting thinner, so add it 1 tablespoon at a time until the frosting has the right consistency.

NUT-FREE OPTION:

Use water rather than almond milk.

NUTRITIONAL INFORMATION

CALORIES: 141 | FAT: 13.2g | CARBS: 1g | PROTEIN: 1.3g

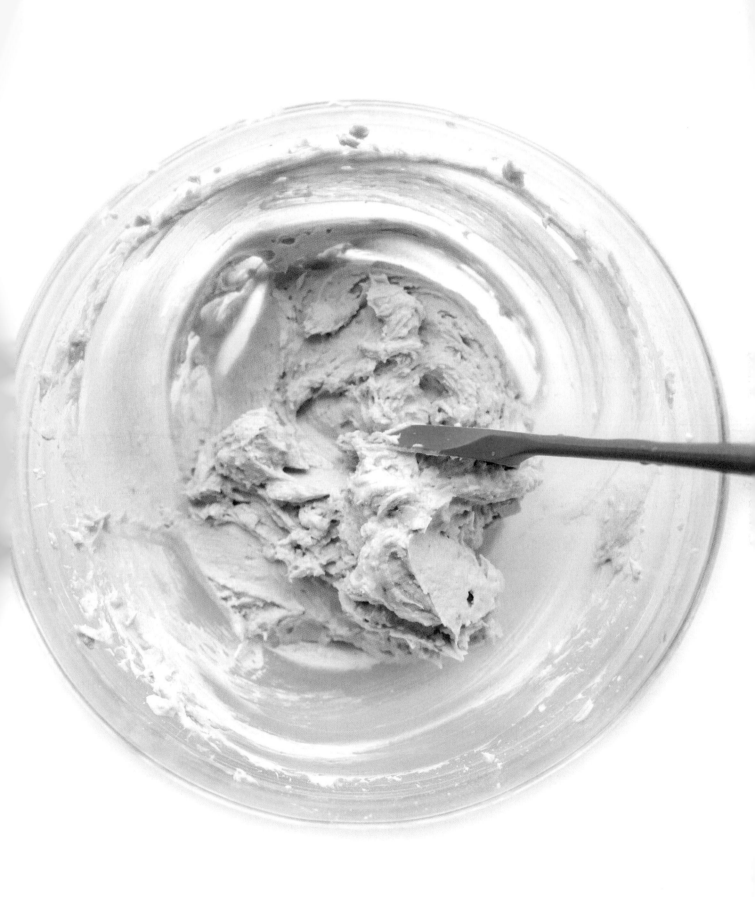

CHOCOLATE BUTTERCREAM FROSTING

OPTION

Yield: About 3 cups (12 servings) Prep Time: 15 minutes Cook Time: —

Many keto dieters find that they lose their taste for overly sweet foods quite quickly. It takes upwards of 2 cups of powdered sugar to give conventional chocolate buttercream the right structure. I started adding a few ounces of cream cheese to my buttercream, which allowed me to reduce the powdered erythritol sweetener and still achieve the right flavor and consistency. The benefits are twofold: it cuts down on expensive sweeteners and keeps the frosting from being tooth-achingly sweet.

2 ounces unsweetened chocolate, chopped

1 tablespoon coconut oil

½ cup (1 stick) unsalted butter, softened

3 ounces cream cheese, softened

⅔ cup powdered erythritol sweetener

2 tablespoons cocoa powder

Pinch of salt

½ teaspoon vanilla extract

⅓ to ½ cup heavy whipping cream

1. Place the chocolate and coconut oil in a medium microwave-safe bowl. Heat on high in 30-second increments, stirring in between, until melted and smooth. Alternatively, you can melt the chocolate and coconut oil in a heatproof bowl set over a pan of barely simmering water. Set aside to cool to lukewarm.

2. In a large bowl, beat the butter and cream cheese with an electric mixer until smooth. Beat in the sweetener, cocoa powder, and salt until well combined.

3. Add the melted chocolate and vanilla and beat until smooth. The mixture will be very thick at this point.

4. Add the cream a few tablespoons at a time until a spreadable consistency is achieved.

5. Spread or pipe on your favorite keto cakes and cupcakes.

COCONUT-FREE OPTION:

I like to melt the chocolate with coconut oil because it melts more smoothly and thinly, but you can use butter or ghee if you prefer.

TIPS: *How much heavy whipping cream you need depends on the other ingredients you use. Certain brands of cream cheese and cocoa powder have more fillers or fiber, which can thicken the frosting and require additional cream.*

A touch of salt in a recipe such as this simply enhances the chocolate flavor. You can leave it out if you prefer.

This recipe makes enough frosting for 12 cupcakes or a 9-inch single layer cake. You may need to multiply the recipe by 1.5 or 2 for a larger cake.

As with the cream cheese frosting, as long as your ingredients are fresh, this buttercream will last in the fridge for up to 5 days or so. Store it in an airtight container.

NUTRITIONAL INFORMATION

CALORIES: 161 | FAT: 15.2g | CARBS: 2.7g | FIBER: 1.1g | PROTEIN: 1.6g

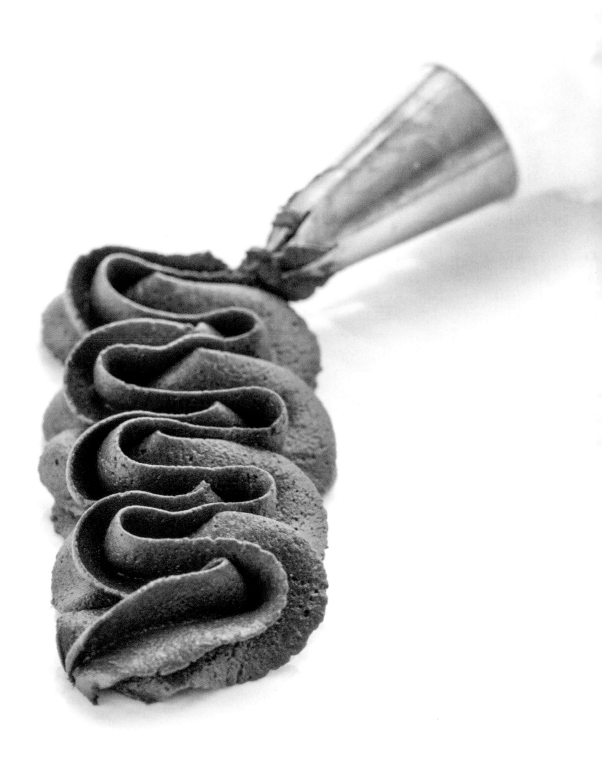

DAIRY-FREE CHOCOLATE FROSTING

Yield: About 3½ cups (12 servings) **Prep Time:** 15 minutes **Cook Time:** —

I wanted to make a really good dairy-free chocolate frosting to pair with the Chocolate Mayonnaise Cake (page 96). I was amazed and delighted by how smooth and creamy this version turned out.

2 ounces unsweetened chocolate, chopped

¾ cup plus 1 tablespoon coconut oil, divided

4 ounces dairy-free cream cheese, softened

1 cup powdered erythritol sweetener

1 teaspoon vanilla extract

⅓ to ½ cup full-fat coconut milk

1. Place the chocolate and 1 tablespoon of the coconut oil in a microwave-safe bowl. Melt on high in 30-second increments, stirring in between, until smooth. Alternatively, you can melt the chocolate and coconut oil in a heatproof bowl set over a pan of barely simmering water. Set aside to cool to lukewarm.

2. Place the remaining ¾ cup of coconut oil in a large bowl. If it's very firm, microwave it for 15 seconds or so. It should be soft without being melted. Add the cream cheese and beat with an electric mixer until smooth. Add the sweetener and vanilla and beat until well combined.

3. Pour in the melted chocolate and beat again until smooth. Add the coconut milk a few tablespoons at a time until a spreadable consistency is achieved.

4. Spread or pipe on your favorite keto cakes and cupcakes.

TIPS: *As with the regular chocolate buttercream (page 382), the dairy-free cream cheese in this recipe helps give the frosting structure without having to add a ridiculous amount of powdered sweetener.*

This frosting can be made ahead and stored in an airtight container in the refrigerator for up to 5 days.

NUTRITIONAL INFORMATION
CALORIES: 158 | FAT: 16.3g | CARBS: 1.7g | FIBER: 0.6g | PROTEIN: 1.4g

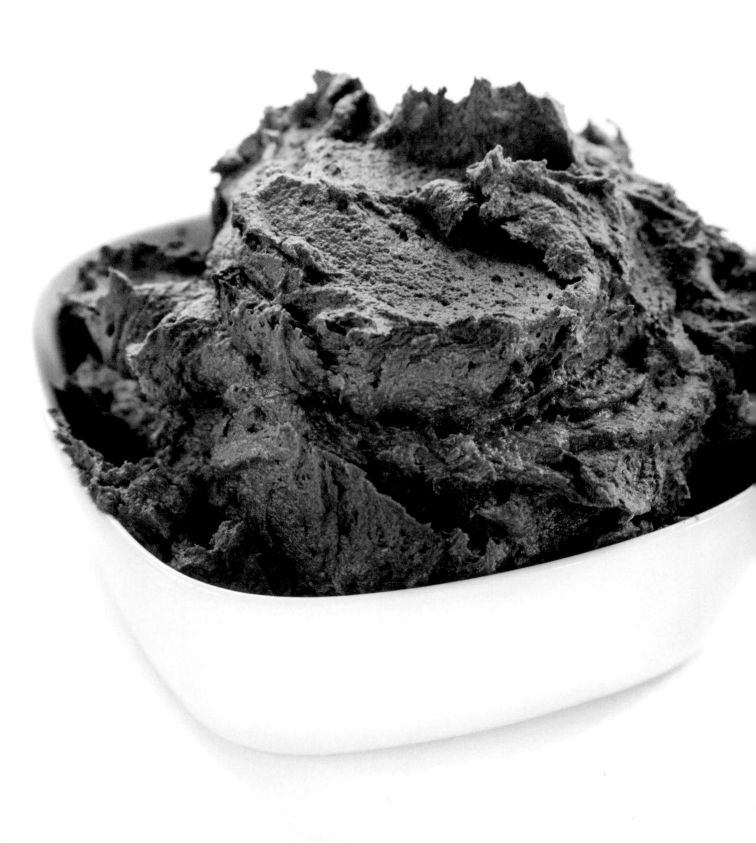

KETO SWEETENED CONDENSED MILK

OPTION

Yield: About 1 cup (8 servings) **Prep Time:** 5 minutes **Cook Time:** 30 minutes

Sweetened condensed milk is a wonderful addition to baked goods, but the "real" stuff has a sky-high carb count. I decided long ago to take matters into my own hands and make sweetened condensed cream. Perfect in the Magic Cookie Bars (page 194)!

1½ cups heavy whipping cream

¼ cup powdered erythritol sweetener

¼ cup Bocha Sweet or allulose (see tips)

2 tablespoons unsalted butter

¼ to ½ teaspoon xanthan gum

1. In a large heavy saucepan, bring the cream to a boil over medium heat. Reduce the heat and simmer gently for 30 minutes. Watch carefully, as you want the cream to simmer but not continue to boil. There should be little bubbles around the edge the whole time.

2. Remove the pan from the heat and whisk in the sweeteners and butter until dissolved. Sprinkle the surface with ¼ teaspoon xanthan gum and whisk vigorously to combine. Let cool for 10 minutes. If the milk is not quite thick enough, whisk in the additional ¼ teaspoon of xanthan gum.

DAIRY-FREE OPTION:

You can omit the butter and make this with full-fat coconut milk, but I've found that it does not reduce and thicken quite as well as the dairy version. You may need to add more xanthan gum to get the syrupy quality of condensed milk.

TIPS: *Because of the liquid nature of this recipe, a mix of sweeteners works best to reduce recrystallization. I like powdered Swerve and Bocha Sweet together. You can do all powdered Swerve, but it may recrystallize in the fridge. However, when the milk is added to a recipe like the Tres Leches Cake (page 110), you won't really notice it.*

As long as the cream you use is fresh, the condensed milk can be stored in the fridge for up to 5 days. I keep mine in a mason jar. It does firm up and thicken, so you may need to gently warm it in a pan before using.

NUTRITIONAL INFORMATION

CALORIES: 182 | FAT: 18.3g | CARBS: 1.3g | PROTEIN: 0.9g

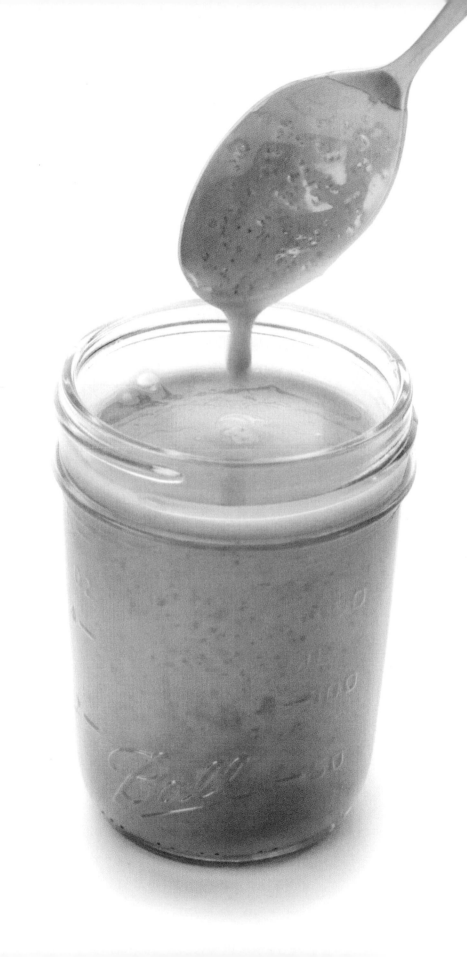

SUGAR-FREE CARAMEL SAUCE

OPTION

Yield: About 1 cup (8 servings) **Prep Time:** 5 minutes **Cook Time:** 10 minutes

Creating a truly amazing caramel sauce was of the utmost importance to me in my early keto days. Over time, I've modified the original recipe, and now it's better than ever.

¼ cup (½ stick) unsalted butter

3 tablespoons Swerve brown sugar substitute (see tips)

3 tablespoons Bocha Sweet or allulose

½ cup heavy whipping cream

¼ teaspoon xanthan gum

¼ teaspoon salt

2 tablespoons water

1. In a medium saucepan over medium heat, bring the butter and sweeteners to a boil. Continue to boil for 3 to 5 minutes, until the mixture turns a deep amber color. (Be careful not to burn it.)

2. Remove the pan from the heat and add the cream. The mixture will bubble vigorously.

3. Sprinkle with the xanthan gum and whisk vigorously to combine. Add the salt and whisk to combine.

4. Return the pan to the heat and boil for 1 more minute. Let cool to lukewarm and stir in the water until well combined.

DAIRY-FREE OPTION:

You can make this sauce with coconut oil and coconut cream, with a few caveats. The coconut oil won't come to a boil with the sweeteners, and you may burn the whole batch if you try to take it there. Simply cook it for 3 minutes in Step 1, watching it carefully. When it's really hot, add the coconut cream. It will be thinner, so skip the water at the end and add ⅛ teaspoon more xanthan gum if it's still too thin.

TIPS: *I highly suggest Swerve Brown here because it is the brown sugar substitute that most closely resembles brown sugar. It has the best color and flavor and helps give the sauce a true caramel flavor. The other brown sugar replacements truly pale in comparison. That said, if you cannot get ahold of Swerve Brown, try a granulated erythritol sweetener with 2 teaspoons of molasses. It will add less than 1 gram of carbs to each serving.*

Just like the condensed milk, this sauce can be stored in a jar in the fridge for up to 5 days. It does thicken and firm up, so you'll need to gently reheat it in a pan before serving.

VARIATION: SALTED CARAMEL SAUCE.

Whisk in an additional ½ teaspoon of salt in Step 3.

NUTRITIONAL INFORMATION

CALORIES: 104 | FAT: 10.6g | CARBS: 0.4g | PROTEIN: 0.4g

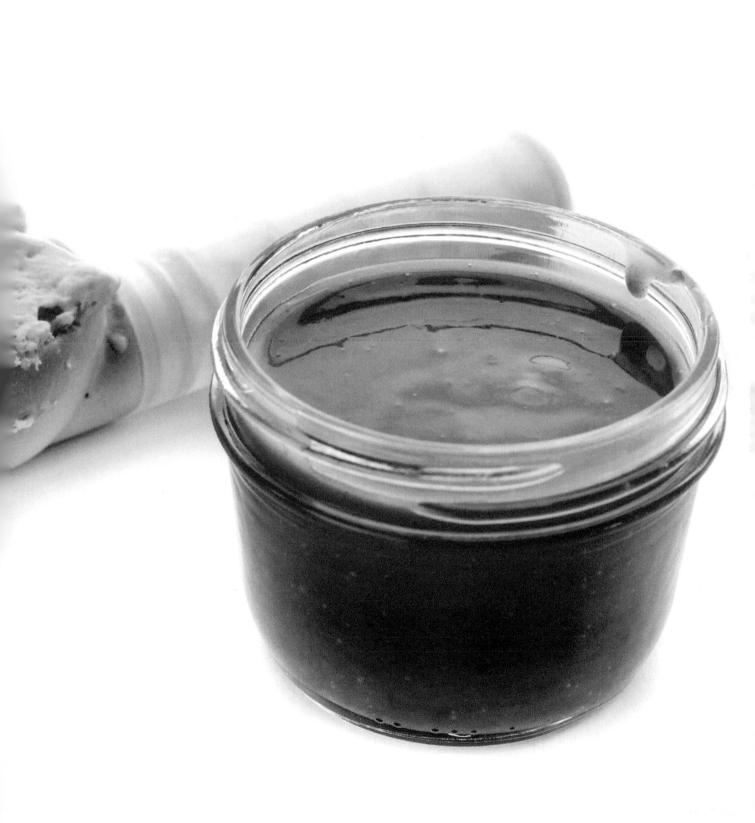

EASY CHOCOLATE GLAZE

OPTION

Yield: ¾ cup (12 servings) **Prep Time:** 10 minutes **Cook Time:** 5 minutes

This is a thinner version of chocolate ganache, and it's delicious drizzled over just about anything.

½ cup heavy whipping cream

2 ounces unsweetened chocolate, finely chopped

¼ cup powdered erythritol sweetener (see tips)

½ teaspoon vanilla extract

1. In a small saucepan over medium heat, bring the cream to a simmer. Remove from the heat and immediately add the chopped chocolate. Let sit for 5 minutes to melt.

2. Add the sweetener and vanilla and whisk until smooth. The glaze will seem very thin at first but should thicken up quite a bit as it cools.

DAIRY-FREE OPTION:

You can use full-fat coconut milk here—or, better yet, coconut cream. But I always find the resulting glaze a little too thin, so I typically add an additional ½ ounce of chopped chocolate.

TIPS: *You can use other sweeteners here, but Bocha Sweet and allulose are much better added to the cream as it heats so that they dissolve properly. They may make the glaze a little softer and stickier. If you do use an erythritol-based sweetener, it really needs to be powdered and should be added after the chocolate is melted so that it recrystallizes less.*

Be sure to watch the cream carefully. Such a small amount can come to a simmer very quickly.

This recipe can be scaled up easily to make more glaze, but I find that this amount is enough to top an 8-inch square pan of brownies or to cover the Flourless Swiss Roll (page 100).

Chocolate is finicky with reheating and this glaze can separate, so it is best made fresh.

NUTRITIONAL INFORMATION

CALORIES: 65 | FAT: 5.8g | CARBS: 1.6g | FIBER: 0.8g | PROTEIN: 0.9g

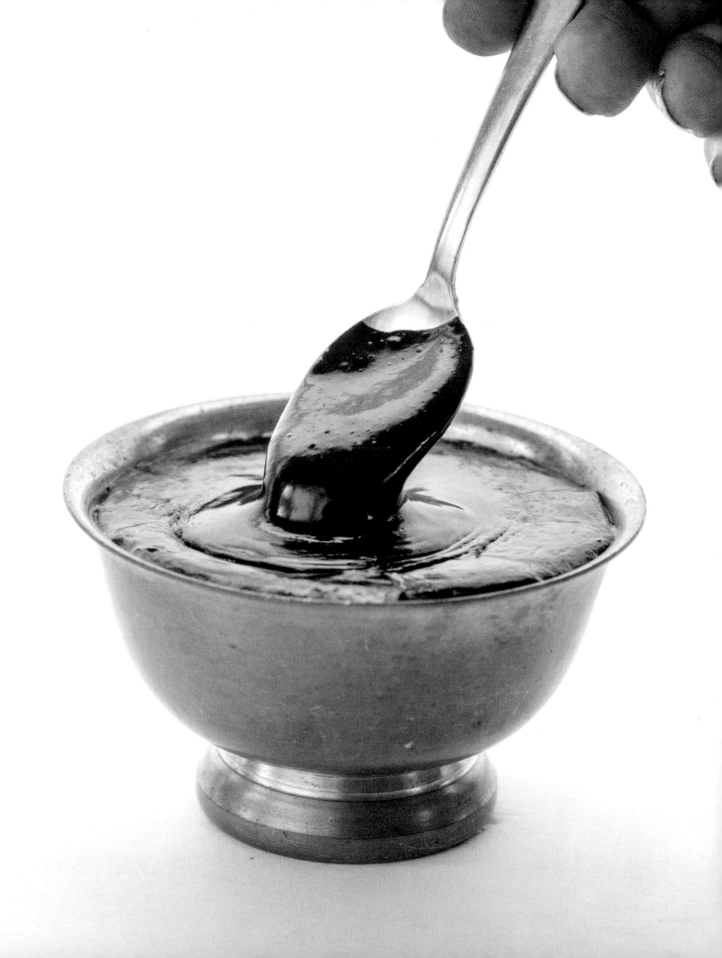

PASTRY CREAM

Yield: About 1 cup (6 servings) Prep Time: 10 minutes Cook Time: 10 minutes

Pastry cream is a thick custard similar to pudding, but it is usually intended to be a filling for cakes, éclairs, and other pastries. Still, if you just want to make this as vanilla pudding, I am not going to stop you! It would also be a lovely filling for the Pavlova (page 354), in place of the whipped cream.

1 cup heavy whipping cream

3 large egg yolks

¼ cup plus 2 tablespoons powdered erythritol sweetener

Pinch of salt

3 tablespoons unsalted butter, cut into 3 pieces

1½ teaspoons vanilla extract

¼ teaspoon glucomannan or xanthan gum

1. In a medium saucepan over medium heat, bring the cream to a simmer. In a medium bowl, whisk the egg yolks with the sweetener and salt.

2. Slowly whisk about half of the hot cream into the yolks, then slowly return the yolk/cream mixture to the saucepan and gently cook, whisking constantly, until thickened, 4 to 5 minutes. Watch it carefully and do not let it curdle, as it can heat up and thicken quickly.

3. Remove the pan from the heat and whisk in the butter and vanilla. Sprinkle the surface with the glucomannan and whisk to combine. Transfer to a blender or food processor and blend until perfectly smooth.

4. Use as directed in the specific recipe. If you aren't going to use the cream right away or the recipe requires you to chill it first, press plastic wrap flush to the surface to keep the cream from developing a "skin." Chill for 3 hours, or until firm.

TIPS: *Don't walk away from the pastry cream while it's on the stove—not even for a second. It can go from almost liquid to a thick pudding state surprisingly quickly, and there's no telling when that will happen.*

Traditional pastry cream recipes usually have you press the cream through a strainer to catch any bits of curdled egg and make it perfectly smooth. But I find this step unnecessary, and I lose too much of the good thick cream that way. I simply transfer it to my blender and blend it until it's smooth; this takes care of any bits of egg that may have curdled in the heating process.

The pastry cream can be stored in a bowl in the fridge, with plastic wrap pressed to the surface, for up to 2 days.

The nutritional info assumes that you are eating this cream as a dessert unto itself. When used as a filling, such as in the Boston Cream Poke Cake (page 112), it's spread over 12 to 16 servings.

NUTRITIONAL INFORMATION

CALORIES: 221 | FAT: 21.4g | CARBS: 1.6g | PROTEIN: 2.2g

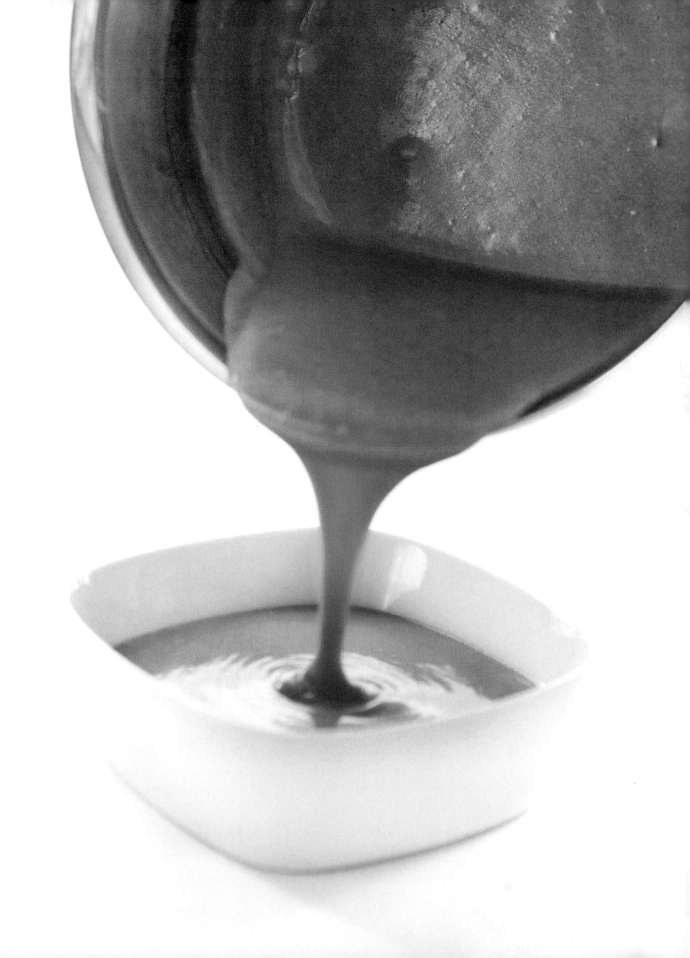

KETO VANILLA ICE CREAM

Yield: About 4 cups (8 servings) **Prep Time:** 40 minutes, plus 1 hour to chill base and 4 hours to freeze ice cream (not including time to make condensed milk) **Cook Time:** —

This is, of course, not a baked recipe at all, and it's not used in any of the baked goods in this book. But because I showcased so many of my desserts with a scoop of delicious vanilla ice cream, I felt it would be cruel not to include the recipe!

1 recipe Keto Sweetened Condensed Milk (page 386), cooled

1½ cups heavy whipping cream

3 tablespoons powdered erythritol sweetener

1½ tablespoons vodka (optional; see tips)

½ teaspoon vanilla extract

⅛ teaspoon salt

1. In a large bowl, whisk together all of the ingredients. Taste the mixture and adjust the sweetener as desired, keeping in mind that frozen foods can taste less sweet to the palate.

2. Chill the mixture for at least 1 hour or up to overnight, then pour into the canister of an ice cream maker and churn according to the manufacturer's directions. Transfer to an airtight container and freeze until firm, at least 4 hours.

TIPS: *For best results, you really want to use both Swerve and Bocha Sweet or allulose in the condensed milk. This is the best combination I've found for softer, scoopable ice cream. All erythritol and it's rock-hard right out of the freezer. All Bocha Sweet and it stays like soft-serve. If you do use only erythritol-based sweeteners, let the ice cream sit out on the counter for 15 minutes to soften before serving.*

Alcohol lowers the temperature at which liquids freeze, so adding a little vodka to an ice cream recipe can help keep it softer and reduce iciness. The amount of alcohol in this recipe adds up to only about ½ teaspoon per serving.

If you have the kind of ice cream maker that requires you to freeze the canister, remember to do that at least 12 hours in advance!

As long as it's stored in an airtight container in the freezer, the ice cream will be good for up to 3 months.

NUTRITIONAL INFORMATION

CALORIES: 319 | FAT: 31.4g | CARBS: 2.4g | PROTEIN: 1.7g

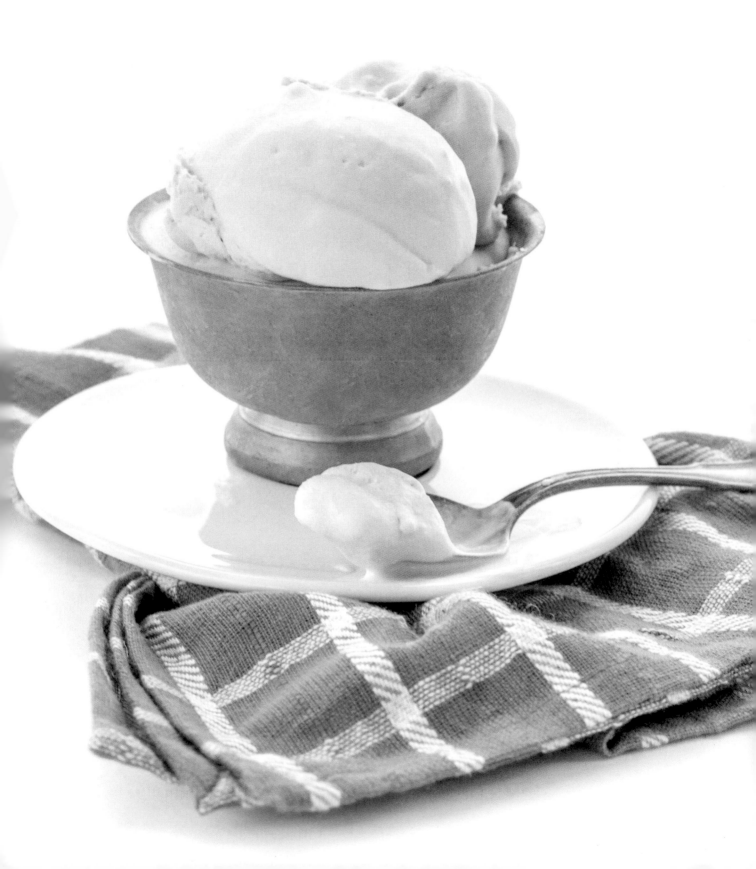

CHOCOLATE SHARDS

Yield: 2 ounces (12 servings) **Prep Time:** 15 minutes **Cook Time:** 3 minutes

This is a fun and easy way to make a pretty chocolate decoration for the tops of cakes and pies.

2 ounces sugar-free dark chocolate, chopped

1. Lay a 10-inch length of waxed paper on a flat work surface.

2. In a small microwave-safe bowl, heat the chocolate on high in 30-second increments, stirring in between, until smooth.

3. Use an offset spatula to spread the chocolate over the waxed paper as evenly as possible, leaving a 1-inch border.

4. Top with another piece of waxed paper and roll up from one end. Place on a large plate or a baking sheet and freeze for at least 1 hour.

5. Unroll the waxed paper. The chocolate will break into shards as you do so. Use them to decorate desserts as desired.

TIPS: *You can keep the shards in an airtight container and refrigerate or freeze for several months. This recipe can easily be doubled, tripled, etc. Just use a larger piece of waxed paper.*

The number of servings really depends on the recipe for which you are using the shards. Eight is a reasonable number of servings when using them as a decoration on a cake or pie.

NUTRITIONAL INFORMATION

CALORIES: 18 | FAT: 1.8g | CARBS: 1.9g | FIBER: 0.9g | PROTEIN: 0.2g

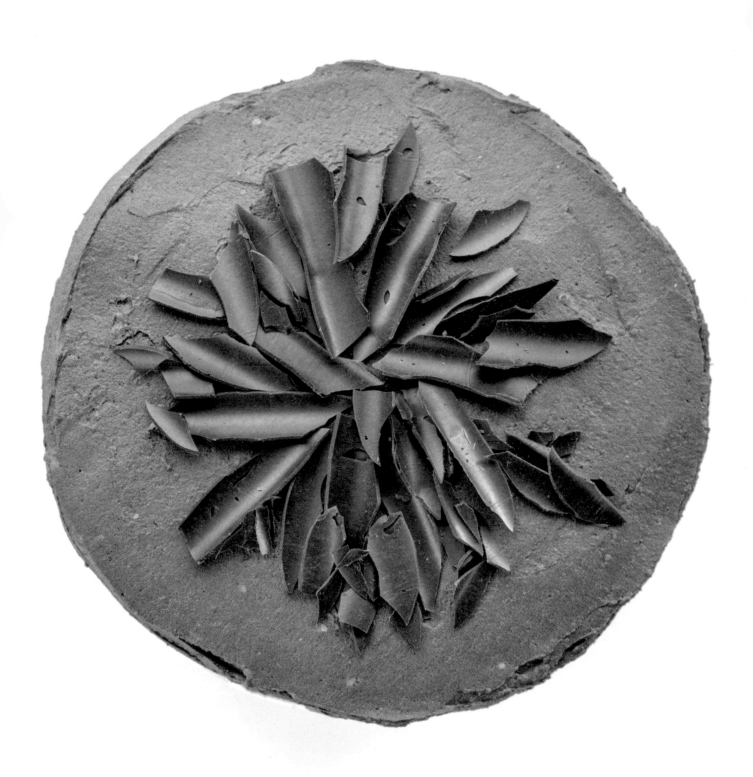

METRIC EQUIVALENCY CHART

I spent a full afternoon making quite a mess in my kitchen, measuring and weighing the ingredients used most frequently in this cookbook. While most packaging will give you both the volume and the weight of a single serving of the product, those numbers are not always accurate for real-life keto baking.

I found that the flours and meals were the most inaccurate. I used the scoop-and-level method and several different sets of measuring cups, weighing each several times. And almost without fail, my weight measurements ended up lower than what the packaging indicated. If you choose to use metric equivalents when making the recipes in this book, you would do well to follow the amounts here rather than those on the packaging.

The sweeteners tended to be more in line with the packaging and weighed out relatively consistently with each other as well. Additionally, being off by a few grams for the sweeteners will have less of an impact on the outcome of your baked goods.

Dry Ingredients

FLOURS AND MEALS
(equivalent to 1 cup)

Almond flour (blanched)	100g
Coconut flour	110g
Hazelnut flour	100g
Peanut flour (defatted)	105g
Pecan meal	100g
Sunflower seed meal	100g
Pumpkin seed meal	100g
Lupin flour	105g
Oat fiber	105g
Ground pork rinds	65g

SWEETENERS
(equivalent to 1 cup)

Blended Sweeteners

Swerve Granular	180g
Swerve Confectioners	130g
Swerve Brown	190g
Lakanto Classic (granular)	190g
Bocha Sweet	192g

Pure Sweeteners

Allulose	196g
Plain erythritol	192g
Plain xylitol	192g

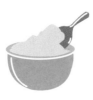

Semisolid Fats and Oils

Butter: ½ cup	114g
Ghee: ½ cup	112g
Coconut oil: ½ cup	112g

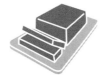

All Other Liquids (Including Liquid Oils)

1 cup	250ml
½ cup	125ml
¼ cup	60ml
1 tablespoon	15ml
1 teaspoon	5ml

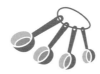

Other Useful Conversions

1 cup	16 tablespoons
½ cup	8 tablespoons
⅓ cup	5 tablespoons plus 1 teaspoon
1 tablespoon	3 teaspoons
1 ounce	28g

Pans

8 x 4 inch	20 x 10 cm
9 x 5 inch	23 x 12.75 cm
13 x 9-inch	33 x 23 cm
15 x 10 x 1 inch	38 x 25 x 2.5 cm
11 x 17 x 1 inch	28 x 43 x 2.5 cm

4-inch round	10-cm round
8-inch round/square	20-cm round/square
9-inch round/square	23-cm round/square
10-inch round	25-cm round

Fahrenheit to Celsius

200°F	95°C
300°F	150°C
325°F	163°C
350°F	177°C
375°F	190°C
400°F	205°C
425°F	220°C
450°F	232°C

RESOURCE GUIDE

I want you to be the most successful keto baker you can be. That means knowing where to source the best ingredients and equipment and where to turn for a little extra guidance when you need it. To that end, I've compiled a list of all my favorite websites and sources to help you out.

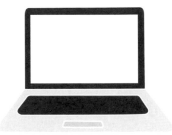

Keto Baking Websites

All Day I Dream About Food (alldayidreamaboutfood.com): I would be remiss if I didn't mention my own website. I have thousands of recipes, most of which are not included in this book. I also try to give readers plenty of tips and information about each recipe and about keto baking and cooking in general.

Gnom Gnom (gnom-gnom.com): Paola is a well regarded keto baker who, like me, gives plenty of tips and tricks for each recipe she creates.

Low Carb Maven (lowcarbmaven.com): Tons of delicious cakes and other baked goods from Kim!

My Sweet Keto (mysweetketo.com): A newer keto blog on the scene, with lots of delicious-looking recipes and plenty of tips and articles on keto baking.

Sugar-Free Mom (sugarfreemom.com): Brenda loves to bake and create sweets, and because she has a child with a nut allergy, many of her baked goods are nut-free.

Other Baking Websites

America's Test Kitchen (americastestkitchen.com): This is one of my favorite resources for general baking and cooking advice. In fact, I tried to model this book after the America's Test Kitchen *Family Baking Book.* They are incredibly comprehensive and test a number of ways to approach any baking dilemma. And, while it doesn't always apply to keto baking, I am often able to find a nugget of wisdom from their articles. It is a subscription-based website but well worth it.

King Arthur Flour (kingarthurflour.com): Another fabulous website for general baking advice. I used some of their advice when researching the tips and tricks for this book.

Serious Eats (seriouseats.com): Great articles by culinary wizards like J. Kenji Lopez-Alt and Stella Parks that always have clear and concise instructions. It was the tips by Stella Parks (the pastry chef behind *Brave Tart: Iconic American Desserts*) that gave me the courage to try a keto version of Swiss meringue buttercream.

Where to Buy Specialty Ingredients

The keto diet is increasing in popularity so quickly that many grocery store chains now carry quite a number of keto baking products. However, some of the less commonly used ingredients are often only available online. I usually purchase from Amazon or Thrive Market, but other places to look include Vitacost, Netrition, and Nuts.com. Also, many brands have commercial websites where they sell their products.

Keto dieters who reside in Canada should check lowcarbcanada.ca or naturamarket.ca. And iHerb ships to over 100 countries and provides services in several different languages.

Keto flours: Almond flour and coconut flour are widely available in most grocery store chains, and many also carry hazelnut meal. Check the healthy eating or gluten-free aisles to see what your local stores carry.

Other nut and seed meals, such as pecan meal and sunflower seed meal, and non-nut flours, like lupin flour or preground pork rinds, are best purchased online. Amazon carries all of these products.

Note: If you need to be nut-free, be sure to read whether the brand of sunflower seed meal, pumpkin seed meal, or sesame seed flour is processed in a facility that also processes nuts. I know that the GERBS brand, which I purchase on Amazon, is completely nut-free.

Keto sweeteners: Most grocery store chains have some alternative sweeteners in among the sugars in the baking aisle and usually carry some erythritol- and/or xylitol-based sweeteners as well as stevia. Swerve and Lakanto are both carried in Whole Foods, Natural Grocers, and many independent health food stores.

Neither Bocha Sweet nor allulose is widely available; these brands are best purchased online. Bocha Sweet is often less expensive when purchased directly from the company.

Sugar-free chocolate: Lily's chocolate has made huge inroads into the regular grocery market, and I've been surprised to see the bars in many large chains and independent grocers. The chocolate chips aren't quite as widely available, but Whole Foods and other health stores tend to carry them. And the new Bake Believe chocolate chips are available at many Walmart stores.

Other brands of keto-friendly chocolate, such as ChocZero and Explorado Market, are available mostly online, either through their own websites or on Amazon.

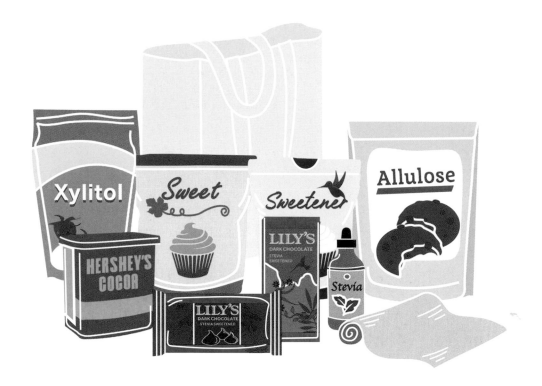

White chocolate chips: What an amazing development that two companies have decided to make keto white chocolate chips. Bake Believe chips can only be found in Walmart stores. I haven't seen the ChocZero chips on Amazon yet, although I am sure that they will be there. They do sell them online through their own website, but at the time of writing this book, they were entirely sold out. Demand exceeds supply, I guess!

Extracts and flavorings: Standard flavorings such as vanilla, peppermint, almond, lemon, and orange are typically available in the baking aisle of most grocery stores. Sometimes maple flavor is as well. But for more interesting flavors, it's best to look online.

OOO Flavors (One on One Flavors) creates almost every food flavoring you can possibly imagine and has a specific keto-friendly line that is dairy-free, gluten-free, nut-free, and non-GMO. Seriously, they've thought of everything, from rye bread flavor to graham cracker flavor, and they are the manufacturers of the cornbread flavoring that I use in this book. Some flavors are available on Amazon, but the full range is best viewed and purchased directly from company at www.oooflavors.com. (And good news for my Canadian audience: One on One is a Canadian company and has a Canadian website, www.oooflavours.ca.)

I also like the extracts and flavorings from Olive Nation, which I purchase on Amazon. They offer a fairly extensive range of all-natural flavors, and it's my favorite brand for fruit-flavored extracts like apple, cherry, and pineapple. I also really like their caramel flavoring.

Sugar-free sprinkles: Yes, they do exist! As of a year ago, no one was making anything like this, and now three companies have come out with keto-friendly sprinkles.

My favorite thus far is The Sprinkle Company, for the variety of fun colors and mixes. They carry sparkling "sugars" for decorating as well. The Sprinkle Company is available through Etsy and is run by fellow keto blogger Nicole of *Oh My Keto* and author of *Keto for Foodies.*

Two other companies, Good Dee's and Stoka Bar, have come out with sprinkles. Both are available on their websites and Amazon.

If you can't access any of these brands and are dying to incorporate sprinkles into your recipes, check out my blog for a tutorial on how to make your own. It's surprisingly easy but also quite time-consuming. https://alldayidreamaboutfood.com/keto-sugar-free-sprinkles/

Food coloring: There are quite a few vegetable-based options for food coloring now, and some are even in stores. I've seen both India Tree and Color Kitchen at Whole Foods. Both are also available online from Amazon and Thrive Market.

I use the Color Kitchen powders because they lend a more vibrant color than the India Tree gels, but sometimes they are so strong that they make everything neon bright. Use a light hand with these, adding just a bit of the powder at a time, until you get the color you want.

Watkins makes some vegetable dyes now, too, although I've only seen them on Amazon. I have not tried them out yet.

Sugar-free jam: Don't feel like making your own jam for the Dairy-Free Jam Thumbprints (page 136)? I get it! There are very few no-sugar-added jams that aren't made with sucralose, but the two that I know of are Nature's Hollow (sweetened with xylitol) and Sweet Jam (sweetened with stevia), both available on Amazon. Sweet Jam also appears to be available on naturamarket.ca.

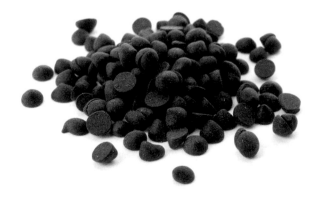

ALLERGEN INDEX

RECIPES	PAGE	🥥	🌾	⚫	🥜	BEG	ADV
Chocolate Zucchini Sheet Cake	66		O		✓	✓	
Dairy-Free Lemon Cake	68	✓	✓			✓	
New York Crumb Cake	70						
Dairy-Free Blueberry Cream Cheese Coffee Cake	72	O	✓				
Rhubarb Almond Skillet Cake	74	✓	O				
Key Lime Pound Cake	76		O			✓	
Chocolate Cupcakes	78		O		✓	✓	
Cream-Filled Chocolate Cupcakes	80				✓		
Cream-Filled Vanilla Cupcakes	84	✓			O		
Confetti Cupcakes	86	✓					
Mini Chocolate Peanut Butter Cheesecakes	88	✓					
Warm Gingerbread Cake	90	✓	O			✓	
Classic Yellow Birthday Cake	94	✓	O				
Chocolate Mayonnaise Cake	96	✓	✓				
Coconut Layer Cake	98						✓
Flourless Swiss Roll	100	✓			✓		✓
Cream Cheese–Filled Carrot Cake	102	✓					
Rum Cake	104		O				
Pecan Pie Pound Cake	106						
Chiffon Cake	108	✓	✓				✓
Tres Leches Cake	110						✓
Boston Cream Poke Cake	112				✓		✓
Marble Cheesecake	114	✓			O		✓
Ricotta Cheesecake with Fresh Berries	116						
Cannoli Icebox Cake	118	✓					
Chocolate Hazelnut Torte	120	✓	✓				✓
Soft and Chewy Chocolate Chip Cookies	124				✓		
Soft and Chewy Snickerdoodles	126				✓		
Classic Peanut Butter Cookies	128	✓				✓	
Cowboy Cookies	130						
Brownie Cookies	132	✓	O		O		
Chewy Ginger "Molasses" Cookies	134	✓	O				
Dairy-Free Jam Thumbprints	136		✓				
Pecan Snowballs	138		O			✓	
Italian Sesame Seed Cookies	140	✓					
Dairy-Free Chocolate Chip Skillet Cookie	142	O	✓			✓	
Chocolate Wafers	146	✓	O		O		

RECIPES	PAGE	🥥	🥛	⊙	🥜	BEG	ADV
Mint Chocolate Thins	148	✓	O		O		
Chocolate Sandwich Cookies (aka No-Reos)	150	✓			O		
Cream Cheese Cutout Cookies	152	✓	O	✓			
Cinnamon Roll Cookies	154						✓
Scottish Shortbread	156	✓		✓			
Slice-and-Bake Mocha Shortbread	158	✓		✓			
Classic Almond Biscotti	160	✓	O				
Chocolate Hazelnut Biscotti	162	✓	✓				
Classic Whoopie Pies	164				✓		
Frosted Lemon Sugar Cookies	166	✓					
"Oatmeal" Lace Cookies	168						
Sugar-Free Meringues	170	✓	✓		✓		✓
Coconut Macaroons	172		✓		✓		
Ladyfingers	174	✓	O				✓
Chewy Keto Brownies	178	✓	O		O	✓	
Peanut Butter Swirl Brownies	180	✓	O		O	✓	
Dairy-Free Peppermint Patty Brownies	182		✓		O		
White Chocolate Macadamia Nut Blondies	184	✓	O				
Butterscotch Bars	186	✓					
Zucchini Spice Bars with Brown Butter Glaze	188				✓		
Maple Walnut Bars	190	✓					
Classic Lemon Bars	192		O				
Magic Cookie Bars	194			✓			
Key Lime Pie Bars	196	✓					
Dairy-Free Coconut Caramel Bars	198		✓	✓			
Dairy-Free Fudge Crumb Bars	200		✓	✓			
Flag Sugar Cookie Bars	202					✓	
Triple Chocolate Cheesecake Bars	204	✓			O		
Granola Bars	206			✓			
Peanut Butter "Oatmeal" Bars	208		O			✓	
Basic Almond Flour Muffins	212	✓	O			✓	
Hazelnut Chocolate Chip Muffins	214	✓	✓			✓	
Double Chocolate Almond Butter Muffins	216		✓		O		
Lemon Ricotta Muffins	218						
Raspberry Coconut Muffins	220		✓		✓	✓	
Piña Colada Muffins	222		✓				
Pizza Muffins	224				✓		

RECIPES	PAGE	⊘	⊘	⊘	⊘	BEG	ADV
Cheesy Garlic Bread Muffins	226	✓					
Mini Corndog Muffins	228				✓	✓	
Blueberry Vanilla Donuts	230		✓		✓	✓	
Chocolate Donuts with Peanut Butter Glaze	232	✓					
Maple-Glazed Donuts	234						
Pumpkin Spice Donut Holes	236				✓		
Cream Cheese Biscuits	240	✓	O				
Cheddar Garlic Drop Biscuits	242	✓				✓	
Classic Cream Scones	244		O			✓	
Cinnamon Roll Scones	246	✓					
Fresh Herb and Ricotta Scones	248	✓					
Toasted Coconut Chocolate Chunk Drop Scones	250		✓				
Popovers	252	✓			✓		
Cranberry Orange Loaf	256	✓	O			✓	
Classic Pumpkin Bread	258		O			✓	
Brown Butter Banana Bread	260						
Cinnamon Swirl Bread	262				✓		
Sweet Alabama Pecan Bread	264	✓				✓	
Rosemary Olive Oil Bread	266		✓				
Cheddar Jalapeño Zucchini Bread	268	O					
Garlic Parmesan Cauliflower Bread	270	O					
Keto Yeast Bread	272	✓	O				✓
Cheesy Pork Rind Breadsticks	274	✓			✓	✓	
Cracklin' Cornbread	276		O		✓	✓	
Chewy Keto Bagels	278				✓		
Spinach Feta Pinwheels	280				✓		✓
Cloverleaf Dinner Rolls	282				✓		
Classic Pepperoni Pizza	286				✓		
Jalapeño Popper Pizza	288				O		
Sausage and Broccoli Calzone	290				✓		
Smoked Salmon Flatbread	292				✓		
Socca Flatbread	294	O	✓		✓		
Rosemary Pecan Crackers	296	✓	✓				
Toasted Sesame Crackers	298	✓	✓				
Graham Crackers	300	✓	O			✓	
Buttery Cheese Crackers	302				✓		
Parmesan Sage Shortbread	304	✓		✓			
German Chocolate Brownie Pie	308						
Mascarpone Berry Tart	310	O			✓	✓	
Kentucky Chocolate Chip Cookie Pie	312				O		
Blueberry Sour Cream Pie	314				✓		

RECIPES	PAGE	🚫	🚫	🚫	🚫	BEG	ADV
Strawberry Rhubarb Galette	316				✓		
Mini Crustless Pumpkin Pies	318	✓	O		✓	✓	
Raspberry Truffle Tart	320	✓			O		
Salted Caramel Tart with Chocolate Glaze	322	✓		✓			✓
Dairy-Free Coconut Cream Tarts	324		✓				✓
Bacon Spinach Artichoke Quiche	326	✓					
Sausage and Mushroom Tart	328				✓		
Tomato Ricotta Tart	330	✓					✓
Tourtiere	332				✓		
Linzertorte	334						✓
Raspberry Cream Cheese Turnovers	336	✓					
Zucchini Crisp	338			✓			
Old-Fashioned Baked Custard	342	✓			✓	✓	
Crème Brûlée	344	✓			✓		✓
Dairy-Free Caramel Flan	346		✓		✓		✓
Dairy-Free Chocolate Pots de Crème	348		✓		✓		
Classic Chocolate Soufflés	350	✓			✓		✓
Dairy-Free Lemon Soufflés	352	✓	✓				✓
Pavlova	354	✓			✓		✓
Summer Berry Cobbler	356	✓		✓		✓	
Hot Fudge Pudding Cakes	358	✓			✓		
Classic Tiramisu	360	✓					✓
Chocolate Lasagna	362	✓					✓
Easy Almond Flour Pie Crust	366	✓	O	✓		✓	
Coconut Flour Pie Crust	368				✓		
Keto Chocolate Pie Crust	370	✓	O	✓	O	✓	
Shortbread Crust	372	✓	O	✓	O	✓	
Magic Mozzarella Dough	375	O					
Nut-Free Magic Mozzarella Dough	376				✓		
Whipped Cream Frosting	377	✓		✓	✓	✓	
Swiss Meringue Buttercream	378	✓			✓		✓
Cream Cheese Frosting	380	✓	O	✓	O	✓	
Chocolate Buttercream Frosting	382	O		✓	✓	✓	
Dairy-Free Chocolate Frosting	384		✓	✓		✓	
Keto Sweetened Condensed Milk	386	✓	O	✓	✓	✓	
Sugar-Free Caramel Sauce	388	✓	O	✓	✓		
Easy Chocolate Glaze	390	✓	O	✓	✓	✓	
Pastry Cream	392	✓			✓		
Keto Vanilla Ice Cream	394	✓		✓	✓	✓	
Chocolate Shards	396	✓	✓	✓	✓	✓	

RECIPE INDEX

Everyday Cakes

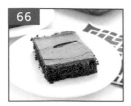
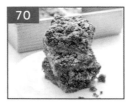
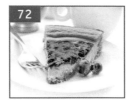
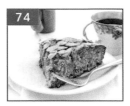
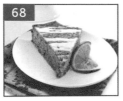
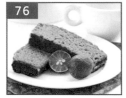
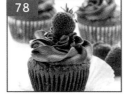
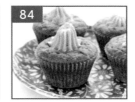
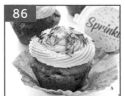
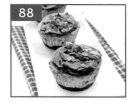
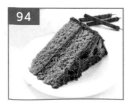
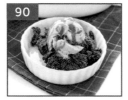
Special Occasion Cakes

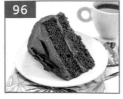
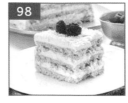
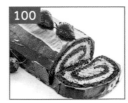
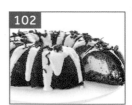

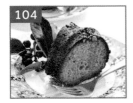
104
Rum Cake

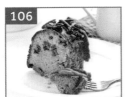
106
Pecan Pie Pound Cake

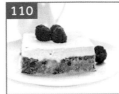
108
Chiffon Cake

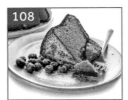
110
Tres Leches Cake

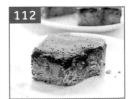
112
Boston Cream Poke Cake

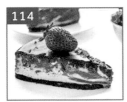
114
Marble Cheesecake

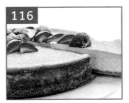
116
Ricotta Cheesecake with Fresh Berries

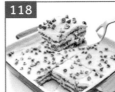
118
Cannoli Icebox Cake

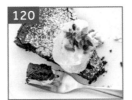
120
Chocolate Hazelnut Torte

Everyday Cookies

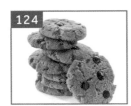
124
Soft and Chewy Chocolate Chip Cookies

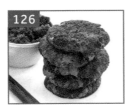
126
Soft and Chewy Snickerdoodles

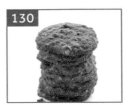
128
Classic Peanut Butter Cookies

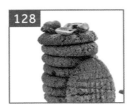
130
Cowboy Cookies

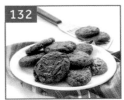
132
Brownie Cookies

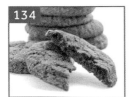
134
Chewy Ginger "Molasses" Cookies

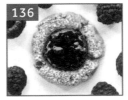
136
Dairy-Free Jam Thumbprints

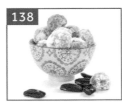
138
Pecan Snowballs

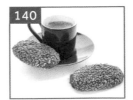
140
Italian Sesame Seed Cookies

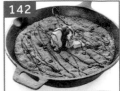
142
Dairy-Free Chocolate Chip Skillet Cookie

Fancy Cookies

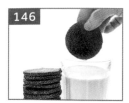
146 Chocolate Wafers

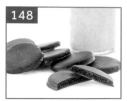
148 Mint Chocolate Thins

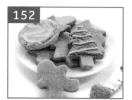
150 Chocolate Sandwich Cookies (aka No-Reos)

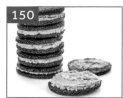
152 Cream Cheese Cutout Cookies

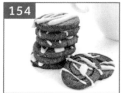
154 Cinnamon Roll Cookies

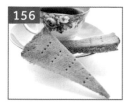
156 Scottish Shortbread

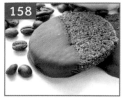
158 Slice-and-Bake Mocha Shortbread

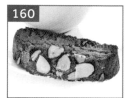
160 Classic Almond Biscotti

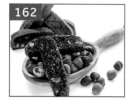
162 Chocolate Hazelnut Biscotti

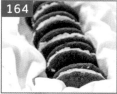
164 Classic Whoopie Pies

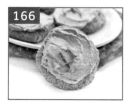
166 Frosted Lemon Sugar Cookies

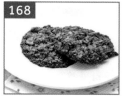
168 "Oatmeal" Lace Cookies

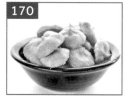
170 Sugar-Free Meringues

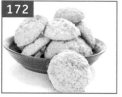
172 Coconut Macaroons

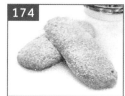
174 Ladyfingers

Brownies & Bars

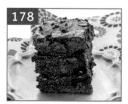
178 Chewy Keto Brownies

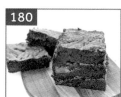
180 Peanut Butter Swirl Brownies

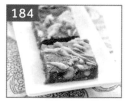
182 Dairy-Free Peppermint Patty Brownies

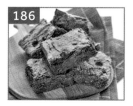
184 White Chocolate Macadamia Nut Blondies

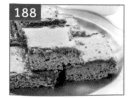
186 Butterscotch Bars

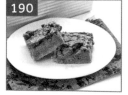
188 Zucchini Spice Bars with Brown Butter Glaze

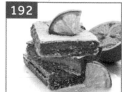
190 Maple Walnut Bars

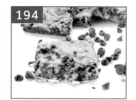
192 Classic Lemon Bars

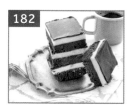
194 Magic Cookie Bars

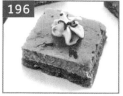
196 Key Lime Pie Bars

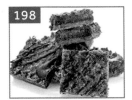
198
Dairy-Free Coconut
Caramel Bars

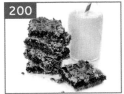
200
Dairy-Free Fudge
Crumb Bars

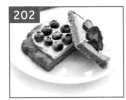
202
Flag Sugar Cookie
Bars

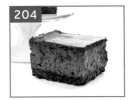
204
Triple Chocolate
Cheesecake Bars

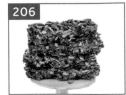
206
Granola Bars

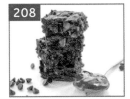
208
Peanut Butter
"Oatmeal" Bars

Muffins & Donuts

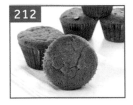
212
Basic Almond Flour
Muffins

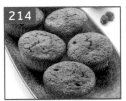
214
Hazelnut Chocolate
Chip Muffins

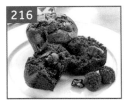
216
Double Chocolate
Almond Butter
Muffins

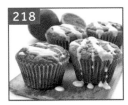
218
Lemon Ricotta
Muffins

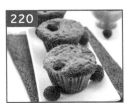
220
Raspberry Coconut
Muffins

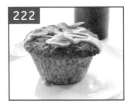
222
Piña Colada Muffins

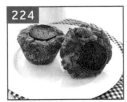
224
Pizza Muffins

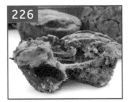
226
Cheesy Garlic Bread
Muffins

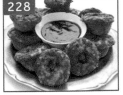
228
Mini Corndog
Muffins

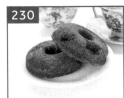
230
Blueberry Vanilla
Donuts

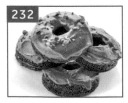
232
Chocolate Donuts
with Peanut Butter
Glaze

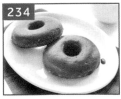
234
Maple-Glazed
Donuts

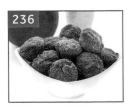
236
Pumpkin Spice
Donut Holes

Biscuits & Scones

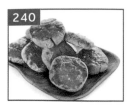
240
Cream Cheese Biscuits

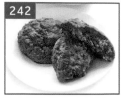
242
Cheddar Garlic Drop Biscuits

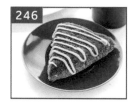
244
Classic Cream Scones

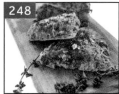
246
Cinnamon Roll Scones

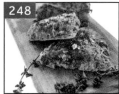
248
Fresh Herb and Ricotta Scones

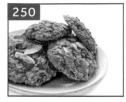
250
Toasted Coconut Chocolate Chunk Drop Scones

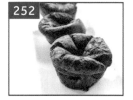
252
Popovers

Breads & Rolls

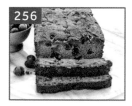
256
Cranberry Orange Loaf

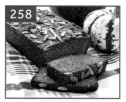
258
Classic Pumpkin Bread

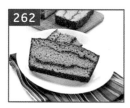
260
Brown Butter Banana Bread

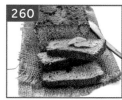
262
Cinnamon Swirl Bread

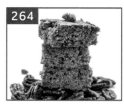
264
Sweet Alabama Pecan Bread

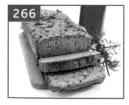
266
Rosemary Olive Oil Bread

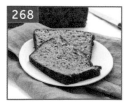
268
Cheddar Jalapeño Zucchini Bread

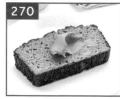
270
Garlic Parmesan Cauliflower Bread

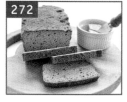
272
Keto Yeast Bread

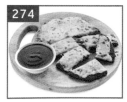
274
Cheesy Pork Rind Breadsticks

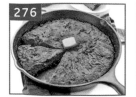
276
Cracklin' Cornbread

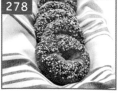
278
Chewy Keto Bagels

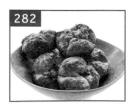
280
Spinach Feta Pinwheels

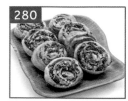
282
Cloverleaf Dinner Rolls

Flatbreads, Pizza & Crackers

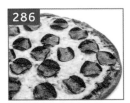
286
Classic Pepperoni Pizza

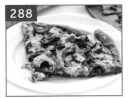
288
Jalapeño Popper Pizza

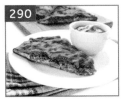
290
Sausage and Broccoli Calzone

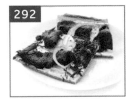
292
Smoked Salmon Flatbread

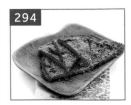
294
Socca Flatbread

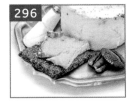
296
Rosemary Pecan Crackers

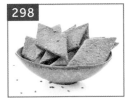
298
Toasted Sesame Crackers

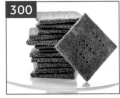
300
Graham Crackers

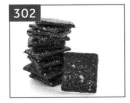
302
Buttery Cheese Crackers

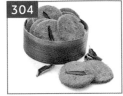
304
Parmesan Sage Shortbread

Pies & Tarts

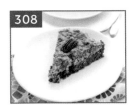
308
German Chocolate Brownie Pie

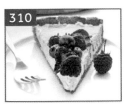
310
Mascarpone Berry Tart

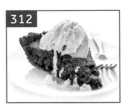
312
Kentucky Chocolate Chip Cookie Pie

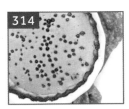
314
Blueberry Sour Cream Pie

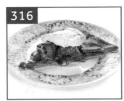
316
Strawberry Rhubarb Galette

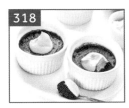
318
Mini Crustless Pumpkin Pies

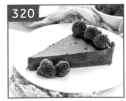
320
Raspberry Truffle Tart

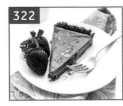
322
Salted Caramel Tart with Chocolate Glaze

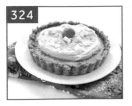
324
Dairy-Free Coconut Cream Tarts

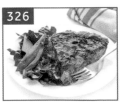
326
Bacon Spinach Artichoke Quiche

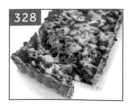
328

Sausage and
Mushroom Tart

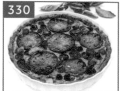
330

Tomato Ricotta Tart

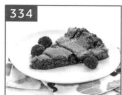
332

Tourtiere

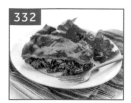
334

Linzertorte

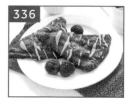
336

Raspberry Cream
Cheese Turnovers

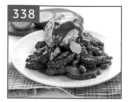
338

Zucchini Crisp

Custards, Soufflés & Other Baked Desserts

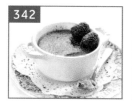
342

Old-Fashioned
Baked Custard

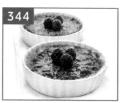
344

Crème Brûlée

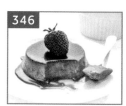
346

Dairy-Free Caramel
Flan

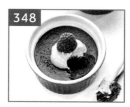
348

Dairy-Free
Chocolate Pots de
Crème

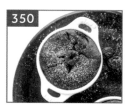
350

Classic Chocolate
Soufflés

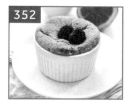
352

Dairy-Free Lemon
Soufflés

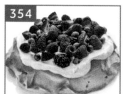
354

Pavlova

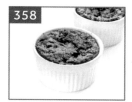
356

Summer Berry
Cobbler

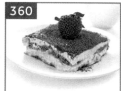
358

Hot Fudge Pudding
Cakes

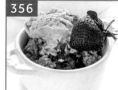
360

Classic Tiramisu

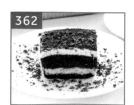
362

Chocolate Lasagna

Extras

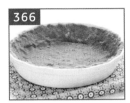

366

Easy Almond Flour
Pie Crust

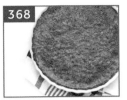

368

Coconut Flour
Pie Crust

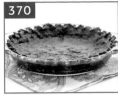

370

Keto Chocolate
Pie Crust

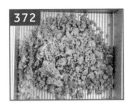

372

Shortbread Crust

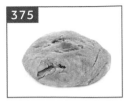

375

Magic Mozzarella
Dough

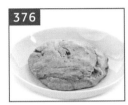

376

Nut-Free Magic
Mozzarella Dough

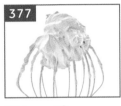

377

Whipped Cream
Frosting

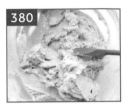

378

Swiss Meringue
Buttercream

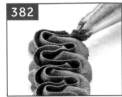

380

Cream Cheese
Frosting

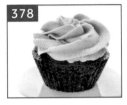

382

Chocolate
Buttercream
Frosting

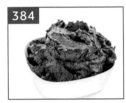

384

Dairy-Free
Chocolate Frosting

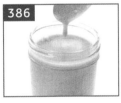

386

Keto Sweetened
Condensed Milk

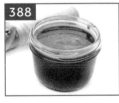

388

Sugar-Free Caramel
Sauce

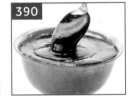

390

Easy Chocolate
Glaze

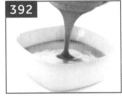

392

Pastry Cream

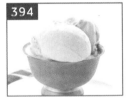

394

Keto Vanilla
Ice Cream

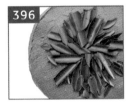

396

Chocolate Shards

GENERAL INDEX